Autoimmune Pancreatitis

Terumi Kamisawa • Jae Bock Chung
Editors

Autoimmune Pancreatitis

Springer

Editors
Terumi Kamisawa, MD, PhD
Department of Internal Medicine
Tokyo Metropolitan Komagome Hospital
Tokyo
Japan

Jae Bock Chung, MD, PhD
Department of Internal Medicine
Severance Hospital, Yonsei University
College of Medicine
Seoul
Korea, Republic of (South Korea)

ISBN 978-3-642-55085-0 ISBN 978-3-642-55086-7 (eBook)
DOI 10.1007/978-3-642-55086-7
Springer Heidelberg New York Dordrecht London

Library of Congress Control Number: 2014955153

Printed on acid-free paper

Springer is part of Springer Science+Business Media (www.springer.com)

Preface

Sarles et al. reported a case of chronic pancreatitis with hypergammaglobulinemia in 1961, and the concept of autoimmune pancreatitis (AIP) was first proposed by Yoshida et al. in 1995. Cases of AIP were initially reported most often from Asia, particularly Japan and Korea; however, AIP has now been described worldwide, with some distinct differences in characteristics between Asian and Western countries. Diagnostic criteria for AIP have been proposed from Japan, Korea, the USA, Germany and Italy. After considering both the full reported spectrum of clinical presentations and the histopathology of AIP, International Consensus Diagnostic Criteria (ICDC) were devised in 2011.

AIP is a unique form of pancreatitis characterized clinically by frequent presentation with obstructive jaundice and dramatic response to steroids, histologically by a lymphoplasmacytic infiltrate with fibrosis, and radiologically by pancreatic enlargement. AIP can be divided into two subtypes, 1 and 2. Type 1 AIP is the prototypical of IgG4-related disease characterized by elevation of serum IgG4 levels and infiltration of IgG4-positive plasma cells, and type 2 AIP is a pancreas-specific disorder not associated with IgG4. As AIP sometimes mimics pancreatic cancer in its presentation, accurate diagnosis is necessary. This book attempts to clarify the current concept of AIP and its subtypes, cover all aspects of clinical, serological, histopathological and imaging features of AIP, illustrate the findings obtained with relevant imaging modalities in both AIP and other organ involvements, serve as an excellent aid to diagnose AIP and allow differentiation of this pathology from pancreatobiliary malignancies, and provide up-to-date therapeutic strategies for AIP.

The goals of this book are both to provide those studying AIP with the opportunity to obtain a complete understanding and to present the practicing physician with the principles for the diagnosis and management of AIP. We are deeply grateful to all the authors for their painstaking writing and contributions in preparing this concise and informative book. The publisher has also made a significant contribution to this book and has turned out an impressive volume with illustrations of the highest quality.

Seoul, Korea — Jae Bock Chung, MD, PhD
Tokyo, Japan — Terumi Kamisawa, MD, PhD

Contents

Contributors

Nazir Ahmed, MD Division of Gastroenterology and Hepatology, Mayo Clinic, Rochester, MN, USA

Norikazu Arakura, MD, PhD Endoscopic Examination Center, Shinshu University School of Medicine, Matsumoto, Japan

Seungmin Bang, MD, PhD Division of Gastroenterology, Department of Internal Medicine, Yonsei University College of Medicine, Yonsei Institute of Gastroenterology, Seodaemun-gu, Seoul, Republic of Korea

Georg Beyer, MD Department of Medicine A, University Medicine, Ernst-Moritz-Arndt-University Greifswald, Greifswald, Germany

Suresh T. Chari, MD Division of Gastroenterology and Hepatology, Mayo Clinic, Rochester, MN, USA

Kazuro Chiba, MD Department of Internal Medicine, Tokyo Metropolitan Komagome Hospital, Tokyo, Japan

Tsutomu Chiba, MD, PhD Department of Gastroenterology and Hepatology, Graduate School of Medicine, Kyoto University, Kyoto, Japan

Jae Bock Chung, MD, PhD Department of Internal Medicine, Yonsei University College of Medicine, Yonsei Institute of Gastroenterology, Seodaemun-gu, Seoul, Republic of Korea

Young Eun Chung, MD, PhD Department of Radiology and Research Institute of Radiological Science, Yonsei University College of Medicine, Seoul, Korea

Phil A. Hart, MD Division of Gastroenterology and Hepatology, Mayo Clinic, Rochester, MN, USA

Masayuki Hijioka, MD, PhD Department of Medicine and Bioregulatory Science, School of Medicine, Graduate School of Medical Sciences, Faculty of Medical Sciences, Kyushu University, Fukuoka City, Japan

Kenji Hirano, MD, PhD Department of Gastroenterology, Graduate School of Medicine, The University of Tokyo, Tokyo, Japan

Kunihiro Hosono, MD, PhD Division of Hepatogastroenterology, Yokohama City University Graduate School of Medicine, Yokohama, Japan

Hisato Igarashi, MD, PhD Department of Medicine and Bioregulatory Science, School of Medicine, Graduate School of Medical Sciences, Faculty of Medical Sciences, Kyushu University, Fukuoka City, Japan

Kazuo Inui, MD, PhD Department of Gastroenterology, Second Teaching Hospital, Fujita Health University, Nagoya, Japan

Tetsuhide Ito, MD, PhD Department of Medicine and Bioregulatory Science, School of Medicine, Graduate School of Medical Sciences, Faculty of Medical Sciences, Kyushu University, Fukuoka City, Japan

Susumu Iwasaki, MD Department of Internal Medicine, Tokyo Metropolitan Komagome Hospital, Tokyo, Japan

Terumi Kamisawa, MD, PhD Department of Internal Medicine, Tokyo Metropolitan Komagome Hospital, Tokyo, Japan

Atsushi Kanno, MD, PhD Division of Hepatogastroenterology, Tohoku University Graduate School of Medicine, Sendai, Japan

Shigeyuki Kawa, MD, PhD Center for Health, Safety, and Environmental Management, Shinshu University, Matsumoto, Japan

Myung-Hwan Kim, MD, PhD Department of Internal Medicine, Asan Medical Center, University of Ulsan College of Medicine, Songpa-Gu, Seoul, South Korea

Yuzo Kodama, MD, PhD Department of Gastroenterology and Hepatology, Graduate School of Medicine, Kyoto University, Kyoto, Japan

Satomi Koizumi, MD Department of Internal Medicine, Tokyo Metropolitan Komagome Hospital, Tokyo, Japan

Kensuke Kubota, MD, PhD Division of Hepatogastroenterology, Yokohama City University Graduate School of Medicine, Yokohama, Japan

Sawako Kuruma, MD Department of Internal Medicine, Tokyo Metropolitan Komagome Hospital, Tokyo, Japan

Kyu Taek Lee, MD, PhD Department of Medicine, Samsung Medical Center, Sungkyunkwan University School of Medicine, Seoul, Korea

Lingaku Lee, MD, PhD Department of Medicine and Bioregulatory Science, School of Medicine, Graduate School of Medical Sciences, Faculty of Medical Sciences, Kyushu University, Fukuoka City, Japan

Markus M. Lerch, MD, FRCP Department of Medicine A, University Medicine, Ernst-Moritz-Arndt-University Greifswald, Greifswald, Germany

Masahiro Maruyama, MD, PhD Department of Gastroenterology, Shinshu University School of Medicine, Matsumoto, Japan

Atsushi Masamune, MD, PhD Division of Gastroenterology, Tohoku University Graduate School of Medicine, Sendai, Japan

Julia Mayerle, MD Department of Medicine A, University Medicine, Ernst-Moritz-Arndt-University Greifswald, Greifswald, Germany

Hironao Miyoshi, MD, PhD Department of Gastroenterology, Second Teaching Hospital, Fujita Health University, Nagoya, Japan

Nobumasa Mizuno, MD, PhD Department of Gastroenterology, Aichi Cancer Center Hospital, Nagoya, Japan

Takashi Muraki, MD, PhD Department of Gastroenterology, Shinshu University School of Medicine, Matsumoto, Japan

Itaru Naitoh, MD, PhD Department of Gastroenterology and Metabolism, Nagoya City University Graduate School of Medical Sciences, Nagoya, Japan

Atsushi Nakajima, MD, PhD Division of Hepatogastroenterology, Yokohama City University Graduate School of Medicine, Yokohama, Japan

Takahiro Nakazawa, MD, PhD Department of Gastroenterology and Metabolism, Nagoya City University Graduate School of Medical Sciences, Nagoya, Japan

Kenji Notohara, MD, PhD Department of Anatomical Pathology, Kurashiki Central Hospital, Kurashiki, Japan

Hirotaka Ohara, MD, PhD Department of Community-based Medical Education, Nagoya City University Graduate School of Medical Sciences, Nagoya, Japan

Kazuichi Okazaki, MD, PhD Division of Gastroenterology and Hepatology, The Third Department of Internal Medicine, Kansai Medical University, Shinmachi, Hirakata, Osaka, Japan

Mi-Suk Park, MD, PhD Department of Radiology and Research Institute of Radiological Science, Yonsei University College of Medicine, Seoul, Korea

Min Jung Park, MD, PhD Department of Radiology and Research Institute of Radiological Science, Yonsei University College of Medicine, Seoul, Korea

Seung Woo Park, MD, PhD Department of Internal Medicine, Institute of Gastroenterology, Yonsei University College of Medicine, Seoul, Korea

Ji Kon Ryu, MD, PhD Division of Gastroenterology, Department of Internal Medicine, Seoul National University College of Medicine, Seoul, Korea

Takako Saeki, MD, PhD Department of Internal Medicine, Nagaoka Red Cross Hospital, Nagaoka, Niigata, Japan

Raghuwansh P. Sah, MD Division of Gastroenterology and Hepatology, Mayo Clinic, Rochester, MN, USA

Kyoko Shimizu, MD, PhD Department of Gastroenterology, Tokyo Women's Medical University, School of Medicine, Tokyo, Japan

Tooru Shimosegawa, MD, PhD Division of Gastroenterology, Tohoku University Graduate School of Medicine, Sendai, Japan

Masahiro Shiokawa, MD, PhD Department of Gastroenterology and Hepatology, Graduate School of Medicine, Kyoto University, Kyoto, Japan

Keiko Shiratori, MD, PhD Department of Gastroenterology, Tokyo Medical Women's University, Tokyo, Japan

Tae Jun Song, MD, PhD Department of Internal Medicine, Asan Medical Center, University of Ulsan College of Medicine, Songpa-Gu, Seoul, South Korea

Taku Tabata, MD Department of Internal Medicine, Tokyo Metropolitan Komagome Hospital, Tokyo, Japan

Tadashi Takeuchi, MD, PhD Department of Gastroenterology, Tokyo Medical Women's University, Tokyo, Japan

Kazushige Uchida, MD, PhD Division of Gastroenterology and Hepatology, The Third Department of Internal Medicine, Kansai Medical University, Shinmachi, Hirakata, Osaka, Japan

Takayuki Watanabe, MD, PhD Department of Gastroenterology, Shinshu University School of Medicine, Matsumoto, Japan

Young Sik Woo, MD, PhD Department of Medicine, Samsung Medical Center, Sungkyunkwan University School of Medicine, Seoul, Korea

Satoshi Yamamoto, MD, PhD Department of Gastroenterology, Second Teaching Hospital, Fujita Health University, Nagoya, Japan

Kenji Yamao, MD, PhD Department of Gastroenterology, Aichi Cancer Center Hospital, Nagoya, Japan

Junji Yoshino, MD, PhD Department of Gastroenterology, Second Teaching Hospital, Fujita Health University, Nagoya, Japan

Part I

Introduction, Epidemiology and Pathology

Overview of Type 1 and Type 2 AIP

1

Terumi Kamisawa, Tadashi Takeuchi, and Keiko Shiratori

Introduction

Autoimmune pancreatitis (AIP) is a peculiar form of pancreatitis that has been known for the last two decades. Sarles et al. [1] first reported pancreatitis associated with hypergammaglobulinemia in 1961. They suggested that autoimmunity was one of the etiologies of pancreatitis. The first case that led researchers to suggest a new concept of AIP was treated with steroids by gastroenterologists (led by Professor Tadashi Takeuchi) in Tokyo Medical Women's University, and the concept was proposed by Yoshida, a member of that group, in 1995 [2]. The characteristic histological feature of the AIP is lymphoplasmacytic sclerosing pancreatitis (LPSP) [3]. AIP has been increasingly seen over the last decade and is now considered a distinct entity [4, 5]. Based on histological and immunohistochemical examinations of various organs and extrapancreatic lesions of AIP patients, a new clinicopathological entity called "IgG4-related systemic disease" was proposed [4, 6]. AIP is now considered to be a pancreatic manifestation of IgG4-related disease [4, 5, 7].

Following retrospective, histological examinations of pancreases resected due to suspicion of pancreatic cancer from patients with mass-forming chronic pancreatitis, American and European pathologists described another unique histological pattern, which was described as idiopathic duct-centric pancreatitis (IDCP) [8] or AIP with granulocytic epithelial lesion (GEL) [9]. Presently, AIP related to IgG4 is called type 1 AIP, and the later AIP reported from Europe is called type 2 AIP [5, 10, 11]. However, different historical paths have been followed to that designation (Table 1.1) [1–3, 6, 8–20]. Many diagnostic criteria for AIP have been published [13–16]. Following several international symposia, international consensus diagnostic criteria, which can be used to diagnose type 1 and type 2 AIP separately, were published in 2011 [18].

T. Kamisawa, MD, PhD (✉)
Department of Internal Medicine,
Tokyo Metropolitan Komagome Hospital,
3-18-22 Honkomagome, Bunkyo-ku, Tokyo 113-8677, Japan
e-mail: kamisawa@cick.jp

T. Takeuchi, MD, PhD • K. Shiratori, MD, PhD
Department of Gastroenterology,
Tokyo Medical Women's University, Tokyo, Japan

The First Report of AIP

A 68-year-old woman developed jaundice and was admitted to another hospital in 1993. Radiographic examinations showed pancreatic enlargement and common bile duct (CBD) obstruction. A tentative diagnosis of pancreatic cancer was made, and exploratory laparotomy was performed. The intraoperative diagnosis was advanced pancreatic cancer, and surgery was concluded without resecting the tumor or performing a biliary bypass procedure, and no biopsy specimens of the tumor were taken. After discharge, the patient presented at Tokyo Women's Medical University Hospital for further examination and treatment.

The patient had no history of alcohol abuse and no family history of pancreatic disease. She had no manifestations of sicca syndrome or any other collagen diseases. On physical examination, a hard, elastic mass with mild tenderness was palpated in the left upper quadrant of the abdomen in the area of the pancreas. The jaundice remitted spontaneously in the absence of any treatment. Though blood chemistry examinations showed evidence of cholestatic liver dysfunction, the total bilirubin level was normal. The pancreatic enzyme data showed an increased elastase-1 level with a low trypsin level, but she had normal lipase and pancreatic amylase levels. Levels of the tumor markers CA19.9, CEA, and Dupan-II were all within their normal ranges. Antinuclear antibody (ANA), anti-thyroglobulin antibody, and anti-microsomal antibody tests were positive. Her IgG level (2,960 mg/dL) was markedly elevated, with slight elevation of the IgE level (452 IU/mL). Though a 75-g oral glucose tolerance test showed a diabetic pattern, her HbA1c value was normal. An abnormally low value was obtained on the secretin test of exocrine pancreatic function.

T. Kamisawa, J.B. Chung (eds.), *Autoimmune Pancreatitis*,
DOI 10.1007/978-3-642-55086-7_1, © Springer-Verlag Berlin Heidelberg 2015

Table 1.1 Timeline of most important clinical observations in autoimmune pancreatitis

Year	Author	Reported findings
1961	Sarles et al. [1]	Idiopathic chronic pancreatitis associated with hypergammaglobulinemia; suggested an autoimmune mechanism
1991	Kawaguchi et al. [3]	Lymphoplasmacytic sclerosing pancreatitis (LPSP)
1995	Yoshida et al. [2]	Proposal of the concept of autoimmune pancreatitis (AIP)
2001	Hamano et al. [12]	Elevated serum IgG4 levels in AIP patients
2002	Japan Pancreas Society [13]	First diagnostic criteria for AIP
2003	Kamisawa et al. [6]	Proposal of IgG4-related systemic disease
2003	Notohara et al. [8]	Idiopathic duct-centric pancreatitis (IDCP)
2004	Zamboni et al. [9]	AIP with granulocyte epithelial lesion (GEL)
2006	Chari et al. [14]	HISORt criteria for AIP
2006	Kim et al. [15]	Korean diagnostic criteria for AIP
2008	Otsuki et al. [16]	Asian diagnostic criteria for AIP
2009	Kamisawa et al. [17]	Standard steroid treatment for AIP
2010	Chari et al. [10]	International consensus on classification of AIP into type 1 and type 2
2010	Sah et al.[11]	Clinical differences between type 1 and 2 AIP
2011	Shimosegawa et al. [18]	International Consensus Diagnostic Criteria
2011	Kamisawa et al. [19]	International survey of AIP
2013	Hart et al. [20]	International survey about long-term outcomes of AIP

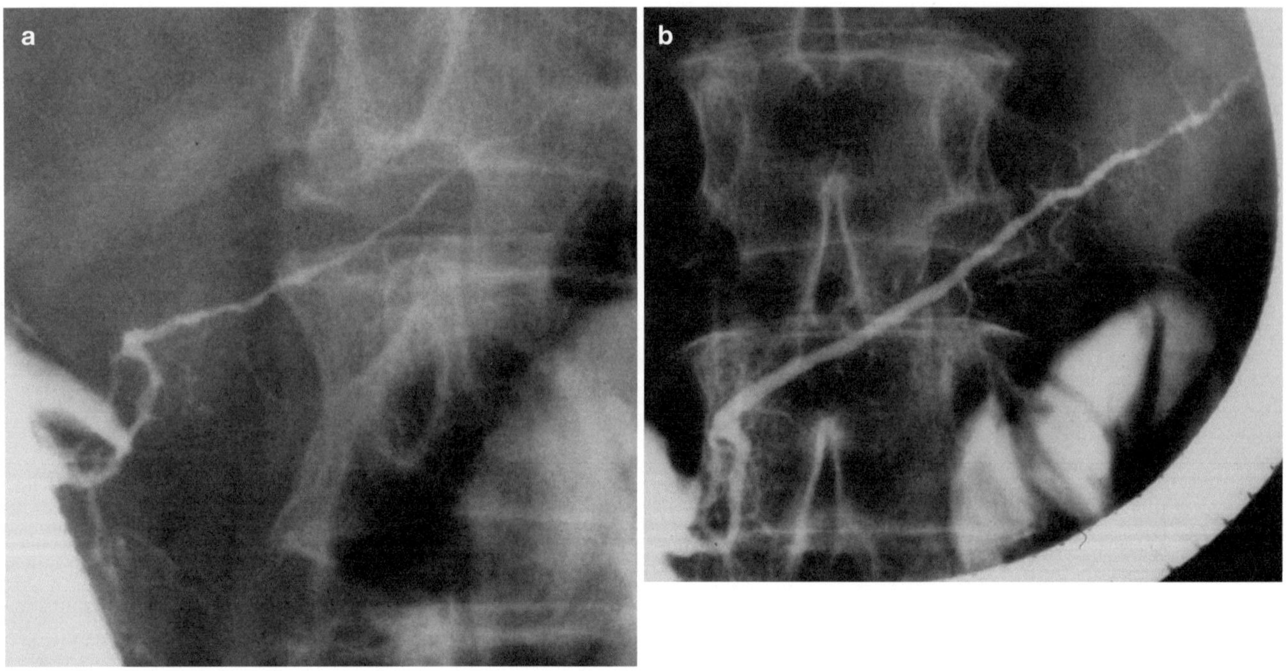

Fig. 1.1 Endoscopic retrograde pancreatography of the first reported case [2]. Diffuse irregular narrowing of the main pancreatic duct (**a**) improved after steroid therapy (**b**)

Ultrasonography showed diffuse enlargement of the pancreas with a slight hypoechoic pattern and CBD dilatation. On CT scans, diffuse pancreatic enlargement was seen, with homogeneous staining of the pancreas on contrast CT. On endoscopic retrograde pancreatography (ERP), the main pancreatic duct showed diffuse narrowing, and the main pancreatic duct wall was irregular (Fig. 1.1a). Histological examination of a needle biopsy specimen of the pancreas showed severe fibrotic change and lymphocyte and plasma cell infiltration.

Based on the above findings, chronic pancreatitis was diagnosed, an autoimmune mechanism was suspected to be involved in its pathogenesis, and it was suggested that steroid therapy would be effective. The patient was given oral prednisolone 40 mg/day for 1 week, followed by gradual tapering. The pancreas showed a dramatic decrease in size 8 weeks after the start of steroid therapy, and the CBD dilatation decreased from 11 to 8 mm. ERP done 4 weeks after the start of steroid therapy showed resolution of the narrowing of the main pancreatic duct, though mild irregularity of its wall remained (Fig. 1.1b). The IgG levels became normal, and the ANA, anti-thyroglobulin antibody, and anti-microsomal antibody titers decreased. The cholestatic liver dysfunction and exocrine pancreatic dysfunction showed complete resolution, and the patient was discharged after an uneventful course.

Based on the findings described above, AIP would have been considered today, but AIP did not exist as a concept at that time. Although the patient had an abdominal mass, pancreatic cancer was unlikely, because her general condition was good, she had no abdominal pain, and spontaneous resolution of her jaundice occurred over a 1-month period in the absence of any treatment. The presence of "diffuse irregular narrowing of the main pancreatic duct" on ERP had been noticed in several previous chronic pancreatitis patients, but its cause was unknown. However, the case reported above suggested that an autoimmune mechanism may have also been involved in the pathogenesis of previous cases.

This is the first case of AIP ever reported, and it was the first case treated with a steroid, and because of the steroid therapy's remarkable efficacy, surgery based on suspicion of pancreatic cancer has become unnecessary in cases with similar findings. Although this was only a report of a single case, the concept of AIP as a new clinical entity was proposed [2].

Type 1 AIP

Clinical Features

AIP is frequent in elderly males. According to a nationwide survey [21] in Japan, the male-to-female ratio of AIP patients was 3.7, with a mean age of 63.0 years. In the USA, the mean age was 61 years, and 85 % was male [22]. Obstructive jaundice induced by sclerosing cholangitis is the predominant initial symptom (74 % in the Komagome Hospital series [23]), and the jaundice sometimes fluctuates. Other symptoms include abdominal or back pain, weight loss, and anorexia. Diabetes mellitus (DM), usually type 2, is found in about half of AIP patients. The diagnoses of DM and AIP are made simultaneously in most patients, but some patients show exacerbation of preexisting DM with the onset of AIP [24, 25]. Mild or moderate pancreatic exocrine dysfunction is frequently detected [24]. Signs of associated extrapancreatic lesions, such as swelling of the salivary glands, hydronephrosis, and lymphadenopathy, are sometimes seen.

Laboratory Features

Liver and biliary enzymes and total bilirubin are frequently increased. Elevation of serum pancreatic enzymes was sometimes detected, but their levels were rarely abnormally high. Peripheral eosinophilia (≥600 cells/mm^3) and elevation of serum IgE levels were present in 11 and 34 %, respectively [26]. Elevation of serum IgG levels, positive antinuclear antibody (ANA), and positive rheumatoid factor (RF) were seen in 56.9, 33.6, and 27.3 %, respectively [21]. Serum IgG4 levels are frequently increased (77 % in the Komagome Hospital series [27], 81 % in the USA [22], and 68 % in Korea [28]). However, serum IgG4 levels are also elevated in some patients with pancreatic cancer (4 % (5/116) in the Komagome Hospital series [27] and 7 % (5/71) in the University of Pittsburgh Medical Center series [29]).

Imaging Features

The typical pancreatic imaging of AIP is diffuse enlargement and effacement of the lobular contour of the pancreas, with enhancement of the enlarged pancreas in the delayed phase of dynamic CT and MRI. A capsule-like rim that surrounds the pancreas is rather specific to AIP patients [30, 31]. On diffusion-weighted magnetic resonance imaging, AIP and pancreatic cancer are seen as high signal intensity areas, which are frequently diffuse or multiple in AIP patients, while they are solitary in pancreatic cancer patients [32].

Ultrasound examination shows an enlarged hypoechoic pancreas with hyperechoic spots [4]. Irregular narrowing (<3 mm in diameter) of the main pancreatic duct is a characteristic pancreatographic finding of AIP. The degree of narrowing of the main pancreatic duct can sometimes differ in the same patient [33–35]. MRCP cannot demonstrate the narrowing of the main pancreatic duct in many cases, but AIP is suggested by the presence of less upstream dilatation of the main pancreatic duct [36]. On fluorine-18 fluorodeoxyglucose positron emission tomography (FDG-PET), both AIP and pancreatic cancer patients showed FDG uptake in the pancreas, but abnormal extrapancreatic FDG uptake, such as extensive lymphadenopathy or swollen salivary gland, is highly suggestive of AIP [37].

Histopathological Features

The histological findings in the pancreas of AIP (LPSP) are abundant infiltration of T lymphocytes and IgG4-positive plasma cells and fibrosis in a periductal and interlobular distribution. The epithelium of the narrowed pancreatic duct is usually well preserved. Obliterative phlebitis is frequently seen in the variably sized pancreatic veins [2, 38, 39].

Diagnostic Criteria and Differential Diagnosis

Recently, the ICDC [18] for AIP were developed to diagnose AIP safely, avoid misdiagnosing pancreatic cancer as AIP, and diagnose AIP when it presents acutely. The criteria for type 1 and type 2 AIP were developed independently, and the diagnosis of AIP is made based on one or more of the following cardinal features: imaging characteristics of the pancreatic parenchyma and pancreatic duct, serology, other organ involvement, pancreatic histology, and the optional criterion of response to steroid therapy. Each feature has been categorized as either level 1 or 2 depending on its diagnostic reliability.

The most important disease to rule out when considering a diagnosis of AIP is pancreatic cancer. CT findings (a capsule-like rim, delayed enhancement of the swollen pancreas, and presence of extrapancreatic lesions) and ERP findings (≥3-cm-long narrowed main pancreatic duct, maximal upstream main pancreatic duct <5 mm, side branch derivation from the narrowed portion, and skipped lesions) suggest AIP rather than pancreatic cancer [33, 35, 40]. However, especially in segmental-type AIP, a histological approach with endoscopic ultrasound-guided fine-needle aspiration (EUS-FNA) plays an important role in confirming the diagnosis and excluding malignancy [41]. IgG4-immunostaining of biopsy specimens taken from the major duodenal papilla of AIP patients is useful to support the diagnosis of AIP [41–43].

Although a diagnostic trial of steroid therapy is useful in some cases to differentiate AIP from pancreatic cancer, it requires extreme caution and should be only be undertaken by pancreatologists in limited cases after a negative workup for pancreatic cancer, including EUS-FNA [18, 38].

Treatment

Although spontaneous improvement of AIP is seen in some patients, the standard therapy for AIP is oral steroid [17, 44, 45]. It is vitally important to distinguish AIP from pancreatic cancer before steroid therapy is started. In the Japanese standard regimen [44, 45] of steroid therapy for AIP, the indications for steroid therapy are principally symptoms such as obstructive jaundice and hydronephrosis. Before steroid therapy, the blood glucose level should be controlled using insulin in patients with DM, and in patients with obstructive jaundice, the jaundice is usually managed by endoscopic or transhepatic biliary drainage. The recommended initial dose of oral prednisolone is 0.6 mg/kg/day. Morphological and serological evaluations of the effectiveness of steroid treatment are performed 2 weeks after its start. A poor response to steroid therapy should raise the possibility of pancreatic cancer and the need to reevaluate the diagnosis. When steroid therapy is effective, the steroid dose is tapered by 5 mg every 1–2 weeks to a maintenance dose over a period of 3–6 months, while the patient's symptoms, as well as the biochemical, serological, and imaging findings, are carefully monitored. Relapses of AIP are frequent (around 30 %) [19, 20]. To prevent relapse, steroid maintenance therapy (5 mg/day) is recommended for at least about 6 months. Predictors of disease relapse include the presence of proximal bile duct involvement [20, 46] and persistent elevation of serum IgG4 levels [17]. In relapsed cases, re-administration or dose-up of steroid [17, 44, 45] and administration of immunosuppressive drugs such as azathioprine [47, 48] or rituximab [48, 49] are effective.

Prognosis

The short-term prognosis of AIP appears good with steroid therapy. However, the long-term outcome is unclear, because there are many unknown factors, such as relapse, pancreatic exocrine or endocrine dysfunction, and associated malignancy. In 27 % of cases, the pancreas became atrophic 1 or 2 years after the initiation of steroid therapy [50]. Pancreatic duct stones are more likely to occur in patients with at least one relapse (14.4 %), compared with those who have never had a relapse (4.0 %) [20]. Nine cases of pancreatic cancer associated with AIP have been recently reported, but whether there is a relationship between AIP and pancreatic cancer is unclear [45].

Type 2 AIP

Type 2 AIP is defined by the histological features of IDCP or GEL [8, 9]. The characteristic histological finding is ductal epithelial granulocytic infiltration leading to ductal damage, which is not seen in LPSP. Obliterative phlebitis and IgG4-positive cell infiltration are uncommon in IDCP [51]. Type 2 AIP is sometimes found in Western countries, but it appears uncommon in Japan and Korea [20]. Unlike type 1 AIP, type 2 AIP appears not to be a systemic disease, but rather a pancreas-specific disease. Type 2 AIP affects younger patients, and there is no male preponderance. It is not associated with increased serum IgG4 levels or with OOI typically seen in type 1 AIP. Acute pancreatitis and inflammatory bowel disease are sometimes associated with type 2 AIP [11, 20]. Currently, there is no serological biomarker for type 2 AIP, and the need for histological examination to diagnosis makes its clinical diagnosis difficult. Type 2 AIP also responds well to steroids. The relapse rate following steroid therapy was lower in type 2 AIP (15.3 %) than in type 1 AIP (35.8 %). Relapses in type 2 AIP were limited to the pancreas, while relapses occurred in various areas including the pancreas and biliary tree in type 1 AIP [20]. The clinical spectrum and long-term outcomes of medically treated type 2 AIP are still unclear.

Conclusions

Type 1 AIP is a pancreatic lesion of IgG4-related systemic disease, while type 2 AIP is a pancreas-specific disorder that is not associated with IgG4. Both AIPs are clinicopathologically, regionally, and ethnically different entities, sharing a need for accurate differentiation from pancreatic cancer. Further investigation is necessary to clarify the pathogenetic mechanisms including more definite serological markers and identification of the best diagnostic and therapeutic strategies.

Acknowledgment This study was partially supported by the Intractable Disease, supported by the Ministry of Health, Labour, and Welfare of Japan.

References

1. Sarles H, Sarles JC, Muratoren R, Guien C. Chronic inflammatory sclerosing of the pancreas–an autonomous pancreatic disease? Am J Dig Dis. 1961;6:688–98.
2. Yoshida K, Toki F, Takeuchi T, Watanabe S, Shiratori K, Hayashi N. Chronic pancreatitis caused by an autoimmune abnormality. Proposal of the concept of autoimmune pancreatitis. Dig Dis Sci. 1995;40:1561–8.
3. Kawaguchi K, Koike M, Tsuruta K, Okamoto A, Tsuruta K, Fujita N. Lymphoplasmacytic sclerosing pancreatitis with cholangitis: a variant of primary sclerosing cholangitis extensively involving pancreas. Hum Pathol. 1991;22:387–95.
4. Kamisawa T, Takuma K, Egawa N, Tsuruta K, Sasaki T. Autoimmune pancreatitis and IgG4-related sclerosing disease. Nat Rev Gastroenterol Hepatol. 2010;7:401–9.
5. Kamisawa T, Chari ST, Lerch MM, Kim MH, Gress TM, Shimosegawa T. Recent advances in autoimmune pancreatitis: type 1 and type 2. Gut. 2013;62:1373–80.
6. Kamisawa T, Funata N, Hayashi Y, et al. A new clinicopathological entity of IgG4-related autoimmune disease. J Gastroenterol. 2003;38:982–4.
7. Stone JH, Khosroshani A, Deshpande V, et al. Recommendations for the nomenclature of IgG4-related disease and its individual organ system manifestations. Arthritis Rheum. 2012;64: 3061–7.
8. Notohara K, Burgart LJ, Yadav D, Chari S, Smyrk TC. Idiopathic chronic pancreatitis with periductal lymphoplasmacytic infiltration. Clinicopathologic features of 35 cases. Am J Surg Patho. 2003;27:1119–27.
9. Zamboni G, Luttges J, Capelli P, et al. Histopathological features of diagnostic and clinical relevance in autoimmune pancreatitis: a study on 53 resection specimens and 9 biopsy specimens. Virch Arch. 2004;445:552–63.
10. Chari ST, Kloeppel G, Zhang L, et al. Histopathologic and clinical subtypes of autoimmune pancreatitis: the Honolulu consensus document. Pancreatology. 2010;10:664–72.
11. Sah RP, Chari ST, Pannala R, et al. Differences in clinical profile and relapse rate of type 1 versus type 2 autoimmune pancreatitis. Gastroenterology. 2010;139:140–8.
12. Hamano H, Kawa S, Horiuchi A, Unno H, Furuya N, Akamatsu T, et al. High serum IgG4 concentrations in patients with sclerosing pancreatitis. N Engl J Med. 2001;344:732–8.
13. Members of the Criteria Committee for Autoimmune Pancreatitis of the Japan Pancreas Society. Diagnostic criteria for autoimmune pancreatitis by the Japan Pancreas Society (in Japanese). Suizou. 2002;17:585–7.
14. Chari ST, Smyrk TC, Levy MJ, et al. Autoimmune pancreatitis: diagnosis using histology, imaging, serology, other organ involvement and response to steroids. Clin Gastroenterol Hepatol. 2006;4:1010–6.
15. Kim KP, Kim MH, Kim JC, et al. Diagnostic criteria for autoimmune chronic pancreatitis revised. World J Gastroenterol. 2006;12:2487–96.
16. Otsuki M, Chung JB, Okazaki K, et al. Asian diagnostic criteria for autoimmune pancreatitis: consensus of the Japan-Korea symposium on autoimmune pancreatitis. J Gastroenterol. 2008;43:403–8.
17. Kamisawa T, Shimosegawa T, Okazaki K, et al. Standard steroid treatment for autoimmune pancreatitis. Gut. 2009;58:1504–7.
18. Shimosegawa T, Chari ST, Frulloni L, et al. International consensus diagnostic criteria for autoimmune pancreatitis: guidelines of the International Association of Pancreatology. Pancreas. 2011;40:352–8.
19. Kamisawa T, Chari ST, Giday SA, et al. Clinical profile of autoimmune pancreatitis and its histological subtypes: an international multicenter survey. Pancreas. 2011;40:352–8.
20. Hart PA, Kamisawa T, Brugge WR, et al. Long-term outcomes of autoimmune pancreatitis: a multicentre, international analysis. Gut. 2012;62:1771–6.
21. Kanno A, Nishimori I, Masamune A, et al. Nationwide epidemiological survey of autoimmune pancreatitis in Japan. Pancreas. 2011;41:835–9.
22. Chari ST, Takahashi N, Levy MJ, et al. A diagnostic strategy to distinguish autoimmune pancreatitis from pancreatic cancer. Clin Gastroenterol Hepatol. 2009;7:1097–103.
23. Kamisawa T, Okamoto A. IgG4-related sclerosing disease. World J Gastroenterol. 2008;14:3948–55.
24. Kamisawa T, Egawa N, Inokuma S, et al. Pancreatic endocrine and exocrine function and salivary gland function in autoimmune pancreatitis before and after steroid therapy. Pancreas. 2003;27:235–8.
25. Miyamoto Y, Kamisawa T, Tabata T, et al. Short and long-term outcomes of diabetes mellitus in patients with autoimmune pancreatitis after steroid therapy. Gut Liver. 2012;6:501–4.
26. Kamisawa T, Anjiki H, Egawa N, Kubota N. Allergic manifestations in autoimmune pancreatitis. Eur J Gastroenterol Hepatol. 2009;21:1136–9.
27. Tabata T, Kamisawa T, Takuma K, et al. Serum IgG4 concentrations and IgG4-related sclerosing disease. Clin Chim Acta. 2009;408:25–8.
28. Ryu JK, Chung JB, Park SW, et al. Review of 67 patients with autoimmune pancreatitis in Korea. A multicenter nationwide study. Pancreas. 2008;37:377–85.
29. Raina A, Krasinskas AM, Greer JB, et al. Serum immunoglobulin G fraction 4 levels in pancreatic cancer: elevations not associated with autoimmune pancreatitis. Arch Pathol Lab Med. 2008;132:48–53.
30. Kamisawa T, Egawa N, Nakajima H, Tsuruta K, Okamoto A, Kamata N. Clinical difficulties in the differentiation of autoimmune pancreatitis and pancreatic carcinoma. Am J Gastroenterol. 2003;98:2694–9.
31. Takahashi N, Fletcher JG, Fidler JL, Hough DM, Kawashima A, Chari ST. Dual-phase CT of autoimmune pancreatitis: a multicenter study. Am J Roentgenol. 2008;190:280–6.
32. Kamisawa T, Takuma K, Anjiki H, et al. Differentiation of autoimmune pancreatitis from pancreatic cancer by diffusion-weighted MRI. Am J Gastroenterol. 2010;105:1870–5.
33. Kamisawa T, Imai M, Chen PY, et al. Strategy for differentiating autoimmune pancreatitis from pancreatic cancer. Pancreas. 2008;37:e62–7.
34. Sugumar A, Levy MJ, Kamisawa T, et al. Endoscopic retrograde pancreatography criteria to diagnose autoimmune pancreatitis: an international multicenter study. Gut. 2011;60:666–70.
35. Takuma K, Kamisawa T, Tabata T, Inaba Y, Egawa N, Igarashi Y. Utility of pancreatography for diagnosing autoimmune pancreatitis. World J Gastroenterol. 2011;17:2332–7.
36. Kamisawa T, Tu Y, Egawa N, et al. Can MRCP replace ERCP for the diagnosis of autoimmune pancreatitis? Abdom Imaging. 2009;34:381–4.

37. Kamisawa T, Takuma K, Anjiki H, et al. FDG-PET/CT findings of autoimmune pancreatitis. Hepatogastroenterology. 2010;57:447–50.
38. Okazaki K, Kawa S, Kamisawa T, Shimosegawa T, Tanaka M, Research Committee for Intractable Pancreatic Disease and Japan Pancreas Society. Japanese consensus guidelines for management of autoimmune pancreatitis: I. Concept and diagnosis of autoimmune pancreatitis. J Gastroenterol. 2010;45:249–65.
39. Kamisawa T, Shimosegawa T. Pancreas: Histological diagnostic criteria for autoimmune pancreatitis. Nat Rev Gastroenterol Hepatol. 2011;9:8–10.
40. Kawa S, Okazaki K, Kamisawa T, Shimosegawa T, Tanaka M, Research Committee for Intractable Pancreatic Disease and Japan Pancreas Society. Japanese consensus guidelines for management of autoimmune pancreatitis: II. Extrapancreatic lesions, differential diagnosis. J Gastroenterol. 2010;45:355–69.
41. Kamisawa T, Ohara T, Kim MH, Kanno A, Okazaki K, Fujita N. Role of endoscopy in the diagnosis of autoimmune pancreatitis and IgG4-related sclerosing cholangitis. Dig Endosc. (Epub ahead of print).
42. Kamisawa T, Tu Y, Egawa N, et al. A new diagnostic endoscopic tool for autoimmune pancreatitis. Gastrointes Endosc. 2008;68:358–61.
43. Kim MH, Moon SH, Kamisawa T. Major duodenal papilla in autoimmune pancreatitis. Dig Surg. 2010;27:110–4.
44. Kamisawa T, Okazaki K, Kawa S, Shimosegawa T, Tanaka M, Research Committee for Intractable Pancreatic Disease and Japan Pancreas Society. Japanese consensus guidelines for management of autoimmune pancreatitis: III. Treatment and prognosis of AIP. J Gastroenterol. 2010;45:471–7.
45. Kamisawa T, Okazaki K, Kawa S, et al. Amendment of the Japanese Consensus Guidelines for Autoimmune Pancreatitis, 2013 III. Treatment and prognosis of autoimmune pancreatitis. J Gastroenterol. 2014;49:961–70.
46. Ghazale A, Chari ST, Zhang L, et al. Immunoglobulin G4-associated cholangitis: clinical profile and response to therapy. Gastroenterology. 2008;134:706–15.
47. Sandanayake NS, Church NI, Chapman MH, et al. Presentation and management of post-treatment relapse in autoimmune pancreatitis/immunoglobulin G4-associated cholangitis. Clin Gastroenterol Hepatol. 2009;7:1089–96.
48. Hart PA, Topazian MD, Witzig TE, et al. Treatment of relapsing autoimmune pancreatitis with immunomodulators and rituximab: the Mayo Clinic experience. Gut. 2013;62:1607–15.
49. Kamisawa T, Zen Y, Pillai S, Stone JH. IgG4-related disease. Lancet. (in press).
50. Kamisawa T, Egawa N, Nakajima H, Tsuruta K, Okamoto A. Morphological changes after steroid therapy in autoimmune pancreatitis. Scand J Gastroenterol. 2004;39:1154–8.
51. Kamisawa T, Notohara K, Shimosegawa T. Two clinicopathologic subtypes of autoimmune pancreatitis: LPSP and IDCP. Gastroenterology. 2010;139:22–5.

Epidemiology of Autoimmune Pancreatitis

2

Atsushi Kanno, Atsushi Masamune, and Tooru Shimosegawa

Introduction

Autoimmune pancreatitis (AIP) is a rare disease that has recently emerged as a unique type of pancreatitis with a presumed autoimmune etiology. In 1995, Yoshida et al. [1] proposed AIP as a diagnostic entity. They summarized the clinical features of AIP as follows: increased serum γ-globulin or immunoglobulin (Ig)G levels and the presence of autoantibodies; diffuse irregular narrowing of the main pancreatic duct (MPD) and enlargement of the pancreas; occasional association with stenosis of the lower bile duct and other autoimmune diseases; mild symptoms, usually without acute attacks of pancreatitis; effectiveness of steroid therapy; and histological findings of lymphoplasmacytic sclerosing pancreatitis (LPSP) [1, 2]. Thereafter, AIP has been extensively reported worldwide including from Japan, Korea, Europe, and the United States. Because AIP is a relatively new clinical entity and the diagnostic criteria are being established, the epidemiology of AIP is not fully known. In Japan, the Research Committee of Intractable Pancreatic Disease provided by the Ministry of Health, Labour, and Welfare of Japan (RCIPD) has conducted three nationwide epidemiological surveys of AIP according to the diagnostic criteria used at that time. We here describe the epidemiology of AIP, mainly focusing on the results of nationwide surveys in Japan [3, 4].

A. Kanno, MD, PhD (✉) • A. Masamune, MD, PhD
T. Shimosegawa, MD, PhD
Division of Gastroenterology, Tohoku University Graduate School of Medicine, 1-1 Seiryo-machi, Aoba-ku, Sendai 980-8574, Japan
e-mail: atsushih@med.tohoku.ac.jp; tshimosegawa@int3.med.tohoku.ac.jp

First Nationwide Survey of AIP in Japan

With the accumulation of similar cases in Japan, the Japan Pancreas Society (JPS) proposed the world's first clinical diagnostic criteria for AIP in 2002 [5]. The criteria consisted of 3 items: (1) specific imaging findings (a mandatory requirement), along with (2) serological and/or (3) pathological evidence. In the 2002 criteria, the length of MPD narrowing on endoscopic retrograde pancreatography (ERP) was defined as more than 1/3 of the entire pancreas to avoid confusion with short-segment narrowing or stenosis caused by pancreatic cancer. As a result, the 2002 criteria were diagnostic for the typical diffuse type of AIP but failed to diagnose the atypical localized type of AIP, which shows focal or segmental swelling of the pancreas and short-segment narrowing of MPD less than 1/3 of the entire pancreas.

Following the proposed diagnostic criteria for AIP, the RCIPD conducted the first nationwide survey of AIP in 2003 [3]. The departments of internal medicine, gastroenterology, digestive surgery, and surgery in the respective hospitals are listed, and a method of stratified random sampling was used to select the departments to be surveyed. The sampling rates were 5, 10, 20, 40, 80, 100, and 100 % for the stratum of general hospitals with less than 100 beds, 100–199 beds, 200–299 beds, 300–399 beds, 400–499 beds, 500 or more beds, and the affiliated university hospitals, respectively. In order to increase the study efficiency, some departments that were expected to treat many patients with pancreatic diseases were selected. These departments were separately classified into a "special strata" category, and all departments in this category were surveyed. A simple questionnaire was made to determine the number of patients with AIP who visited the departments in 2002. This questionnaire was directly mailed in January 2003 to the heads of 2,971 departments randomly chosen as described above. In the second-stage survey, requests for all individual patients' detailed clinico-

T. Kamisawa, J.B. Chung (eds.), *Autoimmune Pancreatitis*,
DOI 10.1007/978-3-642-55086-7_2, © Springer-Verlag Berlin Heidelberg 2015

epidemiological information were sent to those departments reporting that they had seen patients with AIP in 2002 in the first-stage survey.

Of 2,971 departments, 993 departments responded to the questionnaire in the first-stage survey (response rate: 33.4 %), and 294 patients with AIP were identified according to the JPS diagnostic criteria 2002. The estimated number of AIP patients in 2002 was 900 (95 % confidence interval (CI), 670–1,110), suggesting that AIP was a rare disease. In addition, 800 (95 % CI, 410–1,180) patients were suspected to have AIP, although they did not fulfill the JPS diagnostic criteria 2002. These patients might have had atypical localized type AIP, which shows focal or segmental swelling of the pancreas and short-segment narrowing of MPD less than 1/3 of the entire pancreas. Based on the second questionnaire, a total of 158 cases were confirmed to fulfill the JPS diagnostic criteria for AIP. The male to female ratio was 2.85, and the age of disease onset in 95 % of the patients was over 45 years [3].

Second Nationwide Survey in Japan

The 2002 Criteria were revised in 2006 by the JPS and the RCIPD [6]. Major revisions included the elimination of the dependency on the length of MPD narrowing and the incorporation of IgG4 in the serology criterion. In 2001, Hamano et al. [7] reported that elevated serum IgG4 levels were highly specific and sensitive for the diagnosis of AIP. The revised diagnostic criteria consisted of characteristic radiological findings (diffuse or segmental irregular narrowing of the MPD and enlargement of the pancreas) as an essential factor in combination with serological findings (elevated serum γ-globulin, IgG, IgG4, or the presence of autoantibodies, such as antinuclear antibodies and rheumatoid factor) and/or histopathological findings (marked interlobular fibrosis and prominent infiltration of lymphocytes and plasma cells in the periductal area, occasionally with lymphoid follicles in the pancreas) [6].

In 2008, the RCIPD started the second nationwide survey of AIP according to the revised diagnostic criteria for AIP (JPS2006) [4]. The survey was conducted in a similar manner to the first nationwide survey, and the target subjects were patients diagnosed as having AIP in 2007. The first questionnaire was directly mailed in November 2008 to the heads of 3,015 departments randomly chosen as described earlier.

Of 3,015 departments, 1,114 departments responded to the questionnaire in the first-stage survey (response rate: 36.9 %) and 1,069 patients with AIP were identified (Table 2.1). Among them, 391 (36.6 %) cases were newly diagnosed patients as having AIP in 2007. From these data, we estimated that the total number of patients diagnosed as having AIP in Japan was 2,790 (95 % CI, 2,540–3,040), which means an estimated overall prevalence rate of 2.2 per 100,000 population. The number of patients who were newly diagnosed as AIP in 2007 was estimated to be 1,120 (95 % CI, 1,000–1,240), from which the annual incidence rate was calculated to be 0.9 per 100,000 population. The estimated number of AIP patients in this study, 2,790, was 3.1 times higher than the estimated number of 900 in the first nationwide survey in 2002 [3] and was 1.64 times higher than the 1,700 that included the number of suspected AIP patients. The rapid increase in the number of AIP may be explained by (1) the different diagnostic criteria employed in these two surveys and (2) the increasing recognition of AIP as a disease entity.

In response to the questionnaire in the second-stage survey, we collected detailed clinicoepidemiological information on 546 patients (51.0 %; 418 males, 114 females, and 14 patients of unknown sex) who had been identified by the first questionnaire. One hundred seventy-two patients were newly diagnosed in 2007, and 374 patients had been already diagnosed before 2007. All patients were Japanese. The male to female ratio of the AIP patients was 3.7. The mean age was 63.0 ± 11.4 years (male/female = 63.6 ± 10.8/60.3 ± 12.4), and patients aged 60–69 years formed a peak in the age distribution curve (Fig. 2.1).

Diagnosis

Imaging findings of the reported patients are summarized in Table 2.2. Approximately 90 % of the cases had enlargement of the pancreas. Among them, nearly 30 % of the cases showed localized enlargement, which was not included in the 2002 diagnostic criteria [5]. MPD narrowing was seen in more than 90 % of the cases, but narrowing was within one-third of the entire length in approximately one-third of the cases. These cases, again, did not fulfill the JPS 2002 diagnostic criteria.

The serum IgG4 level was increased (≥135 mg/dl) in 87.6 % of the patients (Table 2.3). The IgG level was increased in 56.9 %, but the positive rates for γ-globulin, antinuclear antibody, rheumatoid factor, and eosinophilia were less than half.

Tissue specimens, including both accurate and inaccurate diagnoses, were obtained from various organs including the

Table 2.1 Patient stratification, hospital selection, and survey results

Stratification	Departments in Japan	Selection rate (%)	Departments nominated	Departments replying	Reply rate (%)	Departments replying	New cases (male/female)	Continuous cases (male/female)	Total (male/female)
Specialty hospital	80	100	80	58	72.5	58	121 (89/32)	255 (201/54)	376 (290/86)
University hospital	294	100	294	184	62.6	184	107 (84/23)	229 (186/43)	336 (270/66)
≥500 beds	679	100	679	241	35.5	241	94 (72/22)	97 (68/29)	191 (140/51)
400–499 beds	633	80	506	166	32.8	166	35 (29/6)	65 (36/29)	100 (65/35)
300–399 beds	1,156	40	462	142	30.7	142	21 (15/6)	22 (16/6)	43 (31/12)
200–299 beds	1,689	20	338	100	29.6	100	6 (4/2)	8 (6/2)	14 (10/4)
100–199 beds	3,903	10	390	128	32.8	128	5 (5/0)	0 (0/0)	5 (5/0)
≤99 beds	5,324	5	266	95	35.7	95	2 (2/0)	2 (1/1)	4 (3/1)
Total	13,758	–	3,015	1,114	36.9	1,114	391 (300/91)	678 (514/164)	1,069 (814/255)

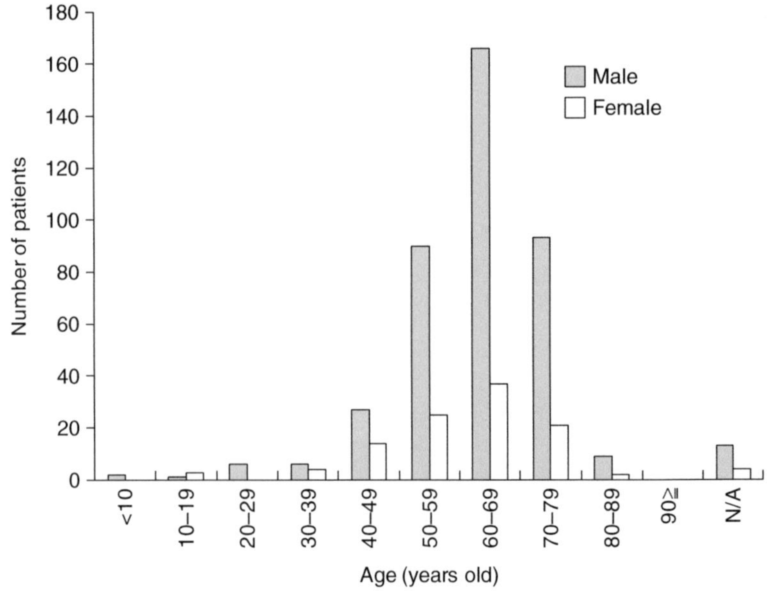

Fig. 2.1 Age distribution of patients with AIP in 2007 (Kanno et al. [4])

Table 2.2 AIP-related imaging findings

Imaging	Number of cases (%)
Enlargement of the pancreas	Enlarged, 478 (87.5 %); not enlarged, 52 (9.5 %)
Area of pancreatic enlargement	Diffuse, 322 (67.4 %); localized, 141 (29.5 %)
Narrowing of the pancreatic duct	Narrowing, 468 (85.7 %); no narrowing, 40 (7.3 %)
Length of the narrowing pancreatic duct	>1/3 of 307 (65.6 %); <1/3 of 151 (32.3 %)

Table 2.3 Serological findings in AIP patients

Serological items	Number of cases (%)
High serum γ-globulin level (≥2.0 g/dL)	153/381 (40.2 %)
High serum IgG level (≥1,800 mg/dL)	292/513 (56.9 %)
High serum IgG4 level (≥135 mg/dL)	388/443 (87.6 %)
ANA (≥80-fold)	154/458 (33.6 %)
RF (≥20)	86/315 (27.3 %)
Eosinophilia (≥8 %)	71/388 (18.3 %)

ANA antinuclear antibody, *IgG* immunoglobulin G, *RF* rheumatic factor

pancreas in 233 (49.1 %) out of 475 cases, whereas histological examination was not performed in 242 cases (Table 2.4). Endoscopic ultrasonography-guided fine-needle aspiration was most frequently performed for obtaining pancreatic tissue samples. Pancreatic resection was performed in 51 cases on suspicion of pancreatic cancer.

Sclerosing cholangitis was the leading extrapancreatic lesion and found in more than half of the patients (Table 2.5). Other relatively common extrapancreatic lesions included sialadenitis, lymphadenopathy, and retroperitoneal fibrosis.

Steroid was used for diagnostic purposes in 36 (6.8 %) of 530 patients. The reasons (52 in total) for steroid trial were as follows: the absence of characteristic imaging findings for AIP in 17 cases, negative serological findings in 19 cases, and lack of typical histological findings in 11 cases.

Table 2.4 Histological examination performed for the diagnosis of AIP

Organs	Procedures	Number of patients[a]
Pancreas	Resection	51/233 (21.9 %)
	EUS-FNA	92/233 (39.5 %)
	EUS-TCB	4/233 (1.7 %)
	Percutaneous biopsy	43/233 (18.5 %)
Salivary gland	Biopsy	18/233 (7.7 %)
Bile duct	Biopsy	35/233 (15.0 %)
Duodenal papilla	Biopsy	6/233 (2.6 %)

EUS-FNA endoscopic ultrasonography-guided fine-needle aspiration, *EUS-TCB* endoscopic ultrasonography-guided trucut biopsy
[a]Including overlapping cases

Table 2.5 Extrapancreatic lesions in the AIP patients

Extrapancreatic lesions	Number of cases (%)
Sclerosing cholangitis	289/546 (52.9 %)
Sialadenitis	76/547 (13.9 %)
Mediastinal/abdominal lymph node swelling	69/548 (12.6 %)
Retroperitoneal fibrosis	44/543 (8.1 %)
Dacryoadenitis	36/545 (6.6 %)
Intestinal pneumonia	20/541 (3.7 %)
Chronic thyroiditis	14/538 (2.6 %)
Intestinal nephritis	14/538 (2.6 %)

Treatment

Four hundred fifty-three (83.0 %) of the 546 patients were treated with steroid, whereas the remaining 17 % patients received no particular medication. No patients received immunosuppressants in this study. Biliary drainage was performed in 41.4 % of the patients due to obstructive jaundice in association with sclerosing cholangitis.

Relapse

Among the 458 patients who had received steroid treatment, 134 (29.6 %) patients relapsed on imaging studies. Relapse occurred in the pancreas in 49 (36.6 %) patients, in extrapancreatic organs in 57 (42.5 %) patients, and in both the pancreas and extrapancreatic organs in 24 (17.9 %) patients.

Third Nationwide Survey in Japan

During the 14th congress of the International Association of Pancreatology held in Fukuoka, Japan, from July 11 through 13, 2010, an international panel of experts met. The working group proposed the International Consensus Diagnostic Criteria (ICDC) [8]. AIP is classified into 2 subtypes on ICDC: type 1 related to IgG4 (LPSP) and type 2 to granulocytic epithelial lesion (idiopathic duct-centric chronic pancreatitis (IDCP)). Criteria for the two types of AIP were independently developed, and AIP is diagnosed based on one or more of the following cardinal features: imaging characteristics of the pancreatic parenchyma (P) and pancreatic duct (D), serology, other organ involvement (OOI), pancreatic histology (H), and the optional criterion of response to steroid therapy. Although the ICDC for AIP firstly enabled us to diagnose independently and compare 2 distinctive subtypes, type 1 and type 2 AIP, the ICDC system is somewhat complicated for a general use. Because cases with type 2 AIP are extremely rare in Japan, the JPS and the RCIPD revised the diagnostic criteria as the clinical diagnostic criteria for AIP 2011 (JPS2011) [9].

The RCIPD is currently conducting the third nationwide survey of AIP according to the JPS2011 diagnostic criteria. Although the details of this survey will be published elsewhere, we here briefly describe the results of the first-stage survey. The survey is being conducted in a similar manner to the previous surveys, and the target subjects are patients diagnosed as having AIP in 2011 in Japan. The first questionnaire was directly mailed in June 2012 to the heads of 4,175 departments randomly chosen as described below. By the end of November 2012, 1,875 departments responded to the questionnaire in the first-stage survey (response rate: 45.1 %), and 1,959 patients with AIP were identified. From these data, we estimated that the total number of patients diagnosed as having AIP in 2011 in Japan was 5,745 (95 % CI, 5,325–6,164), which means an estimated prevalence rate of 4.6 per 100,000 population. The number of patients who were newly diagnosed as AIP in 2011 was estimated to be 1,808 (95 % CI, 1,597–2,018), from which the annual incidence rate was calculated to be 1.4 per 100,000 populations. The estimated number of AIP patients in this study, 5,745, was 2.1 times higher than the estimated number of 2,790 in the second nationwide survey [4].

International AIP Surveys

The prevalence of AIP in other countries is not fully known, with reports limited to case series and description of tertiary referrals. For example, Kamisawa et al. [10] reported the clinicopathological profiles of AIP ($n=731$) and the clinical profiles of LPSP ($n=204$) and IDCP ($n=64$) patients from 15 institutes in 8 countries. They showed that the clinical profiles of non-histologically confirmed AIP from Asia, the United States, and the United Kingdom corresponded to that of LPSP, whereas those from Italy and Germany suggested a mixture of LPSP and IDCP. Similarly, Hart et al. [11] conducted a multicenter, international analysis of patients with AIP diagnosed according to the ICDC. Twenty-three institutions from 10 different countries participated in the study, and a total of 1,064 patients fulfilling the ICDC for type 1 ($n=978$) or type 2 ($n=86$) AIP were included. The proportion of patients diagnosed with type 2 AIP was lower in Asian countries (3.7 %) compared with European (12.9 %, $P<0.001$) and North American countries (13.7 %, $P<0.001$). These studies indeed provide invaluable information about the geographical similarities and differences of AIP. Further epidemiological studies based on the universal diagnostic criteria such as ICDC would facilitate better understanding the clinicopathological characteristics of AIP worldwide.

Summary

We reviewed the results of three nationwide epidemiological surveys of AIP in Japan. To compare the exact distribution and types of AIP worldwide, large-scale epidemiological surveys according to the universal diagnostic criteria are required.

Acknowledgment This work was supported in part by the Research Committee of Intractable Pancreatic Disease (principal investigator: Tooru Shimosegawa) provided by the Ministry of Health, Labour, and Welfare of Japan.

Disclosure

All authors disclosed no financial relationships relevant to this publication.

References

1. Yoshida K, Toki F, Takeuchi T, Watanabe S, Shiratori K, Hayashi N. Chronic pancreatitis caused by an autoimmune abnormality. Proposal of the concept of autoimmune pancreatitis. Dig Dis Sci. 1995;40:1561–8.
2. Kamisawa T, Notohara K, Shimosegawa T. Two clinicopathologic subtypes of autoimmune pancreatitis: LPSP and IDCP. Gastroenterology. 2010;139:22–5.
3. Nishimori I, Tamakoshi A, Otsuki M, Research Committee on Intractable Diseases of the Pancreas, Ministry of Health, Labour and Welfare of Japan. Prevalence of autoimmune pancreatitis in Japan from a nationwide survey in 2002. J Gastroenterol. 2007;42(Suppl. 18):6–8. doi:10.1007/s00535-007-2043-y.
4. Kanno A, Nishimori I, Masamune A, Kikuta K, Hirota M, Kuriyama S, Tsuji I, Shimosegawa T, Research Committee on Intractable Diseases of P. Nationwide epidemiological survey of autoimmune pancreatitis in Japan. Pancreas. 2012;41(6):835–9. doi:10.1097/MPA.0b013e3182480c99.
5. Members of the Criteria Committee for Autoimmune Pancreatitis of the Japan Pancreas Society. Diagnostic criteria for autoimmune pancreatitis by the Japan Pancreas Society (2002). (in Japanese with English abstract) Suizo. 2002;17:585–7.
6. Members of the Autoimmune Pancreatitis Diagnostic Criteria Committee, the Research Committee of Intractable Diseases of the Pancreas supported by the Japanese Ministry of Health, Labor and Welfare, and Members of the Autoimmune Pancreatitis Diagnostic Criteria Committee, the Japan Pancreas Society. Clinical diagnostic criteria of autoimmune pancreatitis 2006. (in Japanese with English abstract) Suizo. 2006;21:395–7.
7. Hamano H, Kawa S, Horiuchi A, Unno H, Furuya N, Akamatsu T, et al. High serum IgG4 concentrations in patients with sclerosing pancreatitis. N Engl J Med. 2001;344:732–8.
8. Shimosegawa T, Chari ST, Frulloni L, et al. International consensus diagnostic criteria for autoimmune pancreatitis: guidelines of the International Association of Pancreatology. Pancreas. 2011;40:352–8.
9. Okazaki K, Shimosegawa T, The Working Group Members of the Japan Pancreas Society and the Research Committee for Intractable Pancreatic Disease by the Ministry of Labor, Health and Welfare of Japan. The Amendment of the clinical diagnostic criteria in Japan (JPS2011) in response to the proposal of the international consensus of diagnostic criteria (ICDC) for autoimmune pancreatitis. Pancreas. 2012;41:1341–2.
10. Kamisawa T, Chari ST, Giday SA, Kim MH, Chung JB, Lee KT, Werner J, Bergmann F, Lerch MM, Mayerle J, Pickartz T, Lohr M, Schneider A, Frulloni L, Webster GJ, Reddy DN, Liao WC, Wang HP, Okazaki K, Shimosegawa T, Kloeppel G, Go VL. Clinical profile of autoimmune pancreatitis and its histological subtypes: an international multicenter survey. Pancreas. 2011;40(6):809–14. doi:10.1097/MPA.0b013e3182258a15.
11. Hart PA, Kamisawa T, Brugge WR, Chung JB, Culver EL, Czako L, Frulloni L, Go VL, Gress TM, Kim MH, Kawa S, Lee KT, Lerch MM, Liao WC, Lohr M, Okazaki K, Ryu JK, Schleinitz N, Shimizu K, Shimosegawa T, Soetikno R, Webster G, Yadav D, Zen Y, Chari ST. Long-term outcomes of autoimmune pancreatitis: a multicentre, international analysis. Gut. 2013;62(12):1771–6. doi:10.1136/gutjnl-2012-303617.

3 Pathophysiology of Autoimmune Pancreatitis

Kazuichi Okazaki and Kazushige Uchida

Introduction

Recent studies suggested the existence of two subtypes of autoimmune pancreatitis (AIP) [1–5]: type 1 AIP (IgG4-related pancreatitis as the pancreatic manifestation of IgG4-related disease (IgG4-RD)) and type 2 AIP (idiopathic duct-centric chronic pancreatitis or AIP with a granulocytic epithelial lesion). The characteristic features of type 1 AIP are swelling of the pancreas, increased serum IgG4 levels, abundant infiltration of IgG4+ plasmacytes with storiform fibrosis, obliterative phlebitis, and other organ involvements (OOIs) such as sclerosing cholangitis, sclerosing sialadenitis, and retroperitoneal fibrosis [4, 6]. The OOIs appear synchronously or metachronously with the pancreatic lesion(s), share the same pathological conditions, and show favorable response to steroid therapy [7]. The lesions are usually detected by imaging and blood tests (CT, MRI, gallium scintigraphy, FDG-PET, and IgG4); however, these should be confirmed by histological findings. The OOIs sometimes mimic, or are misdiagnosed as, primary lesions of the corresponding organs: lachrymal and salivary gland lesions for Sjögren's syndrome, respiratory lesions for sarcoidosis, and sclerosing cholangitis for primary sclerosing cholangitis (PSC) [7, 8].

On the other hand, type 2 AIP, extremely rarely observed in Japan, is not associated with either serum IgG4 elevation or with OOIs seen in LPSP. Type 2 AIP has swelling of the pancreas, but none or very few IgG4-positive plasma cells and clinical features show a distinctly different profile associated with no biomarkers such as serum IgG4, IgG, and autoantibodies, or OOIs except for inflammatory bowel disease [1, 4]. Different from type 1 AIP, very few studies of pathogenic mechanisms in type 2 AIP have been reported except for deposition of C3c and IgG at the basement membrane of pancreatic ducts and acini, which suggests immune complex-mediated destruction of ducts and acini in type 2 AIP [9]. In this chapter, recent advances in the pathophysiology of type 1 AIP are mainly mentioned.

K. Okazaki, MD, PhD (✉) • K. Uchida
Division of Gastroenterology and Hepatology, The Third Department of Internal Medicine, Kansai Medical University, Shinmachi, Hirakata, Osaka 573-1197, Japan
e-mail: okazaki@hirakata.kmu.ac.jp; uchidak@takii.kmu.ac.jp

Immunogenic Backgrounds

Based on immunogenic backgrounds, abnormal conditions of immune responses may be involved in the development of AIP [8]. However, immunogenic factors have been in a few series, mainly from Asian countries, and then not conclusive. As type 2 AIP is rare in Asia, these data are deemed to reflect immunogenic factors in type 1 AIP. Susceptibility to AIP may be associated with the class II antigen of the major histocompatibility complex (MHC), polymorphism of nuclear factor (NF)-kB, and Fc-receptor-like (FCRL) 3 genes expressed on B cells [10, 11]. Two studies of HLA association with AIP have been reported from the Japanese [10] and Korean group [11]. In the Japanese patients with AIP, HLA haplotype DRB1*0405-DQB1*0401 (class II) and ABCF1 proximal to C3-2-11, telomeric of HLA-E (class I) are susceptibility to AIP, but not in the Korean patients. However, substitution of aspartic acid to nonaspartic acid at DQβ1 may be a predictive factor for relapse of AIP in Korean patients [11]. FCRL3 polymorphisms are linked to various autoimmune diseases, such as rheumatoid arthritis, autoimmune thyroid disease, and systemic lupus erythematosus

T. Kamisawa, J.B. Chung (eds.), *Autoimmune Pancreatitis*,
DOI 10.1007/978-3-642-55086-7_3, © Springer-Verlag Berlin Heidelberg 2015

(SLE) in the Japanese population [12, 13]. However, Fc-receptor-like 3 gene polymorphisms is not correlated with the DRB1*0405-DQB1*0401 haplotype, suggesting that while both are related to AIP susceptibility in the Japanese population, they are part of distinct underlying mechanisms of disease development [12, 13].

Innate immunity is important in the development of acquired immunity or autoimmune diseases. Although polymorphisms in toll-like receptor (TLR)-4 gene have been linked with several autoimmune and allergic diseases, it seems not to play an important role in AIP [14]. On the other hand, an inhibitory molecule, cytotoxic T lymphocyte antigen-4 (*CTLA-4*; CD152) expressed on the activated memory T cells and CD4+CD25+ regulatory T cells (Tregs) was independently reported as a susceptibility factor for AIP in the Taiwanese [15] and Japanese population [16]. CTLA-4 acts as a negative regulator of T-cell responses by competing with the CD28 molecule for engagement with the B7 molecules CD80 and CD86 on antigen-presenting cells [17]. Umemura T et al. [16] reported that the 3′ untranslated region of *CTLA-4*+6230 SNP plays a pivotal role for both susceptibility (+6230G/G genotype) to and protection (haplotype of the +6230A allele) from AIP, while exon 1+49 SNP is not associated with AIP in the Japanese patients. They also found that +49A/A or +6230A/A genotypes may be associated with the recurrence of the disease, which is observed in Graves' disease, type 1 diabetes, and clearance of hepatitis B virus [16]. On the other hand, Chan MC et al. [15] have reported that *CTLA-4* SNPs have shown significantly higher frequencies of the +49G allele in patients with AIP than in controls, but not with other subtypes of chronic pancreatitis. TNF-alpha promoter 863A was significantly associated with higher risk of AIP. Racial and geographical differences may be associated with SNPs of the different locus of CTLA-4 [15]. Soluble isoform of CTLA4 (sCTLA4) is reported to be elevated in patients with autoimmune diseases, such as autoimmune thyroid disease, SLE, and myasthenia gravis [17]. Therefore, the sCLTA4 molecule may have a dual role of maintaining self-tolerance and enhancing immune responses by blocking the interaction of CD80 on antigen-presenting cells and CTLA4 on T cells.

Innate Immunity

Recently, abnormal innate immunity has been demonstrated in type 1 AIP. Activation of NOD-2 and TLR ligands on monocytes or basophils from patients with type 1 AIP enhances IgG4 production by B cells through signaling pathways mediated by B-cell-activating factor family (BAFF) and IL-13 and thereby induce systemic IgG4 responses [18, 19]. Although specific microorganisms still remain unclear, several candidates have been reported. Molecular mimicry among microbes and target antigens may be a possible mechanism to break down immune tolerance. The hypothesis is based on the concept that infectious agents share one or more epitopes with self-components or infectious agents cause bystander activation of immune cells with autoaggressive potential [20–23]. Guarneri and colleagues showed significant homology between human CA-II and alpha-CA of *H. pylori*, a fundamental enzyme for bacterial survival and proliferation in the stomach [21]. Moreover, the homologous segments contain the binding motif of DRB1*0405, which confers a risk for AIP development [21]. The plasminogen-binding protein (PBP) peptide newly identified in European patients with AIP shows homology with an amino acid sequence of PBP of *H. pylori* and with ubiquitin-protein ligase E3 component n-recognin 2 (UBR2), an enzyme highly expressed in acinar cells of the pancreas [20], while European patients with AIP did not necessarily show LPSP as the typical histopathology in IgG4-related diseases. These findings suggest that gastric *H. pylori* infection might trigger AIP in genetically predisposed subjects. Although no previous data of viral factors in human IgG4-RD, animal models suggested possible roles of the innate immune system in the development of immune-mediated cholangiopancreatitis and sialadenitis through activation of TLR3/TLR4 by infiltrating pathogen-associated molecular patterns (PAMP) and/or antigen(s) derived from virus or commensal bacteria in addition to virulent bacteria [24–26].

Possible Roles of IgG4 in Type 1 AIP

Although the association of IgE-mediated allergy and IgG4 antibodies is well known, IgG4 characteristics are still poorly understood. IgG4 is involved in an immune process referring to as "Fab-arm exchange," which is a swapping of a heavy chain and attached light chain (half-molecule) with a heavy-light chain pair from another molecule; this usually results in asymmetric antibodies with two different antigen-combining sites (Fig. 3.1a) [27]. While these modified antibodies are heterobivalent, they behave as monovalent antibodies. Another aspect of IgG4 is that it mimics IgG rheumatoid factor (RF) activity by interacting with IgG, namely, Fc-mediated aggregation (Fig. 3.1b) [28]. IgG4 seems to be associated with a pathogenic effect in a few situations. In pemphigus, recognition of skin autoantigens (desmogleins) by IgG4 is at the origin of the disease process [29]. A most recent study of structural determinants of human IgG4-Fc using crystalliza-

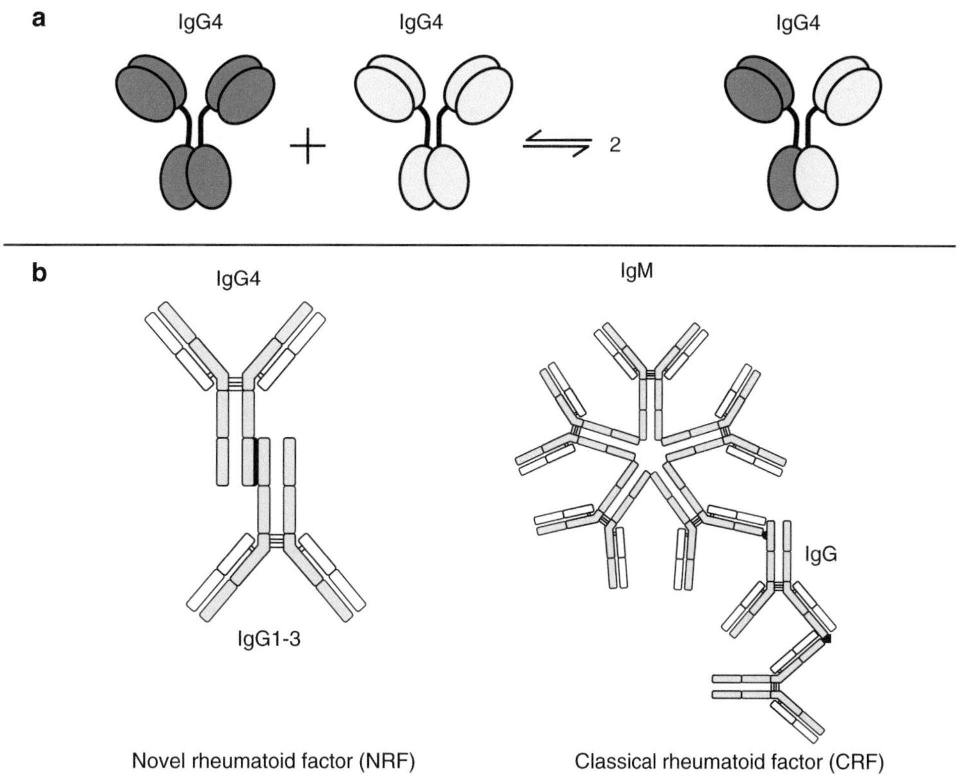

Fig. 3.1 Characteristic forms of IgG4. (**a**) Schematic representation of the generation of bispecific IgG4 antibodies by the exchange of half-molecules ("Fab-arm exchange") (With permission from the publisher of van der Neut Kolfschoten et al. [27]). IgG4 Fab-arm exchange occurs by the exchange of a heavy chain-light chain pair (half-molecule) of one IgG4 molecule with that of another IgG4 molecule. The IgG4 molecule may thereby acquire two distinct Fab arms and become bispecific. The Fc structure remains essentially unchanged apart from potential changes due to differences in glycosylation or allotype. Fab-arm exchange is proposed to be stochastic and dynamic. (**b**) *On the left*: IgG4 Fc interacts with Ig Fc. *On the right*: IgM RF recognizes IgG in a "classical" Fab-Fc recognition (With permission from Kawa et al. [28])

tion suggested that Fc-Fc interactions are compatible with intact IgG4 molecules and may provide a model for the formation of aggregates of IgG4 that can cause disease pathology in the absence of antigen [30].

Another recent data on regulating IgG4 showed that IgG4-related diseases may reflect an excessive production of anti-inflammatory cytokines such as IL-10 that triggers an overwhelming expansion of IgG4-producing plasma cells [31–35]. Increased peripheral inducible memory Tregs are positively correlated with serum levels of IgG4 [33]. In addition, prominent infiltration of Tregs upregulated IL-10 in livers of patients with IgG4-SC [31]. These findings suggest that IgG4 do not act as a pathogenic factor nor as an anti-inflammatory factor in IgG4-RD. Further studies are necessary to clarify the precise role of IgG4 in IgG4-RD.

The Complement System

Patients with active stage of AIP occasionally show decreased complement (C3, C4) with elevated circulating immune complex as well as serum levels of IgG4 [36]. Both tubulointerstitial nephritis (TIN) and membranous glomerulonephritis are often observed in IgG4-related kidney disease (IgG4-KD), and deposition of immune complex (IgG and C3) was observed on the tubular basement membrane as well as the glomerular basement membrane [37, 38]. As the complements cannot connect at the Fc portion of IgG4, the classical pathway of complement activation through IgG1 may be involved in the development of AIP rather than mannose-binding lectin or alternative pathways through IgG4 [39]. Moreover, IgG4 bound to other isotype such as IgG1, IgG2, and IgG3 with an Fc-Fc interaction immune complex in patients with AIP [28], and then IgG4 may contribute to the clearance of immune complexes or termination of the inflammatory process by preventing the formation of large immune complexes with blocking Fc-mediated effector functions of IgG1.

Autoantibodies and Candidate of Target Antigens

Patients with type 1 AIP generally show several autoantibodies in addition to increased IgG and IgG4 [8]. Although some patients have nonspecific antibodies such as antinuclear antibody (ANA), there is scarcely association of IgG4-RD and well-known autoimmune diseases such as Sjögren's syndrome and SLE. From the view of IgG4 function, a big mystery whether IgG4-related disease is autoimmune or allergic disease is addressed. However, occasional coexistence of

OOIs leads us the concept that there may be common target antigens in the involved organs such as the pancreas, salivary gland, biliary tract, lung, renal tubules, and so on. Although the disease-specific antibodies have not been identified at this moment, several disease-related antibodies such as anti-lactoferrin (LF) [40, 41], anti-carbonic anhydrase (CA)-II [40–43], anti-CA-IV [44], anti-pancreatic secretory trypsin inhibitor (PSTI) [45], anti-amylase-alpha [46], anti-HSP-10 [47], and anti-plasminogen-binding protein (PBP) peptide autoantibodies [20] have been reported. Although the patients show increased serum levels of IgG4, the major subclass of these autoantibody is not necessarily IgG4, but often IgG1 [45]. CA-II, CA-IV, LF, and PSTI are distributed in the ductal cells of several exocrine organs, including the pancreas, salivary gland, biliary duct, lung, and renal tubules [40, 41]. Although all peptides have not been studied, immunization with CA-II or LF-induced systemic lesions such as pancreatitis, sialadenitis, cholangitis, and interstitial nephritis in the mice models similar to human IgG4-related diseases [48, 49]. The high prevalence of these antibodies suggests that these may be the candidates for the target antigens in type 1 AIP. Among the involved organs in IgG4-RD, recent studies suggest an extremely high association of pancreatic and biliary lesions [50]. As both peribiliary glands in the biliary tract and pancreatic duct glands associated with pancreatic ducts in human are intermingled with small amounts of pancreatic exocrine acini [51], and the biliary tree-derived stem cells constitute a pancreatic organogenesis in mice [52], Nakanuma et al. have proposed a new concept of the "biliary diseases with pancreatic counterparts" [53], in which targets of type 1 AIP and IgG4-SC may be periductal glands around the bile and pancreatic ducts.

Diabetes mellitus is complicated with 43 ~ 68 % of the patients with AIP, but autoantibodies against glutamic acid decarboxylase, beta-cell, or tyrosine phosphatase-like protein associated type 1A DM are rarely observed [54]. These findings suggest that islet cells may not be targeted in the development of DM associated with AIP.

Role of B Cells

In addition to steroid and immune modulators, the B-cell depletion by rituximab, which reduces only IgG4, but not IgG1, IgG2, or IgG3, is useful in the therapeutic strategy in IgG4-RD [55, 56]. A recent study showed expansion of IgG4+ B-cell receptor (BCR) clones in blood and tissue of patients with active IgG4-cholangiopathy, and disappearance by corticosteroid treatment [57]. A recent study showed that the increased $CD19^+CD24^{high}CD38^{high}$ Bregs may suppress the disease activity of type 1 AIP, whereas the decreased $CD19^+CD24^{high}CD27^+$ Bregs might be involved in the development of type 1 AIP [58]. These findings suggest that specific B-cell responses may have a pivotal role in the pathogenesis of IgG4-RD such as type 1 AIP and IgG4-SC.

Th1 and Th2 Immune Balance

The effector cells in IgG4-related diseases have been poorly understood. Presence of autoantibodies; infiltration of CD4+/CD8 + T cells, plasmacytes, and B cells; and expression of HLA-DR antigens in the pancreas [41] suggest that acquired immunity may be involved in the development of AIP. The CD4 + T cells differentiate from naïve T cells (Th0) to Th1, Th2, Th17, and regulatory T cells (Treg). IL-12 induces Thl cells, which produce IL-2, tumor necrosis factor (TNF)-alpha, and IFN-gamma; mediate cellular immunity, macrophage activation, and cytotoxicity; and help in B-cell production of opsonizing and complement-fixing antibodies [54]. IL-4 induces Th2 cells which produce IL-4, IL-5, IL-6, and IL-10 and promote humoral and allergic responses [59]. TGF-beta, IL-6, IL-21, and IL-23 induce Th17 cells, which secret IL-17 and may be involved in the inflammation in mice. In some patients with AIP, Th1 cells but not Th17 cells are predominant over Th2-type cells in the periphery. In the livers of IgG4-SC patients, however, a Th2-type immune reaction [60, 61] is induced in addition to a Th1 response [60, 62]. The discrepancy may be explained by the shift of Th2 cells from the periphery to local tissues or different disease stages. The mouse model with depletion of Tregs by neonatal thymectomy (nTx) [62] and the WBN/Kob model (Sakaguchi et al. 2002) support the hypothesis that Th1 cells mainly act as effectors in the initial early stage. Th2 cytokines may be involved in the progression of the disease process, especially the maturation and proliferation of local B cells and plasmacytes.

Regulatory T Cells

From naïve Th0 cells, TGF-beta can induce $CD4^+CD25^+$ regulatory T cells (Tregs), which have potent inhibitory function via the transcription factor Foxp3 to $CD4^+$ T-cell-mediated immune responses such as Th1, Th2, and Th17 [61]. This suppressive function is mediated by transforming growth factor β (TGF-β) and IL-10, and/or cell-to-cell contact via ligation of CTLA-4. Foxp3 is a member of the forkhead/winged-helix family of transcriptional regulators and functions as the master regulator in the development and function of $CD4^+CD25^+$ regulatory T cells (Tregs) classified as naturally occurring $CD4^+CD25^+$ Tregs (nTregs) originating in the thymus and adaptive Tregs (aTregs) induced in the periphery by different antigens [63]. As Tregs expressing Foxp3 are critical in the transfer of immune tolerance, deficient Tregs induce various autoimmune diseases in animal

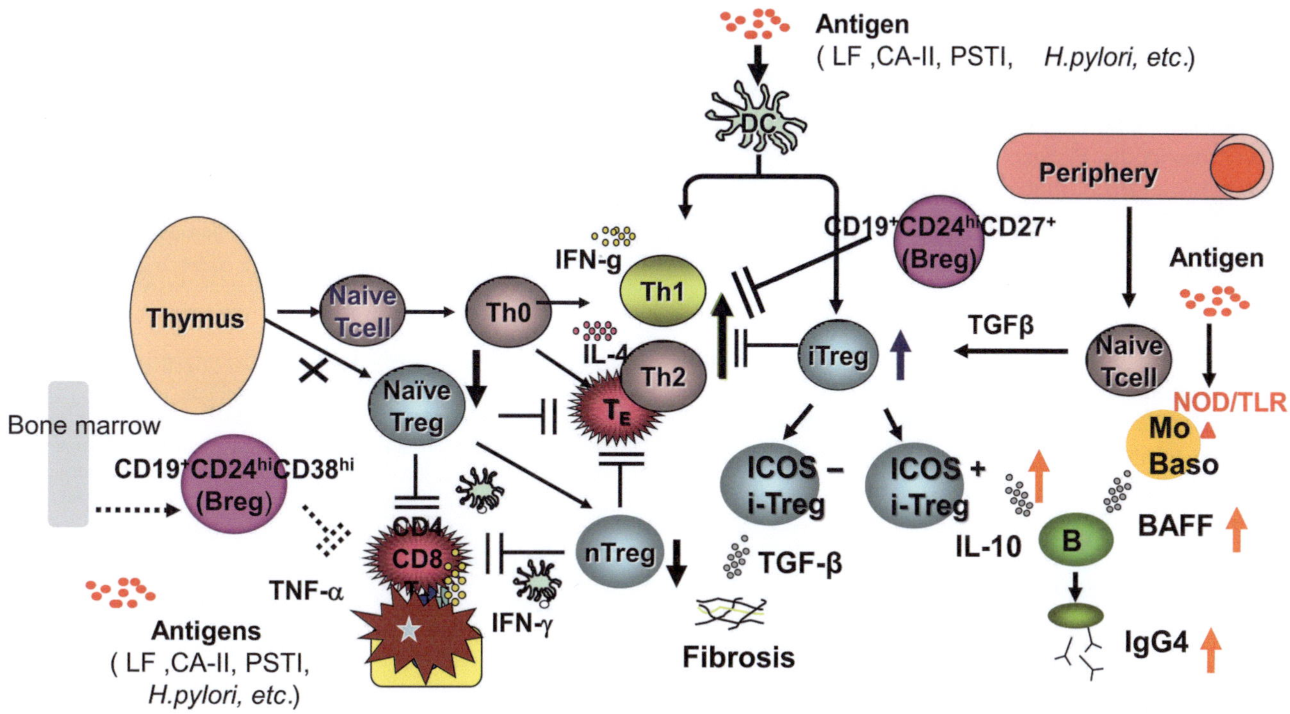

Fig. 3.2 Hypothesis for the pathogenesis of type 1 AIP as an IgG4-related disease (With permission from the publisher of Okazaki et al. [8]). In the central tolerance, naïve and natural regulatory T cells (Tregs) derived from the thymus suppress autoreactive CD4 or CD8 cells in the normal state. The basic concept is the biphasic mechanism of "induction" and "progression." An initial response to unknown disease-specific antigens including self-antigens (LF, CA-II, CA-IV, and PSTI) or microorganisms (bacteria or virus) might be induced by decreased naïve Tregs and/or CD19$^+$CD24^{hi}CD38^{hi} Bregs followed by a Th1-type immune response with the release of proinflammatory cytokines (IFN- γ, IL-1beta, IL-2, TNF-α). In progression, Th2-type immune responses producing IgG, IgG4, and autoantibodies may be involved in pathophysiology. Production of IgG4 may be upregulated by increased IL-10 from ICOS+ inducible aTregs and CD19$^+$CD24^{hi}CD27^{hi} Bregs and BAFF from monocytes and/or basophils. Fibrosis may be induced by TGF-beta secreted from ICOS- inducible aTregs. *iTreg* inducible memory regulatory T cell, *TE* effector T cell, *nTreg* naturally occurring naive regulatory T cell, *BAFF* B-cell-activating factor family, *Breg* regulatory B cell, *ICOS* inhibitory costimulatory molecule

studies [64]. In type 1 AIP, circulatory naïve (CD45RA+) Tregs are significantly decreased in the peripheral blood, whereas memory (CD45RA-) Tregs are significantly increased [33]. In addition, prominent infiltration of Tregs with upregulation of IL-10 is observed in the liver of type 1 AIP and IgG4-SC patients [31, 32]. Moreover, IL-10 and TGF-beta are secreted from ICOS+ and ICOS- inducible aTregs, respectively. These findings suggest that increased memory Tregs in the periphery and local tissues may be an inhibitory immune response against inflammation, although decreased naïve Tregs may be pathogenic.

Hypothesis for the Pathogenesis of Type 1 AIP

The neonatally thymectomized (nTx)-BALB/c mice models showed that immunization with CA-II or LF can induce pancreatitis, cholangitis, and sialadenitis similar to human IgG4-RD [62]. These findings suggest that depletion of naïve Tregs may induce macrophage/T-cell activation and further proinflammatory reactions may occur during the early stage of the disease as direct cytotoxicity effects through Fas ligand expression. WBN/Kob rat models with congenital decreased peripheral Tregs spontaneously develop sclerotic cholangitis, sialadenitis, thyroiditis, and tubulointerstitial nephritis [65]. These animal models suggest that CD4+/CD8+ T cells play major roles in the development of primary lesions similarly to human IgG4-related diseases; however, the counterpart of IgG4 in mice IgG subclasses has not been identified.

Based on these findings, we proposed the pathogenesis of type 1 AIP [8] (Fig. 3.2). The basic concept is the biphasic mechanism of "induction" and "progression." An initial response to unknown disease-specific antigens including self-antigens (LF, CA-II, CA-IV, and PSTI) or microorganisms (bacteria or virus) might be induced by decreased naïve Tregs and/or CD19$^+$CD24^{hi}CD38^{hi} Bregs followed by a Th1-type immune response with the release of proinflammatory cytokines (IFN-γ, IL-1beta, IL-2, TNF-α). In progression, Th2-type immune responses producing IgG, IgG4, and autoantibodies may be involved in pathophysiology. Production of IgG4 may be upregulated by increased IL-10 from ICOS+ inducible aTregs and $CD19^{+}CD24^{hi}CD27^{hi}$ Bregs and BAFF from monocytes and/or basophils. Fibrosis may be induced by TGF-beta secreted from ICOS-inducible aTregs.

Conclusion

Recent advances support the concept of AIP and subtypes, type 1 and type 2 AIP. Type 1 AIP is a pancreatic manifestation of IgG4-RD. Although the pathogenic mechanism remains unclear, innate and acquired immunity, Tregs, and B cells may be involved in the development of type 1 AIP. Further studies are necessary to clarify the pathogenesis including genetic backgrounds, disease-specific antigens, and the role of IgG4.

Acknowledgment This study was partially supported by (1) Grant-in-Aid for Scientific Research (C) of the Ministry of Culture and Science of Japan (20590810, 24591020, 12008507), (2) the Research Program on Intractable Diseases, from the Ministry of Labor and Welfare of Japan, and (3) Grants-in-Aid from the Ministry of Education, Culture, Sports, Science, and Technology of Japan, from CREST Japan Science, and Technology Agency.

References

1. Chari ST, Kloeppel G, Zhang L, et al. Histopathologic and clinical subtypes of autoimmune pancreatitis: the Honolulu consensus document. Pancreas. 2010;39:549–54.
2. Hamano H, Kawa S, Horiuchi A, et al. High serum IgG4 concentrations in patients with sclerosing pancreatitis. New Engl J Med. 2001;344:732–8.
3. Sarles H, Sarles JC, Muratore R, Guien C. Chronic inflammatory sclerosis of the pancreas–an autonomous pancreatic disease? Am J Dig Dis. 1961;6:688–98.
4. Shimosegawa T, Chari ST, Frulloni L, et al. International consensus diagnostic criteria for autoimmune pancreatitis: guidelines of the international association of pancreatology. Pancreas. 2011;40(3):352–8.
5. Yoshida K, Toki F, Takeuchi T, Watanabe S, Shiratori K, Hayashi N. Chronic pancreatitis caused by an autoimmune abnormality. Proposal of the concept of autoimmune pancreatitis. Dig Dis Sci. 1995;40:1561–8.
6. Kawaguchi K, Koike M, Tsuruta K, Fujita N, et al. Lymphoplasmacytic sclerosing pancreatitis with cholangitis: a variant of primary sclerosing cholangitis extensively involving pancreas. Hum Pathol. 1991;22:387–95.
7. Umehara H, Okazaki K, Masaki Y, et al. A novel clinical entity, IgG4-related disease (IgG4RD): general concept and details. Mod Rheumatol. 2012;22:1–14
8. Okazaki K, Uchida K, Koyabu M, et al. Recent advances in the concept and diagnosis of autoimmune pancreatitis and IgG4-related disease. J Gastroenterol. 2011;46:277–88.
9. Klöppel G, Detlefsen S, Chari ST, et al. Autoimmune pancreatitis: the clinicopathological characteristics of the subtype with granulocytic epithelial lesions. J Gastroenterol. 2010;45:787–93.
10. Kawa S, Ota M, Yoshizawa K, et al. HLA DRB10405-DQB10401 haplotype is associated with autoimmune pancreatitis in the Japanese population. Gastroenterology. 2002;122(5):1264–9.
11. Park do H, Kim MH, Oh HB, et al. Substitution of aspartic acid at position 57 of the DQbeta1 affects relapse of autoimmune pancreatitis. Gastroenterology. 2008;134(2):440–6.
12. Kochi Y, Yamada R, Suzuki A, et al. A functional variant in FCRL3, encoding Fc receptor-like 3, is associated with rheumatoid arthritis and several autoimmunities. Nat Genet. 2005;37(5):478–85.
13. Umemura T, Ota M, Hamano H, Katsuyama Y, Kiyosawa K, Kawa S. Genetic association of Fc receptor-like 3 polymorphisms with autoimmune pancreatitis in Japanese patients. Gut. 2006;55(9):1367–8.
14. Umemura T, Katsuyama Y, Hamano H, et al. Association analysis of Toll-like receptor 4 polymorphisms with autoimmune pancreatitis. Hum Immunol. 2009;70(9):742–6.
15. Chang MC, Chang YT, Tien YW, et al. T-cell regulatory gene CTLA-4 polymorphism/haplotype association with autoimmune pancreatitis. Clin Chem. 2007;53(9):1700–5.
16. Umemura T, Ota M, Hamano H, et al. Association of autoimmune pancreatitis with cytotoxic T-lymphocyte antigen 4 gene polymorphisms in Japanese patients. Am J Gastroenterol. 2008;103(3):588–94.
17. Ueda H, Howson JM, Esposito L, et al. Association of the T-cell regulatory gene CTLA4 with susceptibility to autoimmune disease. Nature. 2003;423(6939):506–11.
18. Watanabe T, Yamashita K, Fujikawa S, et al. Involvement of activation of toll-like receptors and nucleotide-binding oligomerization domain-like receptors in enhanced IgG4 responses in autoimmune pancreatitis. Arthritis Rheum. 2012;64:914–24.
19. Watanabe T, Yamashita K, Sakurai T, Kudo M, Shiokawa M, Uza N, et al. Toll-like receptor activation in basophils contributes to the development of IgG4 related disease. J Gastroenterol. 2013;48:247–53.
20. Frulloni L, Lunardi C, Simone R, et al. Identification of a novel antibody associated with autoimmune pancreatitis. N Engl J Med. 2009;361:2135–42.
21. Guarneri F, Guarneri C, Benvenga S. Helicobacter pylori and autoimmune pancreatitis: role of carbonic anhydrase via molecular mimicry? J Cell Mol Med. 2005;9(3):741–4.
22. Kountouras J, Zavos C, Chatzopoulos D. A concept on the role of Helicobacter pylori infection in autoimmune pancreatitis. J Cell Mol Med. 2005;9(1):196–207.
23. Kountouras J, Zavos C, Gavalas E, Tzilves D. Challenge in the pathogenesis of autoimmune pancreatitis: potential role of helicobacter pylori infection via molecular mimicry. Gastroenterology. 2007;133(1):368–9.
24. Haruta I, Yanagisawa N, Kawamura S, et al. A mouse model of autoimmune pancreatitis with salivary gland involvement triggered by innate immunity via persistent exposure to avirulent bacteria. Lab Invest. 2010;90:1757–69.
25. Nishio A, Asada M, Uchida K, et al. The role of innate immunity in the pathogenesis of experimental autoimmune pancreatitis in mice. Pancreas. 2011;40:95–102.
26. Yamashina M, Nishio A, Nakayama S, Okazaki T, Uchida K, Fukui T, et al. Comparative study on experimental autoimmune pancreatitis and its extrapancreatic involvement in mice. Pancreas. 2012;41:1255–62.
27. van der Neut Kolfschoten M, Schuurman J, Losen M, et al. Anti-inflammatory activity of human IgG4 antibodies by dynamic Fab arm exchange. Science. 2007;317(5844):1554–7.
28. Kawa S, Kitahara K, Hamano H, et al. A novel immunoglobulin-immunoglobulin interaction in autoimmunity. PLoS One. 2008;3(2):e1637.
29. Ishii K, Amagai M, Hall RP, et al. Characterization of autoantibodies in pemphigus using antigen-specific enzyme-linked immunosorbent assays with baculovirus-expressed recombinant desmogleins. J Immunol. 1997;159:2010–7.
30. Davies AM, Rispens T, Ooijevaar-de Heer P, et al. Structural determinants of unique properties of human IgG4-Fc. J Mol Biol. 2014;426:630–44.

31. Koyabu M, Uchida K, Miyoshi H, et al. Analysis of regulatory T cells and IgG4-positive plasma cells among patients of IgG4-related sclerosing cholangitis and autoimmune liver diseases. J Gastroenterol. 2010;45:732–41.
32. Kusuda T, Uchida K, Miyoshi H, et al. Involvement of inducible costimulator- and interleukin 10-positive regulatory T cells in the development of IgG4-related autoimmune pancreatitis. Pancreas. 2011;40:1120–30.
33. Miyoshi H, Uchida K, Taniguchi T, et al. Circulating naive and CD4+CD25high regulatory T cells in patients with autoimmune pancreatitis. Pancreas. 2008;36:133–40.
34. Tanaka A, Moriyama M, Nakashima H, et al. Th2 and regulatory immune reactions contribute to IgG4 production and the initiation of Mikulicz disease. Arthritis Rheum. 2012;64:254–63.
35. Zen Y, Fujii T, Harada K, et al. Th2 and regulatory immune reactions are increased in immunoglobin G4-related sclerosing pancreatitis and cholangitis. Hepatology. 2007;45:1538–46.
36. Cornell LD, Chicano SL, Deshpande V, et al. Pseudotumors due to IgG4 immune-complex tubulointerstitial nephritis associated with autoimmune pancreatocentric disease. Am J Surg Pathol. 2007;31(10):1586–97.
37. Kawano M, Mizushima I, Yamaguchi Y, et al. Immunohistochemical characteristics of IgG4-related tubulointerstitial nephritis: detailed analysis of 20 Japanese cases. Int J Rheumatol. 2012;2012:609795.
38. Takeda S, Haratake J, Kasai T, Takaeda C, Takazakura E. IgG4-associated idiopathic tubulointerstitial nephritis complicating autoimmune pancreatitis. Nephrol Dial Transplant. 2004;19:474–6.
39. Muraki T, Hamano H, Ochi Y, et al. Autoimmune pancreatitis and complement activation system. Pancreas. 2006;32:16–21.
40. Okazaki K, Uchida K, Ohana M, et al. Autoimmune-related pancreatitis is associated with autoantibodies and a Th1/Th2-type cellular immune response. Gastroenterology. 2000;118:573–81.
41. Uchida K, Okazaki K, Konishi Y, et al. Clinical analysis of autoimmune-related pancreatitis. Am J Gastroenterol. 2000;95:2788–94.
42. Aparisi L, Farre A, Gomez-Cambronero L, et al. Antibodies to carbonic anhydrase and IgG4 levels in idiopathic chronic pancreatitis: relevance for diagnosis of autoimmune pancreatitis. Gut. 2005;54:703–9.
43. Nishi H, Tojo A, Onozato ML, et al. Anti-carbonic anhydrase II antibody in autoimmune pancreatitis and tubulointerstitial nephritis. Nephrol Dial Transplant. 2007;22:1273–5.
44. Nishimori I, Miyaji E, Morimoto K, et al. Serum antibodies to carbonic anhydrase IV in patients with autoimmune pancreatitis. Gut. 2005;54:274–81.
45. Asada M, Nishio A, Uchida K, et al. Identification of a novel autoantibody against pancreatic secretory trypsin inhibitor in patients with autoimmune pancreatitis. Pancreas. 2006;33:20–6.
46. Endo T, Takizawa S, Tanaka S, et al. Amylase alpha-2A autoantibodies: novel marker of autoimmune pancreatitis and fulminant type 1 diabetes. Diabetes. 2009;58:732–7.
47. Takizawa S, Endo T, Wanjia X, Tanaka S, Takahashi M, Kobayashi T. HSP 10 is a new autoantigen in both autoimmune pancreatitis and fulminant type 1 diabetes. Biochem Biophys Res Commun. 2009;386:192–6.
48. Nishimori I, Bratanova T, Toshkov I, et al. Induction of experimental autoimmune sialoadenitis by immunization of PL/J mice with carbonic anhydrase II. J Immunol. 1995;154(9):4865–73.
49. Ueno Y, Ishii M, Takahashi S, Igarashi T, Toyota T, LaRusso NF. Different susceptibility of mice to immune-mediated cholangitis induced by immunization with carbonic anhydrase II. Lab Invest. 1998;78(5):629–37.
50. Okazaki K, Uchida K, Matsushita M, Takaoka M. How to diagnose autoimmune pancreatitis by the revised Japanese clinical criteria. J Gastroenterol. 2007;42:32–8.
51. Nakanuma Y. A novel approach to biliary tract pathology based on similarities to pancreatic counterparts: is the biliary tract an incomplete pancreas? Pathol Int. 2010;60:419–29.
52. Wang Y, Lanzoni G, Carpino G, et al. Biliary tree stem cells, precursors to pancreatic committed progenitors: evidence for possible life-long pancreatic organogenesis. Stem Cells. 2013;31:1966–79.
53. Nakanuma Y, Harada K, Sasaki M, et al. Proposal of a new disease concept "biliary diseases with pancreatic counterparts". Anatomical and pathological bases. Histol Histopathol. 2014;29:1–10.
54. Okazaki K. Autoimmune pancreatitis: etiology, pathogenesis, clinical findings and treatment. The Japanese experience. JOP. 2005;6(1 Suppl):89–96.
55. Khosroshahi A, Carruthers MN, Deshpande V, et al. Rituximab for the treatment of IgG4-related disease: lessons from 10 consecutive patients. Medicine (Baltimore). 2012;91:57–66.
56. Topazian M, Witzig TE, Smyrk TC, et al. Rituximab therapy for refractory biliary strictures in immunoglobulin G4-associated cholangitis. Clin Gastroenterol Hepatol. 2008;6:364–6.
57. Maillette de Buy Wenniger LJ, Doorenspleet ME, Klarenbeek PL, et al. Immunoglobulin G4+ clones identified by next-generation sequencing dominate the B cell receptor repertoire in immunoglobulin G4 associated cholangitis. Hepatology. 2013;57:2390–8.
58. Sumimoto K, Uchida K, Kusuda T, et al. The role of CD19+CD24highCD38high and CD19+CD24highCD27+ regulatory B cells in patients with type 1 autoimmune pancreatitis. Pancreatology. 2014. http://dx.doi.org/10.1016/j.pan.2014.02.004.
59. Roitt I. Antibodies. In: Roitt I, editor. Roitt's essential immunology. 9th ed. London: Blackwell Science; 1997. p. 43–62.
60. McGeachy MJ, Cua DJ. The link between IL-23 and Th17 cell-mediated immune pathologies. Semin Immunol. 2007; 19(6):372–6.
61. Oukka M. Interplay between pathogenic Th17 and regulatory T cells. Ann Rheum Dis. 2007;66 Suppl 3:iii87–90.
62. Uchida K, Okazaki K, Nishi T, et al. Experimental immune-mediated pancreatitis in neonatally thymectomized mice immunized with carbonic anhydrase II and lactoferrin. Lab Invest. 2002;82:411–24.
63. Valencia X, Lipsky PE. CD4+CD25+FoxP3+ regulatory T cells in autoimmune diseases. Nat Clin Pract Rheumatol. 2007;3(11):619–26.
64. Sakaguchi S, Fukuma K, Kuribayashi K, et al. Organ-specific autoimmune diseases induced in mice by elimination of T cell subset. I. Evidence for the active participation of T cells in natural self-tolerance; deficit of a T cell subset as a possible cause of autoimmune disease. J Exp Med. 1985;161:72–87.
65. Sakaguchi Y, Inaba M, Tsuda M, et al. The Wistar Bonn Kobori rat, a unique animal model for autoimmune pancreatitis with extrapancreatic exocrinopathy. Clin Exp Immunol. 2008;152:1–12.

Pathology

4

Kenji Notohara

General Considerations

Before the entity of autoimmune pancreatitis (AIP) was proposed clinically [1], several disease entities that are now regarded as equivalent to AIP were reported from the pathological standpoint: chronic inflammatory sclerosis [2], lymphoplasmacytic sclerosing pancreatitis (LPSP) [3], and nonalcoholic duct-destructive chronic pancreatitis [4]. Pathologists later recognized that there were at least two different concepts in what had been considered AIP, and these were named LPSP/AIP without granulocytic epithelial lesion (GEL) and idiopathic duct-centric pancreatitis (IDCP)/AIP with GEL [5, 6]. The discovery of elevated serum IgG4 in patients with AIP by Hamano and colleagues motivated further research into AIP [7], and LPSP is now regarded as the pancreatic manifestation of IgG4-related disease (IgG4-RD) in the present consensus [8–10]. In addition, the subclassification of AIP was proposed based on its different demographics and clinical features [11–13], and LPSP and IDCP were designated as type 1 and type 2 AIP, respectively [14]. In fact, the histological features of type 1 and type 2 AIP are distinct, and pathologists can distinguish them with hematoxylin and eosin (HE) stain alone without the aid of IgG4 immunostaining, which was validated by an international interobserver study [15].

Type 1 AIP/LPSP

Type 1 AIP/LPSP is now considered to be the pancreatic manifestation of IgG4-RD. It may be said that type 1 AIP is the prototype of IgG4-RD, because the histological and immunohistochemical features of type 1 AIP contributed to the expansion of the concept of IgG4-RD by providing clues to identify similar lesions in the extrapancreatic organs [16, 17].

The inflammation seen in type 1 AIP involves both the pancreatic parenchyma and nonparenchymal tissues. The histological features found in these locations are characteristic. Storiform fibrosis in particular is unique and can be observed in the entire lesion. In this review article, the histological characteristics of storiform fibrosis are described first, and then the histological features seen in the different anatomical locations as well as the significance of IgG4 immunostaining are elucidated in the later sections.

Storiform Fibrosis

The storiform fibrosis is a haphazard and swirling pattern of fibrosis that consists of small spindle-shaped cells, lymphocytes, and plasma cells. Eosinophils may be seen and are numerous in some cases, whereas neutrophils are essentially absent.

Despite the term "fibrosis" in its name, a portion of storiform fibrosis is cellular and lacks genuine fibrosis (Fig. 4.1a) [18]. This portion gradually transitions into true fibrosis with fewer cellular components (Fig. 4.1b) and finally gives rise to complete fibrosis. This is similar to the ordinal granulation tissue giving rise to fibrosis with time. In most cases, both the cellular and fibrotic components mix in a single lesion, and the degree of genuine fibrosis varies depending among cases.

Storiform fibrosis is most prominent at the border between the pancreas and the peripancreatic adipose tissue. This will be described in detail in a later section.

Pancreatic Parenchymal Inflammation

The pancreatic parenchymal inflammation can be seen in the pancreatic ducts and lobules.

K. Notohara, MD, PhD
Department of Anatomic Pathology, Kurashiki Central Hospital, 1-1-1 Miwa, Kurashiki 710-8602, Japan
e-mail: notohara@kchnet.or.jp

T. Kamisawa, J.B. Chung (eds.), *Autoimmune Pancreatitis*,
DOI 10.1007/978-3-642-55086-7_4, © Springer-Verlag Berlin Heidelberg 2015

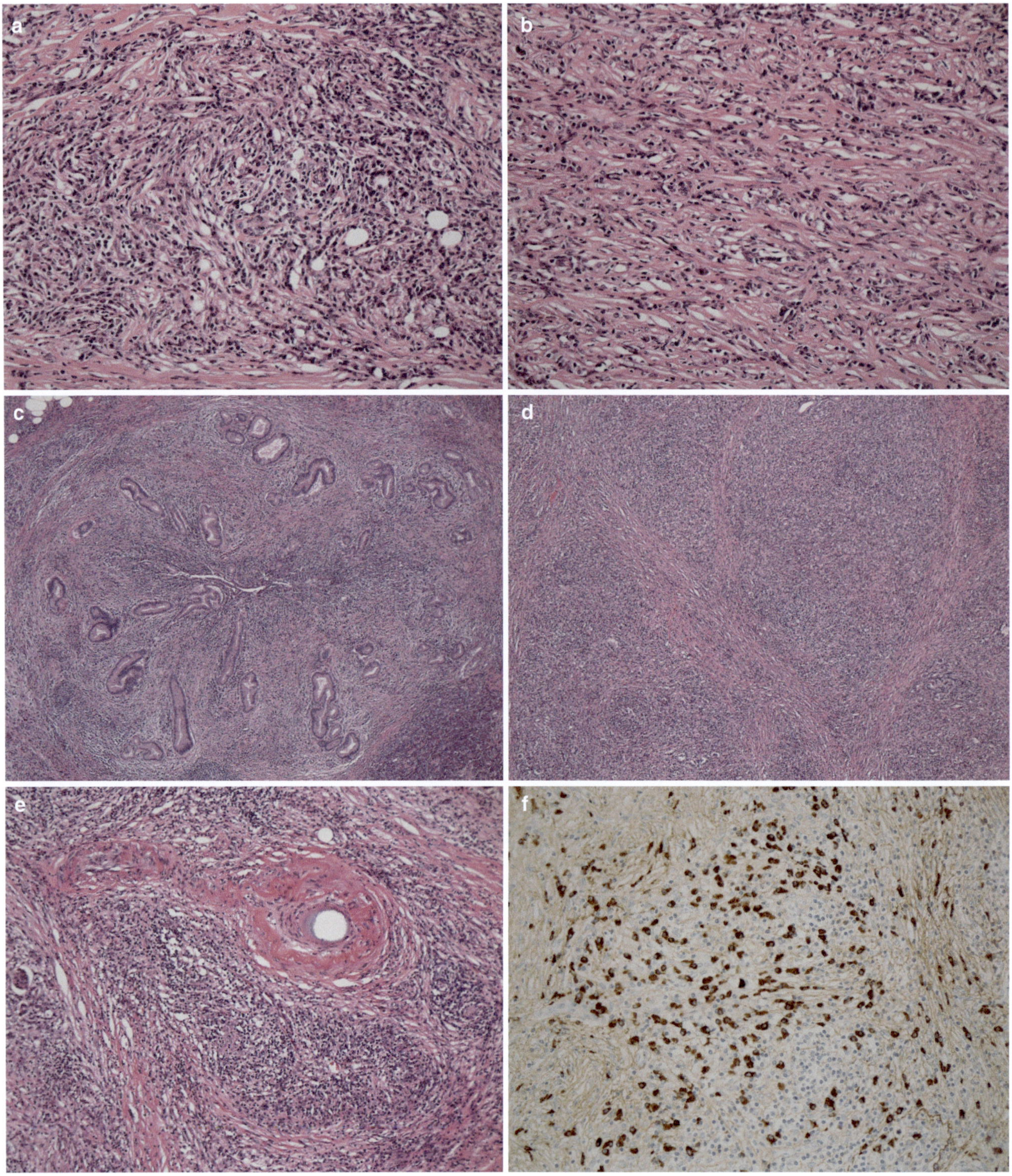

Fig. 4.1 Histological features of type 1 AIP. (**a**, **b**) The cell-rich form (**a**) and transitional form between the cell-rich and fibrotic states (**b**) of storiform fibrosis. (**c**) Ductal inflammation. A thick inflammatory collar with storiform fibrosis surrounds the intact duct epithelium. (**d**) Lobular inflammation. The inflamed lobules show a nodular appearance and maintain their original size. (**e**) Obliterative phlebitis. An inflammatory nodule found adjacent to an arteriole is a clue to identify obliterative phlebitis. (**f**) Immunostaining for IgG4. Numerous IgG4-positive cells are seen

Ductal Inflammation

Although on a pancreatogram the main pancreatic duct looks stenotic and irregular in type 1 AIP, ductal lumens are histologically always open, and the duct epithelium is intact. The ductal inflammation consists of lymphoplasmacytic infiltration that surrounds the epithelium. It can be easily identified in the interlobular pancreatic ducts, but the intralobular ducts are also involved.

The ductal inflammation typically consists of a collar of lymphoplasmacytic infiltration with storiform fibrosis, which looks like a thickened duct wall (Fig. 4.1c). However, there are no structures that are histologically identified as a wall in the normal pancreatic ducts, and thus, they are considered to be a pathological structure caused by the inflammation itself.

The ductal inflammation can also be a thin inflammatory collar of lymphoplasmacytic infiltration just beneath the epithelium, which is surrounded by a fibrotic band. Storiform fibrosis is absent in this pattern.

Lobular Inflammation

Although it has not been emphasized as a significant finding in previous reports, the pancreatic lobules are inflamed in a peculiar way. The lobular inflammation is characterized by acinar cell loss and lymphoplasmacytic infiltration. Interestingly though, this is in a fashion in which the original lobular contour and size are preserved (Fig. 4.1d). This is in contrast to the lobular atrophy or loss seen in pancreatitis due to other causes. The lobular contours are sharply defined by the interlobular fibrosis, giving rise to the nodular appearance of the pancreatic parenchyma. This is especially evident when special stains for fibrosis such as Verhoeff-van Gieson stain are performed. In addition, the lobular appearance may resemble storiform fibrosis with or without true fibrosis. The pancreatic lobules are often destructive at the margin of pancreatic parenchyma, which is explained in the following section. Rarely, the pancreatic lobules are atrophic in cases of type 1 AIP with regressive changes.

The lack of neutrophilic infiltration is a feature that distinguishes type 1 from type 2 AIP. However, in about one-third of cases, neutrophils are observed in the lobules of type 1 AIP. This is most likely due to a secondary inflammation that is caused by ductal strictures. In this instance, the distinction between type 1 and type 2 AIP should be made based on the findings of other histological features in the lobules as well as the inflammation seen in the connective tissues.

Nonparenchymal Tissue Inflammation

Connective tissues such as peripancreatic tissue (adipose tissue), vessels (arteries and veins), and nerves are also involved in type 1 AIP.

Peripancreatic Inflammation

At the border between the pancreas and the surrounding adipose tissue, a collar of inflammation that surrounds the pancreas is formed. At a glance, this looks like the inflammation of the peripancreatic adipose tissue, but in reality both the peripancreatic adipose tissue and the peripheral portion of the pancreas are involved. Involvement of the pancreas can be recognized by identifying residual islets and small ducts within the lesion. As described earlier, storiform fibrosis is most prominent in this area. When the lesion is thick enough, it can be recognized radiologically as a capsule-like rim [19]. The inflammation at this portion may spread to interlobular septa within the pancreas.

Vascular Inflammation

Venous involvement is one of the most well known and unique histological features of type 1 AIP. Venous walls are often infiltrated and destroyed by the inflammatory process, which is histologically similar to that seen around the veins. This inflammatory process further involves venous lumens and finally obliterates them (obliterative phlebitis, Fig. 4.1e). Obliterative phlebitis is common in small veins (venules) that cannot be identified macroscopically. Although obliterated venules are difficult to identify on HE-stained slides, nodular inflammatory lesions adjacent to arterioles are the clue to identify them because the arteries and veins run parallel in the pancreas. In addition, obliterative phlebitis is common and involves relatively larger venules, which makes obliterative phlebitis easily identifiable even on HE-stained slides. According to our study, obliterative phlebitis seen in the larger-sized venules (>100 μm in diameter, as a guide) is more diagnostic for type 1 AIP, and smaller venular lesions are nonspecific [20]. Simple fibrous obstruction without inflammatory cells or only inflammatory cell infiltration without fibrosis in the veins should not be included in obliterative phlebitis in type 1 AIP, because those findings may be seen in pancreatic carcinomas and alcoholic chronic pancreatitis [20]. Obliterative phlebitis with storiform fibrosis is typical for type 1 AIP. When the venous inflammation occurs in a larger vein, such as the splenic vein or portal vein, the luminal occlusion does not occur. This is because they are too large to be occluded completely. Even so, I suggest that this finding is also unique to type 1 AIP. In this situation, it is common to observe a local well-marginated involvement of a vein with storiform fibrosis.

Arteries are also involved in type 1 AIP. This is usually limited to the border between the media and adventitia, and it is thus similar to the periaortitis/periarteritis seen in the larger arteries [21]. Because this involvement is continuous with the surrounding inflammation, it is difficult to determine whether the inflammation is present or not in the arteries themselves. Thus, the true incidence of periarteritis in type 1 AIP has been underestimated. Arteries are not completely occluded by the inflammation, probably due to an anatomical reason, that is, the thicker smooth muscle layer in the arteries.

Nervous Inflammation

Perinervous inflammation is common and may be prominent in type 1 AIP. This finding alone, however, is not specific for type 1 AIP because it can also be observed in alcoholic chronic pancreatitis and pancreatic carcinomas.

IgG4 Immunostaining

IgG4-positive cells are numerous in type 1 AIP (Fig. 4.1f) [22]. This finding is helpful for the diagnosis of type 1 AIP, but there are some pitfalls in the evaluation of IgG4 immunostaining.

It is important to stress that the presence of numerous IgG4-positive cells alone is not specific to type 1 AIP or IgG4-RD, and it should be evaluated in the context of histological findings. In the present diagnostic criteria for type 1 AIP such as the International Consensus Diagnostic Criteria (ICDC) [23] and the clinical diagnostic criteria 2011 in Japan (Japan Pancreas Society (JPS) 2011) [24], the presence of more than 10 IgG4-positive cells in a high-power field (hpf) is considered to be significant. However, this criterion is not entirely specific to type 1 AIP and can be satisfied in pancreatic carcinomas and pancreatitis with other causes including type 2 AIP [22, 25, 26]. In resected tissues of type 1 AIP, there are usually more than 50 IgG4-positive cells/hpf [25]. This finding is more specific to type 1 AIP. However, in the small biopsy tissues, it is rare to observe more than 50/hpf. This is why the criterion of >10/hpf was adopted as part of the abovementioned criteria. In the Consensus Statement regarding the pathology of IgG4-RD, a >40 % IgG4/IgG-positive cell ratio is mandatory to consider the lesion as highly suggestive of IgG4-RD [27]. This finding is also helpful for the diagnosis of type 1 AIP, especially with biopsy samples.

Another pitfall is that numerous IgG4-positive cells are not always found in genuine type 1 AIP cases. This is particularly true in the cases of type 1 AIP with regressive features. I have also encountered some cases in which the IgG4-/IgG-positive cell ratios were under 40 %.

Histological Diagnostic Criteria of Type 1 AIP

As described in the previous section, the finding of numerous IgG4-positive cells is not specific to type 1 AIP. It is now acknowledged that, for the histological diagnosis of type 1 AIP or IgG4-RD, characteristic histological findings such as storiform fibrosis and obliterative phlebitis are important. This way of thinking is adopted in the ICDC and the JPS 2011.

In the ICDC and JPS 2011 guidelines, type 1 AIP can be definitively diagnosed from the histological features alone. In addition to the lymphoplasmacytic infiltration and numerous (>10/hpf) IgG4-positive cells, storiform fibrosis and/or obliterative phlebitis are mandatory to make a definitive diagnosis of type 1 AIP. If only two of the four findings are satisfied, then the diagnosis should be determined with clinical findings. In the Consensus Statement regarding the pathology of IgG4-RD, a different approach is adopted, and histological findings and IgG4 immunostaining alone are not considered to be diagnostic for IgG4-RD. This is due to the fact that the frequency of the appearance and the specificity of storiform fibrosis and obliterated phlebitis may be different among different organs. In the pancreas, however, it is conceivable to consider that those cases with at least three out of four major histological findings are diagnostic for type 1 AIP, because pancreatitis due to other causes almost never satisfies the criteria.

Special Conditions That Could Be Associated with Type 1 AIP

Some cases of type 1 AIP show some regressive features and are difficult to diagnose histologically. In such cases, the diagnostic features should be identified by conducting a thorough sampling of the resection specimen. Understandably, the biopsy diagnosis of type 1 AIP is very difficult in this situation.

Type 1 AIP may be associated with neoplasms. Pancreatic ductal carcinoma associated with type 1 AIP is such an example [28, 29]. There are also anecdotal reports that type 1 AIP and biliary carcinomas [30, 31] or intraductal papillary mucinous neoplasm of the pancreas [32–34] coexisted. These cases are instructive because even if type 1 AIP is diagnosed with a biopsy, the coexistence of a neoplastic disease cannot be excluded. The reason why such combinations happen is as yet unknown. Some authors suggest that such neoplasms correspond to postinflammatory carcinogenesis as a result of type 1 AIP, because some pancreatic carcinomas become clinically evident after the treatment of type 1 AIP [35]. Other authors have proposed that type 1 AIP is a paraneoplastic condition, because the occurrence of neoplastic diseases is common within 1 year after the treatment of type 1 AIP [36].

Type 2 AIP/IDCP

The inflammation of type 2 AIP is centered on the exocrine pancreas (Fig. 4.2a). In contrast to type 1 AIP with its unique stromal changes such as storiform fibrosis and obliterative phlebitis, in type 2 AIP the findings in the stroma are nonspecific, and they usually consist of myofibroblastic proliferation and fibrosis.

The histological feature that characterizes type 2 AIP is the duct-centric inflammation centered on the epithelium [5, 6, 14]. Neutrophils are seen within the lumens and/or epithelium (GEL, Fig. 4.2b). Involvement of interlobular ducts is a diagnostic hallmark, but intralobular ducts and the entire pancreatic lobules are also involved. Type 2 AIP can be seen

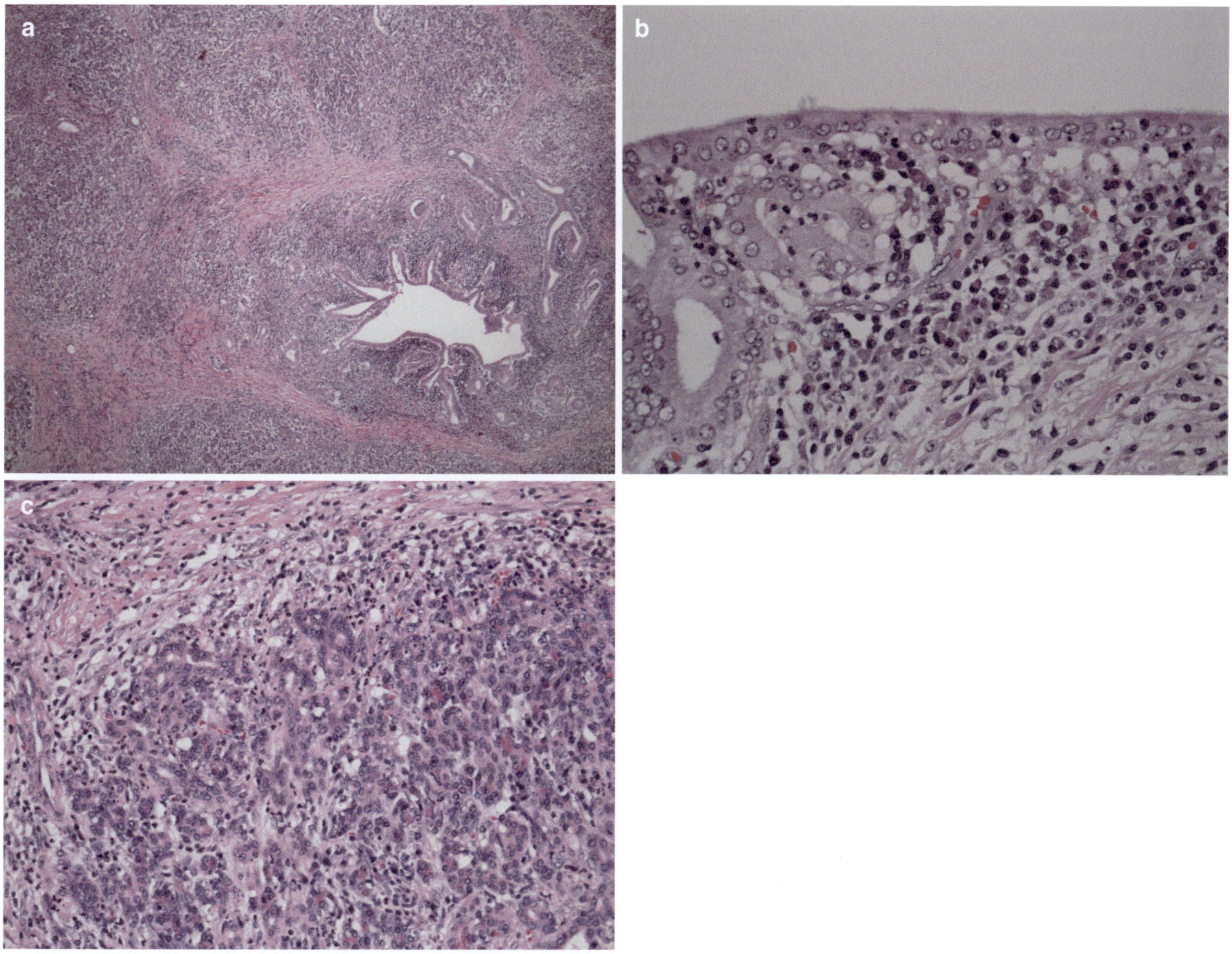

Fig. 4.2 Histological features of type 2 AIP. (**a**) The inflammation centered on the exocrine pancreas (an interlobular duct in the right lower area and surrounding pancreatic lobules). The entire duct appears entrapped by the densely packed inflammatory cells. (**b**) Neutrophilic infiltration within the duct epithelium (GEL). There is also a collar of lymphoplasmacytic infiltration around the epithelium. (**c**) Lobular inflammation. Neutrophils are numerous within the lobules

in the setting of inflammatory bowel disease (IBD). From the pathological viewpoint, this seems reasonable because type 2 AIP and IBD (especially ulcerative colitis) share many histological features. In short, GEL in type 2 AIP corresponds to crypt abscess or neutrophilic infiltration within the epithelium seen in IBD.

Ductal Inflammation

The inflammation in the ducts may be similar to but apparently different from that of type 1 AIP. Although the presence and absence of GEL in type 2 and type 1 AIP, respectively, is an important histological feature, there are other clues that distinguish the two subtypes. Because the duct epithelium itself is inflamed in type 2 AIP, the epithelial cells may be degenerative or may contain enlarged and vesicular nuclei which reflect a regenerative nature of the epithelium. Such epithelial changes are usually absent in type 1 AIP. Though there is typically a collar of lymphoplasmacytic infiltration surrounding the duct epithelium in type 2 AIP, it lacks storiform fibrosis. In some cases of type 2 AIP, the entire ducts appear to be entrapped by the densely packed inflammatory cells (Fig. 4.2a). This does not happen in type 1 AIP. In addition, the inflamed ducts in type 2 AIP seem tortuous and star shaped rather than the straight- or round-shaped ducts typically seen in type 1 AIP.

Lobular Inflammation

Inflammation in the interlobular ducts is usually associated with inflammation in the entire lobules consisting of acinar cell loss and neutrophilic infiltration (Fig. 4.2c). Lymphocytes and/or plasma cells may also be present. The lobules are well demarcated with fibrous stroma, which may contain plump fibroblasts or may be rather fibrotic depending on the specific cases. Some lobules are normal in size, but others are atrophic, and the lobular distribution is sparse in some cases because the inflammation destroys the structure.

Histological Diagnostic Criteria of Type 2 AIP

In contrast to type 1 AIP, which has unique serological features and extrapancreatic manifestations, the clinical findings of type 2 AIP are nonspecific or nondiscriminating against type 1 AIP. Thus, the histological diagnosis is considered mandatory in making the diagnosis of type 2 AIP. In the ICDC [23], the diagnostic criteria for type 2 AIP are adopted. According to these criteria, GEL in inter- and/or intralobular ducts and few or absent (<10/hpf) IgG4-positive cells are definitively diagnostic for type 2 AIP. In cases with acinar neutrophilic infiltration with few or absent IgG4-positive cells, the diagnosis is definite only in patients with IBD.

Biopsy Diagnosis of AIP

In order to avoid unnecessary pancreatic resections, the definitive diagnosis of type 1 or type 2 AIP with biopsy specimens is desired. This approach is now becoming a common practice with the technical advance of endoscopic ultrasound-guided fine-needle aspiration (EUS-FNA).

In general, the diagnosis of AIP with EUS-FNA cytology is almost impossible, because the histological patterns that are important for the diagnosis are lost in the cytology specimens. Even so, EUS-FNA cytology is a sensitive and specific tool to diagnose pancreatic carcinomas, and thus in cases in which the exclusion of pancreatic carcinomas is mandatory, this is a promising test.

An EUS-FNA biopsy is a useful test for the diagnosis of AIP [37]. This is especially true if an EUS-guided Trucut biopsy is conducted [38, 39]. For the diagnosis of type 1 AIP, a biopsy diagnosis is promising because the characteristic histological features such as storiform fibrosis and/or lobular inflammation can be obtained. For the purpose of identifying obliterative phlebitis, elastic stains such as Verhoeff-van Gieson stain is useful. Immunostaining for IgG4 is mandatory when the diagnosis of type 1 AIP is made with biopsy tissues.

In contrast, the definitive diagnosis of type 2 AIP with biopsy samples may be difficult because interlobular ducts are difficult to obtain in such tissues. In cases of type 2 AIP, lobular inflammation with neutrophils is usually obtained in biopsy samples, but this should be interpreted with caution because, as mentioned in the previous section, lobular neutrophilic infiltration can also be seen in type 1 AIP. In this situation, histological features that suggest type 1 AIP should be carefully examined in and around the lobules.

Concluding Remarks

Two subtypes of AIP, type 1 and type 2, are distinct from the pathological viewpoint. It is important, however, to remember that the difference does not depend solely on different immunoreactivities for IgG4 and that the histomorphological features are more unique. The histological diagnosis of AIP with biopsy tissues may be challenging, but it can be achieved for cases of type 1 AIP. Even if the diagnosis of type 1 AIP can be rendered, there is a possibility that an unsampled neoplastic disease may coexist in the same lesion.

Acknowledgment This work was supported in part by the Health and Labour Sciences Research Grants (Intractable Diseases) from the Japanese Ministry of Health, Labour, and Welfare.

References

1. Yoshida K, Toki F, Takeuchi T, Watanabe S, Shiratori K, Hayashi N. Chronic pancreatitis caused by an autoimmune abnormality. Proposal of the concept of autoimmune pancreatitis. Dig Dis Sci. 1995;40(7):1561–8.
2. Sarles H, Sarles JC, Muratore R, Guien C. Chronic inflammatory sclerosis of the pancreas–an autonomous pancreatic disease? Am J Dig Dis. 1961;6:688–98.
3. Kawaguchi K, Koike M, Tsuruta K, Okamoto A, Tabata I, Fujita N. Lymphoplasmacytic sclerosing pancreatitis with cholangitis: a variant of primary sclerosing cholangitis extensively involving pancreas. Hum Pathol. 1991;22(4):387–95.
4. Ectors N, Maillet B, Aerts R, Geboes K, Donner A, Borchard F, Lankisch P, Stolte M, Luttges J, Kremer B, Kloppel G. Non-alcoholic duct destructive chronic pancreatitis. Gut. 1997;41(2):263–8.
5. Notohara K, Burgart LJ, Yadav D, Chari S, Smyrk TC. Idiopathic chronic pancreatitis with periductal lymphoplasmacytic infiltration: clinicopathologic features of 35 cases. Am J Surg Pathol. 2003;27(8):1119–27.
6. Zamboni G, Luttges J, Capelli P, Frulloni L, Cavallini G, Pederzoli P, Leins A, Longnecker D, Kloppel G. Histopathological features of diagnostic and clinical relevance in autoimmune pancreatitis: a study on 53 resection specimens and 9 biopsy specimens. Virchows Arch. 2004;445(6):552–63.
7. Hamano H, Kawa S, Horiuchi A, Unno H, Furuya N, Akamatsu T, Fukushima M, Nikaido T, Nakayama K, Usuda N, Kiyosawa K. High serum IgG4 concentrations in patients with sclerosing pancreatitis. N Engl J Med. 2001;344(10):732–8.
8. Kamisawa T, Funata N, Hayashi Y, Tsuruta K, Okamoto A, Amemiya K, Egawa N, Nakajima H. Close relationship between autoimmune pancreatitis and multifocal fibrosclerosis. Gut. 2003;52(5):683–7.
9. Umehara H, Okazaki K, Masaki Y, Kawano M, Yamamoto M, Saeki T, Matsui S, Yoshino T, Nakamura S, Kawa S, Hamano H, Kamisawa T, Shimosegawa T, Shimatsu A, Nakamura S, Ito T,

Notohara K, Sumida T, Tanaka Y, Mimori T, Chiba T, Mishima M, Hibi T, Tsubouchi H, Inui K, Ohara H. Comprehensive diagnostic criteria for IgG4-related disease (IgG4-RD), 2011. Mod Rheumatol. 2012;22(1):21–30.

10. Stone JH, Khosroshahi A, Deshpande V, Chan JK, Heathcote JG, Aalberse R, Azumi A, Bloch DB, Brugge WR, Carruthers MN, Cheuk W, Cornell L, Castillo CF, Ferry JA, Forcione D, Kloppel G, Hamilos DL, Kamisawa T, Kasashima S, Kawa S, Kawano M, Masaki Y, Notohara K, Okazaki K, Ryu JK, Saeki T, Sahani D, Sato Y, Smyrk T, Stone JR, Takahira M, Umehara H, Webster G, Yamamoto M, Yi E, Yoshino T, Zamboni G, Zen Y, Chari S. Recommendations for the nomenclature of IgG4-related disease and its individual organ system manifestations. Arthritis Rheum. 2012;64(10):3061–7.
11. Sah RP, Chari ST, Pannala R, Sugumar A, Clain JE, Levy MJ, Pearson RK, Smyrk TC, Petersen BT, Topazian MD, Takahashi N, Farnell MB, Vege SS. Differences in clinical profile and relapse rate of type 1 versus type 2 autoimmune pancreatitis. Gastroenterology. 2010;139(1):140–8.
12. Kamisawa T, Chari ST, Giday SA, Kim MH, Chung JB, Lee KT, Werner J, Bergmann F, Lerch MM, Mayerle J, Pickartz T, Lohr M, Schneider A, Frulloni L, Webster GJ, Reddy DN, Liao WC, Wang HP, Okazaki K, Shimosegawa T, Kloeppel G, Go VL. Clinical profile of autoimmune pancreatitis and its histological subtypes: an international multicenter survey. Pancreas. 2011;40(6):809–14.
13. Song TJ, Kim JH, Kim MH, Jang JW, Park do H, Lee SS, Seo DW, Lee SK, Yu E. Comparison of clinical findings between histologically confirmed type 1 and type 2 autoimmune pancreatitis. J Gastroenterol Hepatol. 2012;27(4):700–8.
14. Chari ST, Kloeppel G, Zhang L, Notohara K, Lerch MM, Shimosegawa T. Histopathologic and clinical subtypes of autoimmune pancreatitis: the Honolulu consensus document. Pancreas. 2010;39(5):549–54.
15. Zhang L, Chari S, Smyrk TC, Deshpande V, Kloppel G, Kojima M, Liu X, Longnecker DS, Mino-Kenudson M, Notohara K, Rodriguez-Justo M, Srivastava A, Zamboni G, Zen Y. Autoimmune pancreatitis (AIP) type 1 and type 2: an international consensus study on histopathologic diagnostic criteria. Pancreas. 2011;40(8):1172–9.
16. Zen Y, Harada K, Sasaki M, Sato Y, Tsuneyama K, Haratake J, Kurumaya H, Katayanagi K, Masuda S, Niwa H, Morimoto H, Miwa A, Uchiyama A, Portmann BC, Nakanuma Y. IgG4-related sclerosing cholangitis with and without hepatic inflammatory pseudotumor, and sclerosing pancreatitis-associated sclerosing cholangitis: do they belong to a spectrum of sclerosing pancreatitis? Am J Surg Pathol. 2004;28(9):1193–203.
17. Kitagawa S, Zen Y, Harada K, Sasaki M, Sato Y, Minato H, Watanabe K, Kurumaya H, Katayanagi K, Masuda S, Niwa H, Tsuneyama K, Saito K, Haratake J, Takagawa K, Nakanuma Y. Abundant IgG4-positive plasma cell infiltration characterizes chronic sclerosing sialadenitis (Kuttner's tumor). Am J Surg Pathol. 2005;29(6):783–91.
18. Notohara K, Wani Y, Fujisawa M. Pathologic findings of autoimmune pancreatitis and IgG4-related disease. Curr Immunol Rev. 2011;7(2):212–20.
19. Irie H, Honda H, Baba S, Kuroiwa T, Yoshimitsu K, Tajima T, Jimi M, Sumii T, Masuda K. Autoimmune pancreatitis: CT and MR characteristics. AJR Am J Roentgenol. 1998;170(5):1323–7.
20. Miyabe K, Notohara K, Nakazawa T, Hayashi K, Naitoh I, Okumura F, Shimizu S, Yoshida M, Yamashita H, Takahashi S, Ohara H, Joh T. Histological evaluation of obliterative phlebitis for the diagnosis of autoimmune pancreatitis. J Gastroenterol. 2013;49(4):715–26.
21. Kasashima S, Zen Y, Kawashima A, Konishi K, Sasaki H, Endo M, Matsumoto Y, Kawakami K, Kasashima F, Moriya M, Kimura K, Ohtake H, Nakanuma Y. Inflammatory abdominal aortic aneurysm: close relationship to IgG4-related periaortitis. Am J Surg Pathol. 2008;32(2):197–204.
22. Zhang L, Notohara K, Levy MJ, Chari ST, Smyrk TC. IgG4-positive plasma cell infiltration in the diagnosis of autoimmune pancreatitis. Mod Pathol. 2007;20(1):23–8.
23. Shimosegawa T, Chari ST, Frulloni L, Kamisawa T, Kawa S, Mino-Kenudson M, Kim MH, Kloppel G, Lerch MM, Lohr M, Notohara K, Okazaki K, Schneider A, Zhang L. International consensus diagnostic criteria for autoimmune pancreatitis: guidelines of the International Association of Pancreatology. Pancreas. 2011;40(3):352–8.
24. Shimosegawa T. The amendment of the clinical diagnostic criteria in Japan (JPS2011) in response to the proposal of the international consensus of diagnostic criteria (ICDC) for autoimmune pancreatitis. Pancreas. 2012;41(8):1341–2.
25. Dhall D, Suriawinata AA, Tang LH, Shia J, Klimstra DS. Use of immunohistochemistry for IgG4 in the distinction of autoimmune pancreatitis from peritumoral pancreatitis. Hum Pathol. 2010;41(5):643–52.
26. Suda K, Takase M, Fukumura Y, Kashiwagi S. Pathology of autoimmune pancreatitis and tumor-forming pancreatitis. J Gastroenterol. 2007;42 Suppl 18:22–7.
27. Deshpande V, Zen Y, Chan JK, Yi EE, Sato Y, Yoshino T, Kloppel G, Heathcote JG, Khosroshahi A, Ferry JA, Aalberse RC, Bloch DB, Brugge WR, Bateman AC, Carruthers MN, Chari ST, Cheuk W, Cornell LD, Fernandez-Del Castillo C, Forcione DG, Hamilos DL, Kamisawa T, Kasashima S, Kawa S, Kawano M, Lauwers GY, Masaki Y, Nakanuma Y, Notohara K, Okazaki K, Ryu JK, Saeki T, Sahani DV, Smyrk TC, Stone JR, Takahira M, Webster GJ, Yamamoto M, Zamboni G, Umehara H, Stone JH. Consensus statement on the pathology of IgG4-related disease. Mod Pathol. 2012;25(9):1181–92.
28. Motosugi U, Ichikawa T, Yamaguchi H, Nakazawa T, Katoh R, Itakura J, Fujii H, Sato T, Araki T, Shimizu M. Small invasive ductal adenocarcinoma of the pancreas associated with lymphoplasmacytic sclerosing pancreatitis. Pathol Int. 2009;59(10):744–7.
29. Witkiewicz AK, Kennedy EP, Kennyon L, Yeo CJ, Hruban RH. Synchronous autoimmune pancreatitis and infiltrating pancreatic ductal adenocarcinoma: case report and review of the literature. Hum Pathol. 2008;39(10):1548–51.
30. Oh HC, Kim JG, Kim JW, Lee KS, Kim MK, Chi KC, Kim YS, Kim KH. Early bile duct cancer in a background of sclerosing cholangitis and autoimmune pancreatitis. Intern Med. 2008;47(23):2025–8.
31. Ohtani H, Ishida H, Ito Y, Yamaguchi T, Koizumi M. Autoimmune pancreatitis and biliary intraepithelial neoplasia of the common bile duct: a case with diagnostically challenging but pathogenetically significant association. Pathol Int. 2011;61(8):481–5.
32. Naitoh I, Nakazawa T, Notohara K, Miyabe K, Hayashi K, Shimizu S, Kondo H, Yoshida M, Yamashita H, Umemura S, Ohara H, Joh T. Intraductal papillary mucinous neoplasm associated with autoimmune pancreatitis. Pancreas. 2013;42(3):552–4.
33. Urata T, Naito Y, Izumi Y, Takekuma Y, Yokomizo H, Nagamine M, Fukuda S, Notohara K, Hifumi M. Localized type 1 autoimmune pancreatitis superimposed upon preexisting intraductal papillary mucinous neoplasms. World J Gastroenterol. 2013;19(47):9127–32.
34. Tabata T, Kamisawa T, Hara S, Kuruma S, Chiba K, Kuwata G, Fujiwara T, Egashira H, Koizumi S, Endo Y, Koizumi K, Fujiwara J, Arakawa T, Momma K, Horiguchi S, Hishima T, Kurata M, Honda G, Kloppel G. Intraductal papillary mucinous neoplasm of the pancreas and IgG4-related disease: a coincidental association. Pancreatology. 2013;13(4):379–83.
35. Fukui T, Mitsuyama T, Takaoka M, Uchida K, Matsushita M, Okazaki K. Pancreatic cancer associated with autoimmune pancreatitis in remission. Intern Med. 2008;47(3):151–5.
36. Shiokawa M, Kodama Y, Yoshimura K, Kawanami C, Mimura J, Yamashita Y, Asada M, Kikuyama M, Okabe Y, Inokuma T, Ohana M, Kokuryu H, Takeda K, Tsuji Y, Minami R, Sakuma Y, Kuriyama K, Ota Y, Tanabe W, Maruno T, Kurita A, Sawai Y, Uza

N, Watanabe T, Haga H, Chiba T. Risk of cancer in patients with autoimmune pancreatitis. Am J Gastroenterol. 2013;108(4):610–7.

37. Kanno A, Ishida K, Hamada S, Fujishima F, Unno J, Kume K, Kikuta K, Hirota M, Masamune A, Satoh K, Notohara K, Shimosegawa T. Diagnosis of autoimmune pancreatitis by EUS-FNA by using a 22-gauge needle based on the International Consensus Diagnostic Criteria. Gastrointest Endosc. 2012;76(3):594–602.
38. Levy MJ, Reddy RP, Wiersema MJ, Smyrk TC, Clain JE, Harewood GC, Pearson RK, Rajan E, Topazian MD, Yusuf TE, Chari ST, Petersen BT. EUS-guided trucut biopsy in establishing autoimmune pancreatitis as the cause of obstructive jaundice. Gastrointest Endosc. 2005;61(3):467–72.
39. Mizuno N, Bhatia V, Hosoda W, Sawaki A, Hoki N, Hara K, Takagi T, Ko SB, Yatabe Y, Goto H, Yamao K. Histological diagnosis of autoimmune pancreatitis using EUS-guided trucut biopsy: a comparison study with EUS-FNA. J Gastroenterol. 2009;44(7):742–50.

Pancreatic Endocrine and Exocrine Functions in Patients with Autoimmune Pancreatitis

5

Tetsuhide Ito, Lingaku Lee, Masayuki Hijioka, and Hisato Igarashi

Introduction

Autoimmune pancreatitis (AIP) is a distinctive type of pancreatitis, and it is considered that the pathogenesis of AIP involves autoimmune mechanisms [1–6]. Recently, AIP has been considered as a systemic disease because it is often accompanied by various extrapancreatic lesions including cholangitis, sialadenitis, retroperitoneal fibrosis, hilar lymphadenopathy, and chronic thyroiditis [7–11]. Furthermore, AIP is often associated with pancreatic exocrine and endocrine dysfunction. Recently, AIP is known to have two clinical and histological subtypes [12, 13], and the international consensus diagnostic criteria (ICDC) published in 2012 [14] enabled us to classify these subtypes into type 1 and type 2. Patients with type 1 AIP often show accompanying extrapancreatic lesions but seldom reveal abdominal pain. On the other hand, patients with type 2 AIP commonly have abdominal pain and sometimes accompany acute pancreatitis. In the present manuscript, we focus on the endocrine and exocrine functions associated with type 1 AIP according to the revised Japanese consensus guideline for management of AIP [15–17].

Endocrine Dysfunction Associated with Type 1 AIP

Diabetes mellitus with pancreatic disorders (pancreatic diabetes) is closely related to the progression of a primary disease such as pancreatitis or pancreatic cancer because diabetes mellitus occurs due to pancreatic endocrine dysfunction caused by the progression of a pancreatic disorder [18–21]. From endocrinologic aspects, both insulin and glucagon synthesis/secretion are affected by the primary disease [20, 21]. Therefore, the pathology and clinical features of pancreatic diabetes are often different from those of types 1 and 2 diabetes, and its treatment method should be different [20].

A nationwide epidemiological survey on pancreatic diabetes to determine the incidence, pathology, clinical features, and current treatment status was conducted in Japan [22]. According to this survey, the causal factors of pancreatic diabetes were chronic pancreatitis (40.0 %), pancreatic cancer (24.6 %), pancreatectomy (10.2 %), acute pancreatitis (7.5 %), and AIP (6.1 %) (Table 5.1) [22]. On the other hand, 77.0 % of patients with AIP were reported to be associated with diabetes mellitus [23]. Studies by individual medical facilities reported that 83–88 % of the cases were associated with secretion dysfunction and 42–78 % with diabetes mellitus [11, 24, 25]. The diabetes mellitus accompanying AIP was analyzed in detail in the nationwide survey conducted in Japan in 2006 [26]. Among those AIP patients who sought

Table 5.1 Prevalence of pancreatic diabetes by causal factor and relationship with onset of diabetes

Etiology	Number of patients	(%)	Onset of diabetes secondary to pancreatic disorder (%)
Chronic pancreatitis	684	40.0	46.3
Acute pancreatitis	129	7.5	47.6
Autoimmune pancreatitis	105	6.1	43.3
Pancreatic injury	13	0.8	66.7
Pancreatic cancer	421	24.6	33.7
Pancreatic endocrine tumor	18	1.1	38.9
Pancreatic cystic tumor	117	6.8	38.6
Other tumors	15	0.9	60.0
After pancreatectomy	174	10.2	65.2
Pancreatic hemochromatosis	8	0.5	71.4
Pancreatic hypoplasia	1	0.1	0
Others	25	1.5	45.8
Total	1,710	100	44.5

Modified from Ref. [22]

T. Ito, MD, PhD (✉) • L. Lee, MD, PhD
M. Hijioka, MD, PhD • H. Igarashi, MD, PhD
Department of Medicine and Bioregulatory Science, School of Medicine, Graduate School of Medical Sciences, Faculty of Medical Sciences, Kyushu University, 3-1-1 Maidashi, Higashi-ku, Fukuoka City 812-8582, Japan
e-mail: itopapa@intmed3.med.kyushu-u.ac.jp

T. Kamisawa, J.B. Chung (eds.), *Autoimmune Pancreatitis*,
DOI 10.1007/978-3-642-55086-7_5, © Springer-Verlag Berlin Heidelberg 2015

medical attention during the 1-year period of 2002, 66.5 % of cases were found to be associated with diabetes mellitus; of those, 33.3 % had diabetes mellitus prior to the onset of AIP, and 51.6 % started developing diabetes mellitus around the same time as the onset of pancreatitis. Among those patients having diabetes mellitus, 14 % developed diabetes after steroid treatment [26], suggesting that such diabetes may be caused by long-term steroid treatment. There are some cases where pancreatic endocrine dysfunction was improved by steroid treatment; however, since not all cases improved, it can be stated that medical conditions that have progressed far enough to cause some degree of organic change cannot be reversed.

Previously, we demonstrated for the first time that endocrine pancreas showed the dysfunction of both insulin secretion from beta cells and glucagon secretion from alpha cells in patients with AIP [27]. These findings mean that endocrine dysfunction in AIP is a secondary pancreatic diabetes mellitus, unlike primary diabetes mellitus, in which glucagon secretion is preserved [27]. Furthermore, the results of histological findings in AIP showed markedly that fibrosis and lymphoplasmacytic cell infiltration were observed strongly around the islet cell, but the islet cell was revealed to be almost intact [27]. Therefore, the onset mechanism of endocrine dysfunction in AIP is considered to be as follows: At first, rapid inflammatory cell infiltration and fibrosis induce the reduction in blood flow in exocrine pancreas, and subsequently, islet cells fall into ischemia because of the reduction in blood flow, and then circulation failure causes the dysfunction of hormone secretion from islet cells, such as alpha cells and beta cells. However, interestingly, Tanaka et al. [28] reported that the volume of beta cells was reduced in patients with AIP, but the volume of alpha cells in AIP did not differ from that of type 2 diabetes by immunohistologic examination. Accordingly, exocrine dysfunction in AIP, especially insulin secretion from beta cells, may be induced not only by circulation failure in islet cells but also by the reduction in the number of beta cells. However, details need to be clarified in the future. After all, the mechanism of pathogenesis of diabetes mellitus is assumed to be affected by both of the following disorders [11, 28]: obstructed blood flow to the endocrine glands (islets of Langerhans) associated with the fibrosis of the exocrine glands and damaged islets of Langerhans due to the spreading of inflammation [11, 28].

Exocrine Dysfunction Associated with Type 1 AIP

AIP is in many cases associated with pancreatic exocrine dysfunction. According to the nationwide survey conducted in Japan in 2000, 80.6 % of patients with AIP showed abnormal pancreatic exocrine function in which the abnormality is defined as 70 % or lower secretion in the BT-PABA (PFD test), and 70.0 % of the cases showed exocrine dysfunction (as determined by the secretin test), comparable to that in confirmed cases of chronic pancreatitis [15]. From our detailed examination of secretin test, differences of results between chronic pancreatitis and AIP were clarified [27]. Patients with chronic pancreatic exocrine dysfunction examined by secretin test revealed especially the reduction in bicarbonate concentration, whereas main reductions in patients with AIP were in volume and amylase output. The reason for these differences between chronic pancreatitis and AIP was determined by histological examination as follows: Destruction of the basement membranes of the pancreatic duct in chronic pancreatitis was observed. Therefore, as pancreatic ducts assume the responsibility of bicarbonate secretion, bicarbonate secretion in chronic pancreatitis by secretin test may be reduced. On the other hand, most basement membranes in AIP were intact, so bicarbonate secretion was preserved. However, stenoses of pancreatic ducts cause disturbances in pancreatic juice flow in AIP, and therefore, volume and amylase output by secretin test may be reduced. Of course, if the basement membranes were destroyed, bicarbonate secretion would diminish even in AIP. On this point, Otsuki et al. [29] and Yamaguchi et al. [30, 31] reported certain interesting facts. They examined 2 models of pancreatitis in rats – irreversible pancreatitis induced by intraductal infusion of oleic acid and reversible pancreatitis induced by retrograde intraductal infusion of sodium taurocholate – and noted that the difference between irreversible pancreatitis and reversible pancreatitis depended on the degree of injury of the pancreatic duct, especially injury of the pancreatic ductal basement membranes [29–31]. These experimental studies have clearly indicated that the difference between reversible and irreversible pancreatitis depended on the degree of damage of the duct epithelium where pancreatic progenitor cells exist. If the epithelial cells were severely injured, the pancreas could not regenerate [29–31]. Furthermore, Song et al. [32] reported that the pattern of fibrosis was mainly loose fibrosis with stromal edema in AIP, whereas it was dense fibrosis in CP. Taken together, it is considered that exocrine function in AIP is reversible to some extent by steroid therapy if the basement membranes of the pancreatic ducts are not destroyed, because the pancreatic ducts are compressed and stenosed by lymphoplasmacytic cell infiltration, which extended from the pancreatic parenchyma to the ducts in most AIP.

After all, in AIP, the mechanism of pathogenesis of pancreatic exocrine dysfunction is assumed to involve the following: decreased secretion of pancreatic enzymes associated with collapsed acinar cells caused by pronounced cellular infiltration mainly of plasmacytes and fibrosis and obstructed flow of pancreatic juice due to inflammatory cell infiltration around the pancreatic ducts and subsequent narrowing of the pancreatic ducts [11, 25, 26, 28]. A recent study suggested that mislocalization of cystic fibrosis transmembrane conductance regulator (CFTR), which plays a central role in pancreatic duct HCO_3– secretion, and upregulation of aquaporin-1 (AQP1) on the plasma membrane and in the cytoplasm of pancreatic duct cells may be involved in the development of AIP [33]. Corticosteroids reduce inflammation and restore both digestive enzyme and HCO_3– secretion in patients with AIP by regenerating acinar cells and correcting CFTR localization in pancreatic duct cells [33].

Pancreatic Exocrine and Endocrine Functions After Steroid Therapy in AIP

Many AIP patients have associated pancreatic exocrine and endocrine dysfunction [11, 24–27, 34]. It has been reported that improvement of pancreatic exocrine and endocrine function was detected after steroid therapy in 38 % [25]–50 % [11] and 25 % [25]–45 % [11] of AIP patients, respectively. It has also been suggested as a mechanism of improvement in pancreatic exocrine and endocrine functions after steroid therapy that steroid suppresses lymphoplasmacytic cell infiltration and fibrosis, permitting the attenuation of blood flow [27] and further regenerating islet cells by suppression of cytokine production [28]. A recent study about the changes in pancreatic tissue before and after steroid therapy in AIP patients revealed regeneration of acinar cells by steroids and suggested that acinar cell regeneration might be associated with CD133-positive pancreatic progenitor cells [33]. Diabetes mellitus control worsens in 75 % of AIP patients with type 2 diabetes mellitus before AIP onset after steroid therapy [11]. DM also develops after steroid therapy in some AIP patients [11, 26]. We should therefore take occurrence of DM into consideration in patients who continuously undergo steroid therapy.

The Management of Pancreatic Exocrine Insufficiency in Patients with AIP Associated with Pancreatic Diabetes

Pancreatic diabetes is frequently complicated with lack or insufficiencies in pancreatic enzymes because of the destruction and reduction of pancreatic exocrine cells due to pancreatic exocrine diseases. Consequently, patients with pancreatic diabetes suffer from excessive malnutrition, such as hypoglycemia, hypoproteinemia, hypoalbuminemia, hypocholesterolemia, and hypotriglycemia, caused by insufficiencies in digestion and absorption of fat, protein, and carbohydrates (Fig. 5.1) [20]. This condition is one of the reasons for the unstable glycemic control and poor prognosis in patients with pancreatic diabetes. Therefore, patients with pancreatic diabetes need to receive sufficient pancreatic exocrine replacement therapy for the supplementation of pancreatic enzymes. The clinical management of pancreatic diabetes is divided into two parts: one is the adequate supplementation of pancreatic diges-

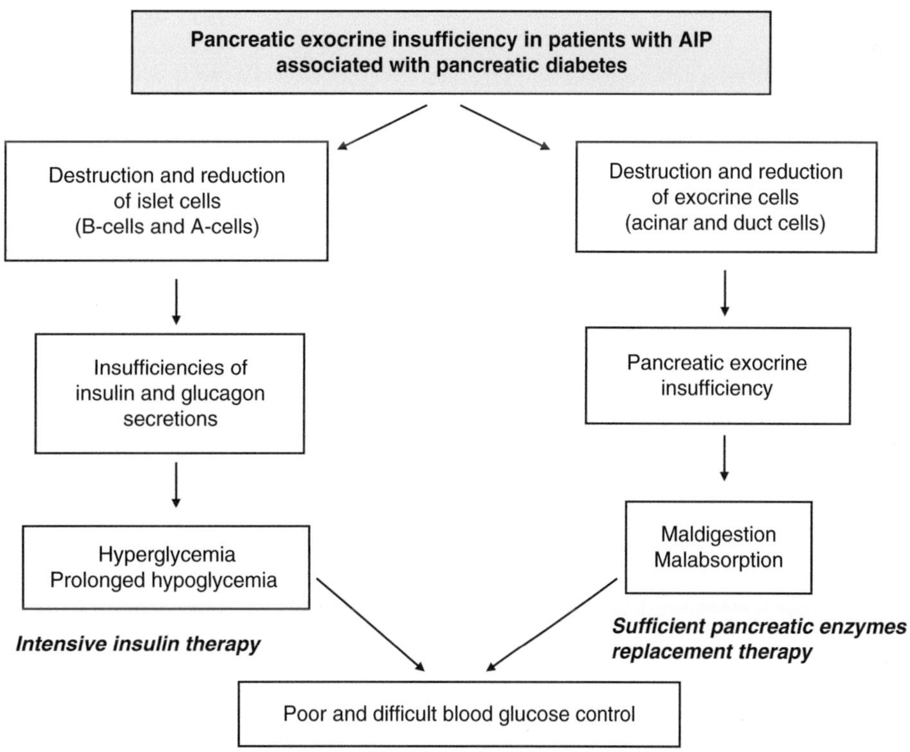

Fig. 5.1 Management of pancreatic exocrine insufficiency in patients with AIP-associated pancreatic diabetes

tive enzymes and the other is the achievement of appropriate glycemic control. The appropriate and sufficient pancreatic exocrine replacement therapy is important for the maintenance of better nutrient conditions for patients with pancreatic diabetes. Furthermore, the intensive insulin therapy combined with short- or ultrashort-acting insulin and long-acting insulin can be achieved for the stable glycemic control and reduction of severe frequent hypoglycemia in patients with pancreatic diabetes. To mimic physiological insulin secretion and achieve appropriate glycemic control in patients with pancreatic diabetes, we should recognize that sufficient basal insulin supplementation is important [20]. These current advanced management techniques against insufficiencies of pancreatic exocrine endocrine functions are beneficial for improving and maintaining the quality of life in patients with AIP-associated pancreatic diabetes.

Conclusion

In this chapter, we focus on the endocrine and exocrine functions associated with type 1 AIP according to the revised Japanese consensus guideline for management of AIP [15–17]. In conclusion, AIP is often associated with pancreatic exocrine and endocrine dysfunctions (diabetes mellitus); occurrence ratios are about 80 % and 70 %, respectively. Pancreatic exocrine and endocrine functions improve after steroid therapy in some AIP patients. Many AIP patients with type 2 diabetes mellitus before AIP onset showed worsening of diabetes mellitus control after steroid therapy [35].

References

1. Yoshida K, Toki F, Takeuchi T, Watanabe S, Shiratori K, Hayashi N. Chronic pancreatitis caused by an autoimmune abnormality. Proposal of the concept of autoimmune pancreatitis. Dig Dis Sci. 1995;40:1561–8.
2. Ito T, Nakano I, Koyanagi S, et al. Autoimmune pancreatitis as a new clinical entity. Three cases of autoimmune pancreatitis with effective steroid therapy. Dig Dis Sci. 1997;42:1458–68.
3. Okazaki K, Chiba T. Autoimmune related pancreatitis. Gut. 2002;51:1–4.
4. Pickartz T, Mayerle J, Lerch MM. Autoimmune pancreatitis. Nat Clin Pract Gastroenterol Hepatol. 2007;4:314–23.
5. Gardner TB, Chari ST. Autoimmune pancreatitis. Gastroenterol Clin North Am. 2008;37:439–60.
6. Okazaki K, Kawa S, Kamisawa T, et al. Japanese clinical guidelines for autoimmune pancreatitis. Pancreas. 2009;38:849–66.
7. Kawabe K, Ito T, Arita Y, et al. Successful treatment of advanced-stage autoimmune pancreatitis-related sclerosing cholangitis. Pancreas. 2006;33:434–7.
8. Kamisawa T, Funata N, Hayashi Y, et al. A new clinicopathological entity of IgG4-related autoimmune disease. J Gastroenterol. 2003;38:982–4.
9. Yamamoto M, Takahashi H, Ohara M, et al. A new conceptualization for Mikulicz's disease as an IgG4-related plasmacytic disease. Mod Rheumatol. 2006;16:335–40.
10. Masaki Y, Dong L, Kurose N, et al. Proposal for a new clinical entity, IgG4-positive multi-organ lymphoproliferative syndrome: analysis of 64 cases of IgG4-related disorders. Ann Rheum Dis. 2009;68:1310–5.
11. Ito T, Nishimori I, Inoue N, et al. Treatment for autoimmune pancreatitis: consensus on the treatment for patients with autoimmune pancreatitis in Japan. J Gastroenterol. 2007;42:50–8.
12. Notohara K, Burgart LJ, Yadav D, et al. Idiopathic chronic pancreatitis with periductal lymphoplasmacytic infiltration: Clinicopathologic features of 35 cases. Am J Surg Pathol. 2003;27:1119–27.
13. Zamboni G, Lüttges J, Capelli P, et al. Histopathological features of diagnostic and clinical relevance in autoimmune pancreatitis: A study on 53 resection specimens and 9 biopsy specimens. Virchows Arch. 2004;445:552–63.
14. Shimosegawa T, Chari ST, Frulloni L, et al. International consensus diagnostic criteria for autoimmune pancreatitis: Guidelines of the international association of pancreatology. Pancreas. 2011;40:352–8.
15. Okazaki T, Kawa S, Kamisawa T, et al. Amendment of the Japanese Consensus Guidelines for Autoimmune Pancreatitis, 2013. I. Concept and diagnosis of autoimmune pancreatitis. J Gastroenterol. 2014;49:567–88.
16. Kawa S, Okazaki K, Kamisawa T, et al. Amendment of Japanese Consensus Guidelines for Autoimmune Pancreatitis, 2013. II. Extra-pancreatic lesions, differential diagnosis. J Gastroenterol. 2014;49:765–84.
17. Kamisawa T, Okazaki T, Kawa S, et al. Japanese Consensus Guideline for Management of Autoimmune Pancreatitis. III. Treatment and prognosis of AIP. J Gastroenterol. 2014;49:961–70.
18. Owyang C. Endocrine changes in pancreatic insufficiency. In: Go VLW, DiMagno EP, editors. The Pancreas: biology, pathobiology and disease. New York: Raven; 1993. p. 8803–13.
19. Angelopoulos N, Dervenis C, Goula A, et al. Endocrine pancreatic insufficiency in chronic pancreatitis. Pancreatology. 2005;5:122–31.
20. Kawabe K, Ito T, Igarashi H, et al. The current managements of pancreatic diabetes in Japan. Clin J Gastroenterol. 2009;2:1–8.
21. Czakó L, Hegyi P, Rakonczay Z, et al. Interactions between the endocrine and exocrine pancreas and their clinical relevance. Pancreatology. 2009;9:351–9.
22. Ito T, Otsuki M, Igarashi H, et al. Epidemiological study of pancreatic diabetes in Japan in 2005: a nationwide study. Pancreas. 2010;39:829–35.
23. Nishimori I, Suda K, Oi I, et al. Nationwide survey for so-called autoimmune pancreatitis in Japan. Annual reports of research committee of intractable pancreatic diseases supported by Ministry of Health, Labour and Welfare of Japan. 2002:125–36. (in Japanese).
24. Kamisawa T, Egawa N, Inokuma S, et al. Pancreatic endocrine and exocrine function and salivary gland function in autoimmune pancreatitis before and after steroid therapy. Pancreas. 2003;27:235–8.
25. Nishino T, Toki F, Oyama H, et al. Long-term outcome of autoimmune pancreatitis after oral prednisolone therapy. Intern Med. 2006;45:497–501.
26. Nishimori I, Tamakoshi A, Kawa S, et al. Influence of steroid therapy on the course of diabetes mellitus in patients with autoimmune pancreatitis: findings from a nationwide survey in Japan. Pancreas. 2006;32:244–8.
27. Ito T, Kawabe K, Arita Y, et al. Evaluation of pancreatic endocrine and exocrine function in patients with autoimmune pancreatitis. Pancreas. 2007;34:254–9.
28. Tanaka S, Kobayashi T, Nakanishi K, et al. Corticosteroid-responsive diabetes mellitus associated with autoimmune pancreatitis. Lancet. 2000;356:910–1.
29. Otsuki M. Regeneration of the pancreas after pancreatitis. J Jpn Pancreas Soc. 2002;17:8–21. (in Japanese).

30. Yamaguchi T, Nakamura H, Kihara Y, et al. Long-term overexpression of membrane type-1 matrix metalloproteinase and matrix metalloproteinase-2 in oleic acid-induced pancreatitis in rats. Pancreas. 2002;24:348–56.
31. Yamaguchi T, Kihara Y, Taguchi M, et al. Persistent destruction of the basement membrane of the pancreatic duct contributes to progressive acinar atrophy in rats with experimentally induced pancreatitis. Pancreas. 2005;31:365–72.
32. Song MH, Kim MH, Jang SJ, et al. Comparison of histology and extracellular matrix between autoimmune and alcoholic chronic pancreatitis. Pancreas. 2005;30:272–8.
33. Ko SB, Mizuno N, Yatabe Y, et al. Corticosteroids correct aberrant CFTR localization in the duct and regenerate acinar cells in autoimmune pancreatitis. Gastroenterology. 2010;138:1988–96.
34. Kamisawa T, Yoshiike M, Egawa N, et al. Treating patients with autoimmune pancreatitis: results from a long-term follow-up study. Pancreatology. 2005;5:234–40.
35. Ito T, Nakamura T, Fujimori N, et al. Characteristics of pancreatic diabetes in patients with autoimmune pancreatitis. J Dig Dis. 2011;12:210–6.

Type 2 AIP

6

Tae Jun Song and Myung-Hwan Kim

Introduction

During the last decade, there has been growing recognition of a peculiar type of chronic pancreatitis known as autoimmune pancreatitis (AIP). AIP consists of two distinct clinical and histopathological forms of pancreatitis: type 1 and type 2 [1–5]. Type 1 AIP refers to the subtype that has the histological pattern known as lymphoplasmacytic sclerosing pancreatitis (LPSP) or granulocytic epithelial lesion (GEL)-negative AIP, whereas type 2 AIP refers to the subtype that has the histological pattern called idiopathic duct-centric pancreatitis (IDCP) or GEL-positive AIP [4]. Since pancreatic histology often may not be available, the terms type 1 and type 2 AIP have been introduced to describe the clinical profiles associated with LPSP and IDCP. The increasing number of reported AIP cases had resulted in the identification of several clinical, serologic, and histopathologic features that distinguish the 2 subtypes of the disease [6].

Although some overlap exists, a number of clinical, serologic, and histopathologic features distinguish the two subtypes of the disease. Type 1 AIP is considered as part of the spectrum of IgG4-related systemic disease, whereas type 2 disease is not. The subtyping of AIP is more than just an academic exercise because different diagnostic criteria and algorithms are applied in the diagnosis of AIP, depending on the subtype of AIP.

Epidemiology of Type 2 AIP

There is a difference in the prevalence of 2 subtypes. Type 2 AIP appears to be relatively common in the United States and Europe but rare in East Asia. Type 2 AIP has been reported to be very rare in Japan, but it accounted for 37 % of cases of resected AIP from the Mayo Clinic and 45 % in Europe [7, 8]. According to the Japanese nationwide survey, 2.8 % cases of histologically confirmed type 2 AIP were reported [5]. In Korea, type 2 AIP was not as rare as previously thought, with an estimated 10 % prevalence rate among total AIP. The plausible explanation for the reason why the ratio of type 2 AIP among total AIP is higher in Korea than it is in Japan is that pancreatic core biopsies (percutaneous transabdominal US-guided or endoscopic ultrasound [EUS]-guided) were more actively performed to confirm the diagnoses. Since the definitive diagnosis of type 2 AIP requires pancreatic histology, under-recognition of type 2 AIP is far more likely than that of type 1 AIP.

Imaging Features of Type 2 AIP

According to a recent study, the typical imaging features seen in type 1 AIP also were seen in type 2 AIP with similar frequencies [5]. Typical parenchymal imaging on CT/MRI is diffuse pancreatic enlargement with delayed enhancement, sometimes associated with rim-like enhancement (Fig. 6.1) [9]. The key ERP findings highly suggestive of AIP include (1) a long stricture involving more than one-third of the duct length, (2) lack of upstream duct dilatation from the stricture, and (3) multifocal strictures (Fig. 6.2) [10]. Type 2 AIP potentially benefits the most from diagnostic ERP because patients with type 2 AIP typically have normal levels of serum IgG4 and no OOI.

Histopathology of Type 2 AIP

Type 1 AIP can be diagnosed on the basis of histological findings that fulfill three or more of the following conditions: periductal lymphoplasmacytic infiltrate without granulocytic infiltration, obliterative phlebitis, storiform fibrosis, and abundant IgG4-positive cells [9]. In contrast, these features are very rarely seen in type 2 AIP in most instances [4]. The definite diagnosis of type 2 AIP can be made based on the presence of granulocytic epithelial lesion (GEL) which is

T.J. Song, MD, PhD • M.-H. Kim, MD, PhD (✉)
Department of Internal Medicine,
Asan Medical Center, University of Ulsan College of Medicine,
Asanbyeongwon-Gil 86, Songpa-Gu, Seoul 138-736, South Korea
e-mail: mhkim@amc.seoul.kr

T. Kamisawa, J.B. Chung (eds.), *Autoimmune Pancreatitis*,
DOI 10.1007/978-3-642-55086-7_6, © Springer-Verlag Berlin Heidelberg 2015

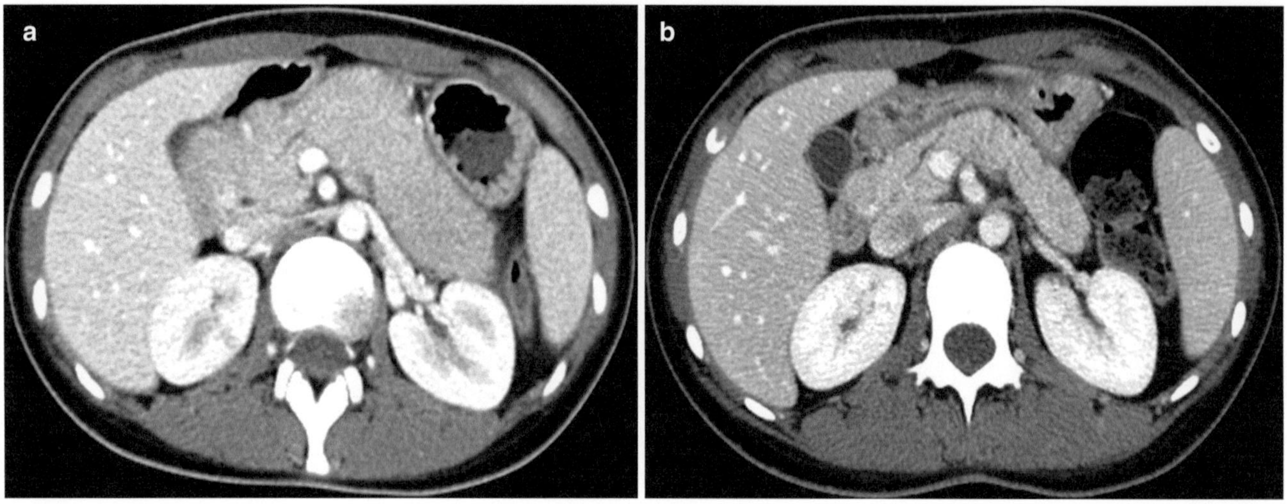

Fig. 6.1 CT findings of type 2 autoimmune pancreatitis. (**a**) CT scan demonstrates diffuse pancreatic enlargement. (**b**) After steroid therapy, diffuse pancreatic enlargement is markedly improved on follow-up CT scan

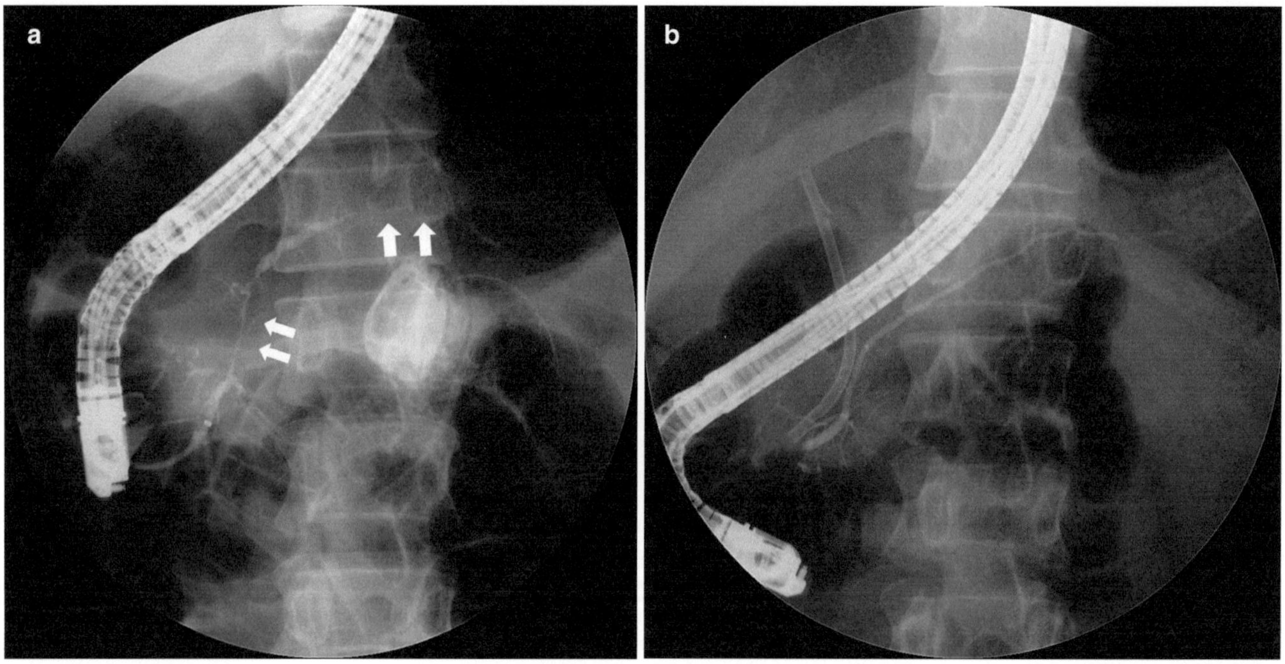

Fig. 6.2 Endoscopic retrograde pancreatography (ERP) findings in type 2 autoimmune pancreatitis. (**a**) ERP demonstrates skipped, multifocal irregular narrowing of the main pancreatic duct (*arrow*). (**b**) After steroid therapy, the narrowing of main pancreatic duct recovered to almost normal

characterized by the infiltration of neutrophils into the lumen or epithelium of the pancreatic duct (Fig. 6.3). The finding of the so-called GEL is known to be specific to type 2 AIP [11]. If GELs are identified in a pancreatic core biopsy (PCB) or resection specimen, it is pathognomonic for type 2 AIP [12]. GEL often cause destruction and obliteration of the pancreatic duct lumen [12].

GEL may not be present exclusively to type 2 AIP. A recent study reported that GEL could be found in up to 27 % of type 1 AIP although it consisted only of intraepithelial neutrophils [4]. In addition, there is a report that typical LPSP coexisted with GEL [13]. GEL seen in type 1 AIP may result from secondary changes developing on the background of LPSP due to a pancreatic ductal stricture. A previous study included GELs present in small intralobular ducts as well as those seen in medium- and large-sized interlobular ducts [14]. However, some experts suggested that GEL in the intralobular duct should not be used as a diagnostic hallmark of type 2 AIP since this finding is not uncommon even in type 1 AIP [15]. Given the some uncertainties surrounding

GELs, a consensus definition of GELs based on more stringent criteria are necessary.

Clinical Manifestations of Type 2 AIP

When the clinical manifestations of patients with these two histological entities were compared, they were distinctly different (Table 6.1). Patients with type 2 are significantly younger than those with type 1, and type 2 AIP may be missed in young patients whom the pancreas is rarely biopsied [16]. While the most frequent presenting symptom of type 1 AIP is obstructive jaundice, patients with type 2 are as likely to present with abdominal pain and pancreatitis [5, 17].

Patients with type 2 AIP have no collateral evidences such as elevated serum IgG4 and OOI which is of great help in nonsurgically diagnosing AIP [16]. Inflammatory bowel disease (IBD), particularly ulcerative colitis, is more common in type 2 than type 1 AIP, although type 1 has a higher prevalence of it compared with the general population [17]. Approximately 30 % of reported cases of type 2 AIP have associated IBD (Fig. 6.4).

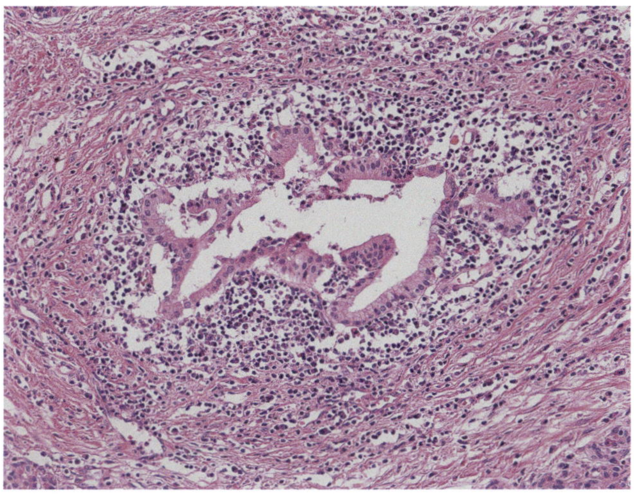

Fig. 6.3 Granulocytic epithelial lesion is seen at interlobular ducts (*arrows*) and moderate mixed inflammatory cell infiltration is in the interlobular connective tissue (H&E, ×400)

Compared with patients with type 2 AIP, patients with type 1 AIP are older, have increased serum IgG4 levels, and frequently show other organ involvement (OOI) such as proximal bile duct involvement, salivary gland involvement, kidney involvement, and retroperitoneal fibrosis [5]. In contrast, patients with type 2 AIP are more than a decade younger, have normal serum IgG4 levels, and show an association with IBD. In seronegative AIP cases without OOI, determination of the AIP subtype may not be possible without the aid of histopathology because a proportion of histologically confirmed type 1 AIP can also show seronegativity and no OOI [6].

Diagnosis of Type 2 AIP

The previous published criteria for AIP were geared toward diagnosing type 1 AIP [2]. The international consensus diagnostic criteria (ICDC) and algorithms are the first diagnostic criteria that enable the diagnosis of type 2 AIP separately (Table 6.2; Fig. 6.5) [9]. According to the ICDC, patients can be diagnosed with definite type 2 AIP if they have histologically confirmed IDCP (both GEL with/without granulocytic acinar inflammation and absent/scant IgG4-positive cells). The diagnosis of definite type 2 AIP can be made even though GELs are not observed on histology, if they show level 2 histology (both granulocytic and lymphoplasmacytic acinar infiltrate and absent/scant IgG4-positive cells) on PCB, clinical IBD and steroid responsiveness. The diagnosis of probable type 2 AIP can be made if they have level 2 histology or clinical IBD, and steroid responsiveness.

Since type 2 AIP patients are seronegative and lack OOI, pancreatic histology is essential for definitive diagnosis. One

Table 6.1 Differences between clinicopathologic profiles of type 1 and type 2 AIP

	Type 1 AIP	Type 2 AIP
Synonym	Lymphoplasmacytic sclerosing pancreatitis (LPSP)	Idiopathic duct-centric chronic pancreatitis (IDCP)
Epidemiology	Asia > United States, Europe	Europe, United States > Asia
Clinical presentation	Obstructive jaundice (painless)	Obstructive jaundice/acute pancreatitis
Age at diagnosis	Old	Young
Serum IgG4 level	Elevated	Normal
Histological hallmarks	Periductal lymphoplasmacytic infiltrate, storiform fibrosis, obliterative phlebitis	Granulocytic epithelial lesion (GEL)
Tissue IgG4 stain	Many IgG4 (+) cells	None or very few IgG4 (+) cells
Other organ involvement	Bile duct, salivary gland, kidney, retroperitoneum	Not seen
Ulcerative colitis	Rare	20–30 %
Steroid responsiveness	Excellent	Excellent
Recurrence	Common	Rare

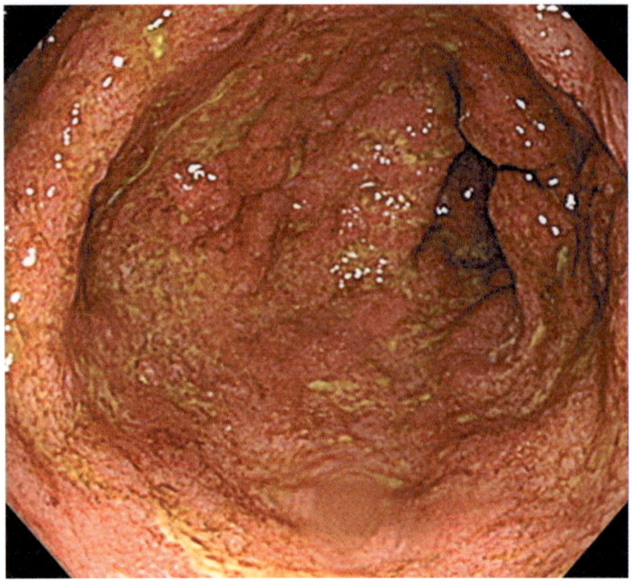

Fig. 6.4 Colonoscopic findings in type 2 autoimmune pancreatitis. Colonoscopy shows friable and erythematous colonic mucosa with loss of the normal vascular markings, which is compatible with ulcerative colitis

can suspect type 2 AIP in young patients with mild acute pancreatitis and obstructive jaundice (with negative investigations for cancer) who are seronegative and have no OOI other than possibly IBD [5]. However, up to 25 % of those with type 1 (histologically confirmed) are seronegative, and 30–40 % of those with type 1 have no discernible OOI [18].

Treatment and Follow-Up

Initial reports of type 2 AIP included only patients who had undergone surgical resection [7, 8]. In such patients, no further treatment was required and no relapses were reported. Type 2 AIP is known to respond dramatically to steroid therapy as in the case of type 1 AIP [5]. The steroid regimen is identical to the case of type 1 AIP. Recent studies demonstrated that none of the histologically confirmed type 2 AIP patients experienced a relapse after steroid therapy during the follow-up period [5, 17]. Therefore, no or less frequent relapse can be considered to form another important clinical feature that distinguishes type 2 from type 1 AIP.

Table 6.2 The international consensus diagnostic criteria for autoimmune pancreatitis

Diagnosis	Imaging evidence	Collateral evidence
Definitive type 1 AIP	Typical/indeterminate	Histologically confirmed LPSP (level 1 H)
	Typical	Any non-D level 1/level 2
	Indeterminate	Two or more from level 1 (+level 2 D)
	Indeterminate	Level 1 S/OOI + Rt or level 1 D + level 2 S/OOI/H + Rt
Probable type 1 AIP	Indeterminate	Level 2 S/OOI/H + Rt
Definitive type 2 AIP	Typical/indeterminate	Histologically confirmed IDCP (level 1 H) or clinical inflammatory bowel disease + level 2 H + Rt
Probable type 2 AIP	Typical/indeterminate	Level 2 H/clinical inflammatory bowel disease + Rt
AIP-not otherwise specified	Typical/indeterminate	D1/2 + Rt

LPSP lymphoplasmacytic sclerosing pancreatitis, *H* histology of the pancreas, *D* ductal imaging, *S* serology, *OOI* other organ involvement, *Rt* steroid responsiveness, *IDCP* idiopathic duct-centric pancreatitis

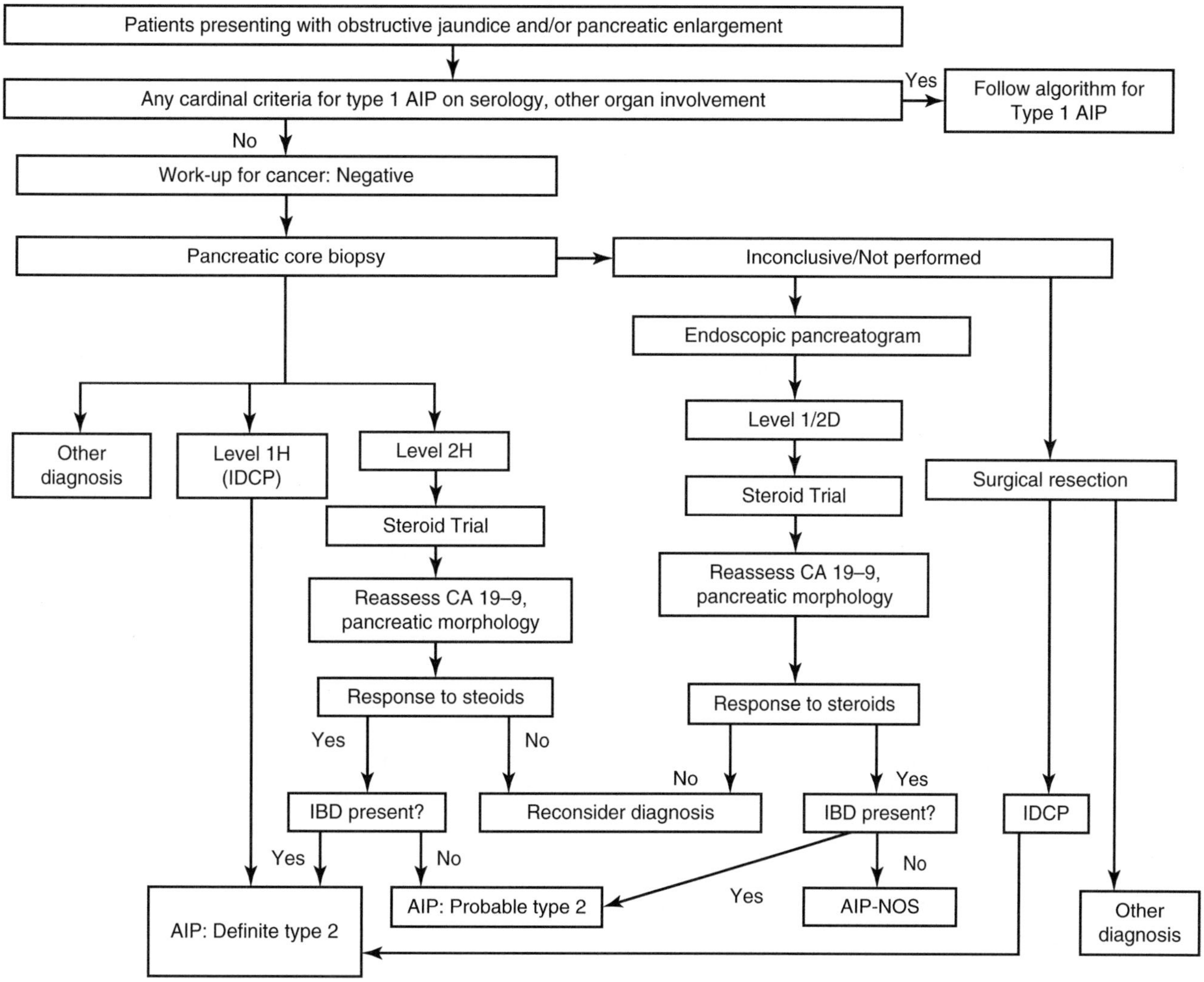

Fig. 6.5 The international consensus diagnostic algorithm for AIP shows a flow to diagnose type 2 AIP with typical/indeterminate (atypical) findings of the pancreas without collateral evidences

Conclusion

Type 2 AIP is a distinct disease entity that shares some common features with type 1 AIP. The two subtypes have different clinical manifestations and histopathology. The radiological findings on CT scan and the typical pancreatographic abnormalities were similar between type 1 and type 2 AIP. Type 2 AIP responded well to steroid therapy as did type 1 AIP. Unlike type 1 AIP, which is recognized as part of IgG4-related systemic disease, type 2 AIP may be an isolated pancreatic disorder. Our understanding of the clinical spectrum of type 2 AIP continues to evolve.

References

1. Chari ST, Kloeppel G, Zhang L, et al. Histopathologic and clinical subtypes of autoimmune pancreatitis: the Honolulu consensus document. Pancreas. 2010;39:549–54.
2. Kamisawa T, Notohara K, Shimosegawa T. Two clinicopathologic subtypes of autoimmune pancreatitis: LPSP and IDCP. Gastroenterology. 2010;139:22–5.
3. Maire F, Le Baleur Y, Rebours V, et al. Outcome of patients with type 1 or 2 autoimmune pancreatitis. Am J Gastroenterol. 2010;106(1):151–6.
4. Deshpande V, Gupta R, Sainani N, et al. Subclassification of autoimmune pancreatitis: a histologic classification with clinical significance. Am J Surg Pathol. 2011;35:26–35.
5. Song TJ, Kim JH, Kim MH, et al. Comparison of clinical findings between histologically confirmed type 1 and type 2 autoimmune pancreatitis. J Gastroenterol Hepatol. 2012;27:700–8.
6. Moon SH, Kim MH. Autoimmune pancreatitis: role of endoscopy in diagnosis and treatment. Gastrointest Endosc Clin N Am. 2013;23:893–915.
7. Notohara K, Burgart LJ, Yadav D, et al. Idiopathic chronic pancreatitis with periductal lymphoplasmacytic infiltration: clinicopathologic features of 35 cases. Am J Surg Pathol. 2003;27:1119–27.
8. Zamboni G, Luttges J, Capelli P, et al. Histopathological features of diagnostic and clinical relevance in autoimmune pancreatitis: a study on 53 resection specimens and 9 biopsy specimens. Virchows Arch. 2004;445:552–63.

9. Shimosegawa T, Chari ST, Frulloni L, et al. International consensus diagnostic criteria for autoimmune pancreatitis: guidelines of the International Association of Pancreatology. Pancreas. 2011;40:352–8.
10. Sugumar A, Levy MJ, Kamisawa T, et al. Endoscopic retrograde pancreatography criteria to diagnose autoimmune pancreatitis: an international multicentre study. Gut. 2010;60(5):666–70.
11. Kloppel G, Detlefsen S, Chari ST, et al. Autoimmune pancreatitis: the clinicopathological characteristics of the subtype with granulocytic epithelial lesions. J Gastroenterol. 2010;45:787–93.
12. Klöppel G. Type 2 Autoimmune Pancreatitis. The Pancreapedia: Exocrine Pancreas Knowledge Base, 2013. DOI: 10.3998/panc.2013.22. (http://www.pancreapedia.org/reviews/type-2-autoimmune-pancreatitis).
13. Ikeura T, Takaoka M, Uchida K, et al. Autoimmune pancreatitis with histologically proven lymphoplasmacytic sclerosing pancreatitis with granulocytic epithelial lesions. Intern Med. 2012;51:733–7.
14. Detlefsen S, Mohr Drewes A, Vyberg M, et al. Diagnosis of autoimmune pancreatitis by core needle biopsy: application of six microscopic criteria. Virchows Arch. 2009;454:531–9.
15. Notohara K, Wani Y, Fujisawa M, Miyabe K, Nakazawa T, Kawa S. Lymphoplasmacytic sclerosing pancreatitis with neutrophilic infiltration: comparison with cases without neutrophilic infiltration. Mod Pathol. 2012;25:447A.
16. Kamisawa T, Chari ST, Lerch MM, et al. Recent advances in autoimmune pancreatitis: type 1 and type 2. Gut. 2013;62:1373–80.
17. Sah RP, Chari ST, Pannala R, et al. Differences in clinical profile and relapse rate of type 1 versus type 2 autoimmune pancreatitis. Gastroenterology. 2010;139:140–8; quiz e12–3.
18. Park DH, Kim MH, Chari ST. Recent advances in autoimmune pancreatitis. Gut. 2009;58:1680–9.

Part II

Diagnosis

Diagnostic Criteria of Autoimmune Pancreatitis

7

Atsushi Kanno, Atsushi Masamune,
and Tooru Shimosegawa

Introduction

Autoimmune pancreatitis (AIP) is a relatively rare disease that has recently emerged as a unique type of pancreatitis with a presumed autoimmune etiology. Sarles et al. [1] first reported a form of idiopathic chronic pancreatitis which might be caused by an autoimmune mechanism in 1961. It is uncertain whether the pancreatitis they reported coincides with AIP as we currently understand it. In 1991, Kawaguchi et al. [2] reported two cases of unusual inflammatory disease, involving the pancreas and biliary tract that were resected on suspicion of pancreatic cancer, and described the histology as lymphoplasmacytic sclerosing pancreatitis (LPSP). In 1992, Toki et al. [3] reported four cases with an unusual type of chronic pancreatitis showing diffuse, irregular narrowing of the entire main pancreatic duct (MPD) on endoscopic retrograde pancreatography (ERP) scans. This type of pancreatitis was described in the marginal notes of the newly established the JPS criteria for chronic pancreatitis in 1995 as "duct-narrowing chronic pancreatitis," a chronic inflammation of the pancreas which may not fulfill the criteria of chronic pancreatitis [4]. In 1995, Yoshida et al. [5] proposed AIP as a diagnostic entity. They summarized the clinical features as follows: increased serum γ-globulin or immunoglobulin (Ig)G levels and the presence of autoantibodies; diffuse irregular narrowing of MPD and enlargement of the pancreas; occasional association with stenosis of the lower bile duct and other autoimmune diseases; mild symptoms, usually without acute attacks of pancreatitis; effectiveness of steroid therapy; and histological findings of LPSP [5, 6]. Thereafter, AIP has been extensively reported worldwide including from Japan, Korea, Europe, and the USA. In this chapter, we will describe the diagnostic criteria of AIP, mainly focusing on the International Consensus Diagnostic Criteria (ICDC) [7] and those proposed by the JPS [8–10].

The JPS Diagnostic Criteria 2002 and 2006

With the accumulation of similar cases in Japan, the JPS proposed the world's first clinical diagnostic criteria for AIP in 2002 [8]. The criteria consisted of 3 items, (1) specific imaging findings (a mandatory requirement), along with (2) serological and/or (3) pathological evidence. In the 2002 criteria, the length of MPD narrowing on ERP was defined as more than 1/3 of the entire pancreas to avoid confusion with short segment narrowing or stenosis caused by pancreatic cancer. As a result, the 2002 criteria were diagnostic for the typical diffuse type of AIP but failed to diagnose the atypical localized type AIP, which shows focal or segmental swelling of the pancreas and short segment narrowing of MPD less than 1/3 of the entire pancreas.

The 2002 criteria were revised in 2006 by the JPS and the Research Committee for Intractable Pancreatic Disease by the Ministry of Labor, Health, and Welfare of Japan [9]. Major revisions included the elimination of the length dependency of MPD narrowing and the incorporation of IgG4 in the serology criteria. In 2001, Hamano et al. [11] reported that elevated serum IgG4 levels were highly specific and sensitive for the diagnosis of AIP. Overall, the basic concepts of the JPS diagnostic criteria were established based on the following minimal consensus: (1) the

A. Kanno, MD, PhD (✉) • A. Masamune, MD, PhD
T. Shimosegawa, MD, PhD
Division of Gastroenterology, Tohoku University Graduate School of Medicine, 1-1 Seiryo-machi, Aoba-ku, Sendai 980-8574, Japan
e-mail: atsushih@med.tohoku.ac.jp; tshimosegawa@int3.med.tohoku.ac.jp

T. Kamisawa, J.B. Chung (eds.), *Autoimmune Pancreatitis*,
DOI 10.1007/978-3-642-55086-7_7, © Springer-Verlag Berlin Heidelberg 2015

criteria are as simple and user-friendly as possible for both general physicians and pancreatologists; (2) the criteria are used to distinguish and exclude malignant disorders such as pancreatic cancer or bile duct cancer as much as possible; (3) the criteria are applied, pathologically, to the clinical cases showing evidence of LPSP; (4) the criteria are used to diagnose pancreatic lesions, although the disease may be systemic; and (5) diagnostic trials of steroid therapy must be avoided [12].

Diagnostic Criteria in South Korea, the USA, and Europe

Because AIP has been extensively reported worldwide, diagnostic criteria for AIP have been proposed in Korea [13], the USA [14, 15], Germany [16], and Italy [17, 18]. With understanding of the full spectrum of clinical presentations of AIP, the American [14, 15] and Korean [13] criteria incorporated additional diagnostic features, including varied appearance on computed tomography (CT), other organ involvement (OOI), and response to steroids. Italian diagnostic criteria for AIP [17] were reported in 2003 based on the histologic findings, comorbidity with other autoimmune diseases, and response to steroid treatment. In 2006, Mayo Clinic investigators proposed diagnostic criteria for AIP, namely, the HISORt criteria, using clinical data from patients with histologically confirmed LPSP [14]. Very importantly, the histopathological features of AIP other than LPSP were reported in Western countries. This type of pancreatitis was also defined as idiopathic duct-centric chronic pancreatitis (IDCP) or granulocytic epithelial lesion (GEL), which is histologically characterized by the infiltration of neutrophils in the pancreatic duct epithelium, associated with destruction of the pancreatic duct epithelium and the accumulation of neutrophils in the pancreatic duct [19–21]. In 2009, the Mayo Clinic group proposed a revised version of the HISORt criteria, which dealt with both LPSP and IDCP/GEL [15].

Establishment of the International Consensus Criteria

The lack of consensus on diagnostic criteria for AIP was mainly due to 2 basic reasons [7]. First, the practice patterns in the usage of various tests and the perceived accuracy of these tests for the diagnosis of AIP vary considerably worldwide. For example, ERP is routinely used for investigating obstructive jaundice in Japan and is a mandatory criterion in the JPS diagnostic criteria [9, 10]. However, Western endoscopists generally avoid injecting the pancreatic duct in patients with obstructive jaundice for fear of causing pancreatitis, and ERP is not required for the diagnosis of AIP in the West. Similarly, core biopsy of the pancreas to diagnose AIP has been championed by the Mayo Clinic group [14, 15] but is not routinely used elsewhere. Another important reason for the lack of consensus was the fact that it has become increasingly clear that the term "AIP" includes two different types of the disease with distinct histopathology and clinical profiles that need different criteria for their diagnoses [19–21]. Whereas the Asian diagnostic criteria have focused on type 1 AIP, American and Italian diagnostic criteria may pertain to both subtypes [15, 17].

As a first step towards the international diagnostic criteria, Japanese and Korean pancreatologists established the Asian diagnostic criteria that included response to steroid therapy as an optional criterion in 2008 [22]. The creation of a consensus between Eastern and Western countries on the diagnostic criteria was debated during the joint meeting on the 40th anniversary of the JPS and the American Pancreatic Association, which was held in Honolulu on November 4, 2009 [23, 24]. At that meeting, all experts agreed that the clinical phenotypes associated with LPSP and IDCP should be nosologically distinguished; however, their terminology was controversial. While most experts agreed that the entities should be referred to as type 1 and type 2 AIP, respectively, others had concerns regarding the use of the term "autoimmune" to describe IDCP [23, 24].

During the 14th congress of the International Association of Pancreatology held in Fukuoka, Japan, from July 11 through 13, 2010, an international panel of experts met. The working group proposed the ICDC, keeping in mind the differences in clinical practice throughout the world [7].

Overview of the ICDC

The goals of the ICDC for AIP are to develop criteria that can be applied worldwide, taking marked differences in practice patterns into consideration, to safely diagnose AIP and avoid misdiagnosis of pancreatic cancer as AIP [7]. AIP is classified into 2 subtypes in the ICDC: type 1 with IgG4 (LPSP) and type 2 with GEL (IDCP). The former is suspected to represent the pancreatic lesions of IgG4-related diseases [25]. Criteria for the two types of AIP were independently developed, and AIP is diagnosed based on one or more of the following cardinal features: imaging characteristics of the pancreatic parenchyma (P) and pancreatic duct (D), serology, other organ involvement (OOI), pancreatic histology (H), and the optional criterion of response to steroid therapy. Depending on the diagnostic reliability, each feature has been categorized as either level 1 or 2. Types 1 and 2 AIP can be diagnosed as definitive or probable, but they are sometimes indistinguishable (AIP-not otherwise specified (NOS)).

Table 7.1 Diagnosis of definitive and probable type 1 AIP using the International Consensus Diagnostic Criteria (ICDC)

Diagnosis	Primary basis for diagnosis	Imaging evidence	Collateral evidence
Definitive type 1 AIP	Histology	Typical/indeterminate	Histologically confirmed LPSP
	Imaging	Typical	Any non-D level 1/level 2
		Indeterminate	Two or more from level 1 (+level 2 D*)
	Response to steroid	Indeterminate	Level 1 S/OOI+Rt or level 1 D+level 2 S/OOI/H+Rt
Probable type 1 AIP		Indeterminate	Level 2 S/OOI/H+Rt

*Level 2 D is counted as level 1 in this setting, *Rt* response to steroid, *D* pancreatic duct findings, *S* serum findings, *OOI* other organ involvement, *LPSP* lymphoplasmacytic sclerosing pancreatitis, *AIP* autoimmune pancreatitis, *H* histological findings

Type 1 AIP

As described earlier, in the ICDC, there is a combination of 5 cardinal features of AIP: pancreatic imaging (parenchyma and duct), serology, OOI, histology, and steroid responsiveness. The first 4 features are graded into levels 1 and 2 depending on their strength of association with type 1 AIP. In patients with typical CT imaging findings for AIP, definitive type 1 AIP can be diagnosed even in the absence of ERCP findings if there is sufficient evidence of elevated IgG4 levels or OOI. However, if pancreatic imaging yields indeterminate findings (segmental or focal enlargement), it is necessary to acquire the findings of irregular narrowing of the pancreatic duct for the diagnosis of definitive AIP through ERCP. If the results of the biopsy of the pancreas or pancreatic tissue indicate LPSP, that is, if 3 of the 4 cardinal histological findings are present, definitive type 1 AIP can be diagnosed without the need for any other findings. The most important point in the diagnosis of type 1 AIP is the combination of these cardinal findings and the comprehensive assessment of some cases (Tables 7.1 and 7.2).

Type 2 AIP

The cardinal histological finding of type 2 AIP is GEL, which is necessary for the diagnosis of definitive type 2 AIP. If the examination of biopsy tissue specimens or pancreatic tissues provides confirmation of GEL, that is, if the major histological findings suggesting type 2 AIP indicate a level 1 finding, definitive type 2 AIP can be diagnosed. Cases that show typical pancreatic imaging findings of AIP with inflammatory bowel disease and responsiveness to steroid therapy can be diagnosed as probable type 2 AIP, even in the absence of the histological finding of GEL. However, it is essential to continue clarifying the pathogenesis of type 2 AIP because of its unknown etiology (Tables 7.3 and 7.4).

AIP-Not Otherwise Specified (NOS)

Cases that exhibit compatible pancreatic imaging findings, without other cardinal factors of type 1 or 2 AIP, and show responsiveness to steroid treatment can be diagnosed as AIP-not otherwise specified (NOS). These cases should be carefully followed up, while considering the possibility of other diseases (Table 7.5).

ICDC and the JPS Diagnostic Criteria 2011

Although the ICDC for AIP enabled us to diagnose and compare 2 distinctive subtypes, type 1 and type 2 AIP, independently, the ICDC is somewhat complicated for general use. Since in Japanese cases with type 2 AIP are extremely rare, the JPS and the Research Committee for Intractable Pancreatic Disease by the Ministry of Labor, Health, and Welfare of Japan revised the diagnostic criteria as the clinical diagnostic criteria for AIP 2011 (JPS2011) [26]. The JPS2011 adopted as much as possible the basic concepts of both the previous Japanese criteria and these concerning type 1 in the ICDC: (1) simple to use by general physicians; (2) diffuse/segmental/focal classification on pancreatic imaging; (3) IgG4 alone as a serological marker; (4) sclerosing cholangitis, sclerosing sialadenitis, and retroperitoneal fibrosis as OOIs; (5) no classifications of level 1/2 in serum IgG4 and OOI; and (6) optional steroid trial only after excluding malignancy by endosonography-guided fine needle aspiration (EUS-FNA) [26]. ERCP is basically required in the focal/segmental type, because the findings of the pancreatic duct are important in the differential diagnosis with pancreatic cancer. In the general clinical practice in Japan, the JPS 2011 criteria are recommended for the diagnosis of AIP; however, the ICDC are required to diagnose cases of AIP-NOS or type 2 AIP.

Comparison of the Different Diagnostic Criteria for AIP

Sumimoto et al. [27] reported a comparison of 5 major sets of diagnostic criteria: the ICDC [7], the Korean diagnostic criteria [13], the JPS diagnostic criteria 2011 [10], the Asian criteria [22], and the HISORt criteria [15]. The study enrolled 61 patients with a confirmed diagnosis of AIP and 56 patients with pancreatic cancer as controls. Pancreatic

Table 7.2 Level 1 and level 2 criteria for type 1 AIP

	Criterion	Level 1	Level 2
P	Parenchymal imaging	*Typical* Diffuse enlargement with delayed enhancement (sometimes associated with rim-like enhancement)	*Indeterminate (including atypical*[b]*)* Segmental/focal enlargement with delayed enhancement
D	Ductal imaging (ERP)	Long (>1/3 length of the mpd) or multiple strictures without marked upstream dilatation	Segmental/focal narrowing without marked upstream dilatation (duct size <5 mm)
S	Serology	IgG4 >2 X upper limit of normal value	IgG4 1–2 X upper limit of normal value
OOI	Other organ involvement	(a) or (b) (a) *Histology of extrapancreatic organs* Any three of the following: (i) Marked lymphoplasmacytic (ii) Infiltration with fibrosis and without granulocytic infiltration (iii) Storiform fibrosis (iv) Obliterative phlebitis (v) Abundant (>10 cells/hpf) IgG4-positive cells (b) *Typical radiological evidence* At least one (i) Segmental/multiple proximal (hilar/intrahepatic) or proximal and distal bile duct stricture (ii) Retroperitoneal fibrosis	(a) or (b) (a) *Histology of extrapancreatic organs including endoscopic biopsies of bile duct*[c] Both of the following: (i) Marked lymphoplasmacytic infiltration without granulocytic infiltration (ii) Abundant (>10 cells/hpf) IgG4-positive cells (b) *Physical or radiological evidence* At least one (i) Symmetrically enlarged salivary/lacrimal glands (ii) Radiologic evidence of renal involvement described in association with AIP
H	Histology of the pancreas	LPSP (core biopsy/resection) At least three of the following: (i) Periductal lymphoplasmacytic infiltrate without granulocytic infiltration (ii) Obliterative phlebitis (iii) Storiform fibrosis (iv) Abundant (>10 cells/hpf) IgG4-positive cells	LPSP (core biopsy) Any two of the following: (i) Periductal lymphoplasmacytic infiltrate without granulocytic infiltration (ii) Obliterative phlebitis (iii) Storiform fibrosis (iv) Abundant (>10 cells/hpf) IgG4-positive cells
Diagnostic steroid trial			
Response to steroid (Rt)[a]		Rapid (≤2 weeks) radiologically demonstrable resolution or marked improvement in pancreatic/extrapancreatic manifestations	

[a]Diagnostic steroid trial should be conducted carefully by pancreatologists with caveats (see text) only after negative work-up for cancer including EUS-FNA

[b]Atypical: some AIP cases may show low-density mass, pancreatic ductal dilatation, or distal atrophy. Such atypical imaging findings in patients with obstructive jaundice and/or pancreatic mass are highly suggestive of pancreatic cancer. Such patients should be managed as pancreatic cancer unless there is strong collateral evidence for AIP and a thorough work-up for cancer is negative (see algorithm)

[c]Endoscopic biopsy of duodenal papilla is a useful adjunctive method because the ampulla is often involved pathologically in AIP

Table 7.3 Diagnosis of definitive and probable type 2 AIP using the International Consensus Diagnostic Criteria (ICDC)

Diagnosis	Imaging evidence	Collateral evidence
Definitive type 2 AIP	Typical/indeterminate	Histologically confirmed IDCP or clinical IBD + level 2 H + Rt
Probable type 2 AIP	Typical/indeterminate	Level 2 H/clinical IBD + Rt

Rt response to steroid, *IBD* inflammatory bowel disease, *IDCP* idiopathic duct-centric chronic pancreatitis, *AIP* autoimmune pancreatitis, *H* histological findings

imaging on CT and ERP were independently evaluated by 3 pancreatologists, and each diagnostic criterion of ICDC was validated with special reference to levels 1 and 2. Of the 5 criteria, the ICDC is the most sensitive and useful for diagnosing AIP; the sensitivities of the 5 major sets of criteria were 95.1 % (ICDC), 90.2 % (Korean), 86.9 % (JPS), 83.6 % (Asian), and 83.6 % (HISORt) with 100 % of specificity in each. In the evaluation of pancreatic imaging, the diagnostic sensitivities of the combination of CT and ERP in segmental/focal type of AIP were significantly higher than those with single imaging (26 % in CT ($P<0.01$) or

Table 7.4 Level 1 and level 2 criteria for type 2 AIP

	Criterion	Level 1	Level 2
P	Parenchymal imaging	*Typical* Diffuse enlargement with delayed enhancement (sometimes associated with rim-like enhancement)	*Indeterminate (including atypical*[b]*)* Segmental/focal enlargement with delayed enhancement
D	Ductal imaging (ERP)	Long (>1/3 length of the mpd) or multiple strictures without marked upstream dilatation	Segmental/focal narrowing without marked upstream dilatation (duct size <5 mm)
OOI	Other organ involvement		Clinically diagnosed inflammatory bowel disease
H	Histology of the pancreas (core biopsy/resection)	IDCP Both of the following: (i) Granulocytic infiltration of duct wall (GEL) with or without granulocytic acinar inflammation (ii) Absent or scant (0–10 cells/hpf) IgG4-positive cells	Both of the following: (i) Granulocytic and lymphoplasmacytic acinar infiltrate (ii) Absent or scant (0–10 cells/hpf) IgG4-positive cells
Diagnostic steroid trial			
Response to steroid (Rt)[a]		Rapid (<2 weeks) resolution or marked improvement in manifestations	

[a]Diagnostic steroid trial should be conducted carefully by pancreatologists with caveats (see text) only after negative work-up for cancer including EUS-FNA

[b]Atypical: some AIP cases may show low-density mass, pancreatic ductal dilatation, or distal atrophy. Such atypical imaging findings in patients with obstructive jaundice and/or pancreatic mass are highly suggestive of pancreatic cancer. Such patients should be managed as pancreatic cancer unless there is strong collateral evidence for AIP and a thorough work-up for cancer is negative (see algorithm)

Table 7.5 Diagnosis of AIP-not otherwise specified using the International Consensus Diagnostic Criteria (ICDC)

Diagnosis	Imaging evidence	Collateral evidence (case with only D1/2)
AIP-not otherwise specified	Typical/indeterminate	D1/2+Rt

Rt response to steroid, *D* pancreatic duct findings, *AIP* autoimmune pancreatitis

35 % in ERP ($P<0.05$) vs. 63 % in CT+ERP), but not significantly different in the diffuse type. Based on this finding, the authors have proposed a diagnostic algorithm with CT for the diffuse type of AIP, and the combination CT+ERP followed by EUS-FNA for the segmental/focal type [27].

Differential Diagnosis Between AIP and Pancreatic Cancer

Cases of AIP with segmental/focal pancreatic enlargement are difficult to differentiate from pancreatic cancer (Fig. 7.1). Certain features such as the clinical symptoms, the findings of serology and imaging, and histological examinations might be useful for the differentiation of these conditions. Obstructive jaundice is a typical symptom of pancreatic head cancer; however, AIP with IgG4-related sclerosing cholangitis often exhibits this symptom [28–30]. The serum IgG4 level is useful for diagnosing type 1 AIP and differentiating this condition from pancreatic cancer [11]. Ghazale et al. [31] reported that the serum IgG4 levels were elevated (>140 mg/dL) in 13/135 (10 %) patients with pancreatic cancer; however, only 1 % had IgG4 levels >280 mg/dL compared with 53 % of AIP. Several imaging modalities can be used to diagnose AIP and pancreatic cancer. CT (Fig. 7.1a), magnetic resonance imaging (MRI), and EUS (Figure 7.1b) are useful for detecting enlargement of the pancreatic parenchyma [32–34]. The utility of diffusion-weighted MRI for differentiating AIP from pancreatic cancer has been reported. The apparent diffusion coefficient values were significantly lower in AIP than in pancreatic cancer [35]. ERCP is necessary for diagnosing the segmental/focal type of AIP according to the JPS 2011 [9] (Fig. 7.1c). EUS-FNA is useful for acquiring a histological sample and diagnosing pancreatic cancer. Although some reports emphasize the usefulness of EUS-FNA for the diagnosis of AIP (Figure 7.1d–g) [36, 37], core biopsy or resection is required for the histological evaluation of the pancreas in ICDC. Nevertheless, EUS-FNA might be useful as a negative work-up for cancer.

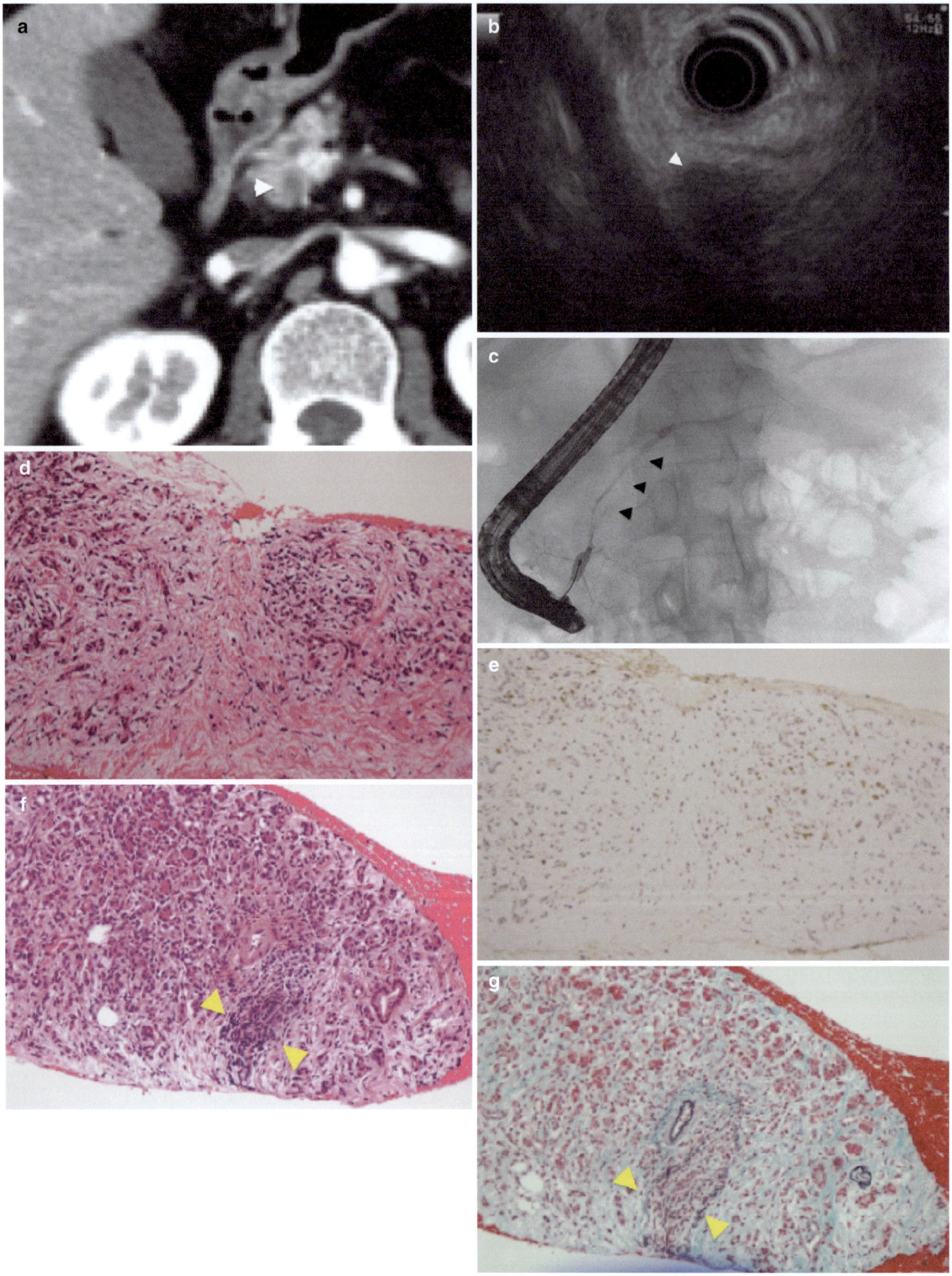

Fig. 7.1 Cases of AIP with focal pancreatic enlargement. (**a**) CT revealed a less enhanced lesion in the pancreatic head (*arrowhead*). (**b**) EUS revealed clearly a low echoic lesion in the pancreatic head (*arrowhead*). (**c**) ERCP revealed diffuse irregular narrowing of the main pancreatic duct (*arrowhead*). (**d**) The findings of high-power fields (×400) show lymphoplasmacytic infiltration and storiform fibrosis (*arrowhead*). (**e**) Immunohistochemical staining for IgG4. Abundant IgG4-positive plasma cells were found in the HPF. (**f**) Obliterative phlebitis (HE) (*arrowhead*). (**g**) Obliterative phlebitis (Elastica-Masson (EM) staining) (*arrowhead*). The finding of obliterative phlebitis is clear in EM staining

Summary

We reviewed the diagnostic criteria for AIP, especially focusing on the ICDC. These diagnostic criteria should contribute to further clarification of the clinical features, pathogenesis, and natural history of AIP throughout the world.

Acknowledgment This work was supported in part by the Research Committee of Intractable Pancreatic Disease (principal investigator: Tooru Shimosegawa) provided by the Ministry of Health, Labor, and Welfare of Japan.

Disclosure All authors disclosed no financial relationships relevant to this publication.

References

1. Sarles H, Sarles JC, Muratoren R, et al. Chronic inflammatory sclerosing of the pancreas–an autonomous pancreatic disease? Am J Dig Dis. 1961;6:688–98.
2. Kawaguchi K, Koike M, Tsuruta K, Okamoto A, Tabata I, Fujita N. Lymphoplasmacytic sclerosing pancreatitis with cholangitis: a variant of primary sclerosing cholangitis extensively involving pancreas. Hum Pathol. 1991;22:387–95.
3. Toki F, Kozu T, Oi I, Nakasako T, Suzuki M, Hanyu F. An unusual type of chronic pancreatitis showing diffuse irregular narrowing of the entire main pancreatic duct on ERCP-a report of four cases. Endoscopy. 1992;24:640.
4. The Criteria Committee for Chronic Pancreatitis of the Japan Pancreas Society. Final report of clinical diagnostic criteria of chronic pancreatitis (in Japanese). Suizo. 1995;10:xxiii–vi.
5. Yoshida K, Toki F, Takeuchi T, Watanabe S, Shiratori K, Hayashi N. Chronic pancreatitis caused by an autoimmune abnormality. Proposal of the concept of autoimmune pancreatitis. Dig Dis Sci. 1995;40:1561–8.
6. Kamisawa T, Notohara K, Shimosegawa T. Two clinicopathologic subtypes of autoimmune pancreatitis: LPSP and IDCP. Gastroenterology. 2010;139:22–5.
7. Shimosegawa T, Chari ST, Frulloni L, et al. International consensus diagnostic criteria for autoimmune pancreatitis: guidelines of the International Association of Pancreatology. Pancreas. 2011;40:352–8.
8. Members of the Criteria Committee for Autoimmune Pancreatitis of the Japan Pancreas Society. Diagnostic criteria for autoimmune pancreatitis by the Japan Pancreas Society (2002). (in Japanese with English abstract) Suizo. 2002;17:585–7.
9. Members of the Autoimmune Pancreatitis Diagnostic Criteria Committee, the Research Committee of Intractable Diseases of the Pancreas supported by the Japanese Ministry of Health, Labor and Welfare, and Members of the Autoimmune Pancreatitis Diagnostic Criteria Committee, the Japan Pancreas Society. Clinical diagnostic criteria of autoimmune pancreatitis 2006. (in Japanese with English abstract) Suizo. 2006;21:395–7.
10. The Japan Pancreas Society, the Ministry of Health and Welfare Investigation Research Team for Intractable Pancreatic Disease. Clinical diagnostic for autoimmune pancreatitis 2011 (in Japanese with English abstract). Suizo. 2012;27:17–25.
11. Hamano H, Kawa S, Horiuchi A, et al. High serum IgG4 concentrations in patients with sclerosing pancreatitis. N Engl J Med. 2001;344:732–8.
12. Okazaki K, Kawa S, Kamisawa T, et al. Japanese consensus guidelines for management of autoimmune pancreatitis: I. Concept and diagnosis of autoimmune pancreatitis. J Gastroenterol. 2010;45: 249–65.
13. Kim KP, Kim MH, Kim JC, et al. Diagnostic criteria for autoimmune chronic pancreatitis revised. World J Gastroenterol. 2006;12:2487–96.
14. Chari ST, Smyrk TC, Levy MJ, et al. Autoimmune pancreatitis: diagnosis using histology, imaging, serology, other organ involvement and response to steroids. Clin Gastroenterol Hepatol. 2006;4:1010–6.
15. Chari ST, Takahashi N, Levy MJ, et al. A diagnostic strategy to distinguish autoimmune pancreatitis from pancreatic cancer. Clin Gastroenterol Hepatol. 2009;10:1097–103.
16. Schneider A, Löhr JM, Singer MV. The M-ANNHEIM classification of chronic pancreatitis: introduction of a unifying classification system based on a review of previous classification of the disease. J Gastroenterol. 2007;42:101–19.
17. Pearson RK, Longnecker DS, Chari ST, et al. Controversies in clinical pancreatology. Autoimmune pancreatitis: does it exist? Pancreas. 2003;27:1–13.
18. Frulloni L, Scattolini C, Falconi M, et al. Autoimmune pancreatitis: differences between the focal and diffuse forms in 87 patients. Am J Gastroenterol. 2009;104:2288–94.
19. Notohara K, Burgart LJ, Yadav D, Chari S, Smyrk TC. Idiopathic chronic pancreatitis with periductal lymphoplasmacytic infiltration: clinicopathologic features of 35 cases. Am J Surg Pathol. 2003;27:1119–27.
20. Zamboni G, Lüttges J, Capelli P, Frulloni L, Cavallini G, Pederzoli P, Leins A, Longnecker D, Klöppel G. Histopathological features of diagnostic and clinical relevance in autoimmune pancreatitis: a study on 53 resection specimens and 9 biopsy specimens. Virchows Arch. 2004;445:552–63.
21. Sugumar A, Klöppel G, Chari ST. Autoimmune pancreatitis: pathologic subtypes and their implications for its diagnosis. Am J Gastroenterol. 2009;104:2308–10.
22. Otsuki M, Chung JB, Okazaki K, et al. Asian diagnostic criteria for autoimmune pancreatitis: consensus of the Japan-Korea symposium on autoimmune pancreatitis. J Gastroenterol. 2008;43:403–8.
23. Chari ST, Klöppel G, Zhang L, et al. Histologic and clinical subtypes of autoimmune pancreatitis: the Honolulu consensus document. Pancreas. 2010;39:549–54.
24. Chari ST, Klöppel G, Zhang L, et al. Histologic and clinical subtypes of autoimmune pancreatitis: the Honolulu consensus document. Pancreatology. 2010;10:664–72.
25. Umehara H, Okazaki K, Masaki Y, et al. Comprehensive diagnostic criteria for IgG4-related disease (IgG4-RD), 2011. Mod Rheumatol. 2012;22:21–30.
26. Okazaki K, Shimosegawa T, The working Group Members of the Japan Pancreas Society and the Research Committee for Intractable Pancreatic Disease by the Ministry of Labor, Health and Welfare of Japan. The Amendment of the clinical diagnostic criteria in Japan (JPS2011) in response to the proposal of the international consensus of diagnostic criteria (ICDC) for autoimmune pancreatitis. Pancreas. 2012;41:1341–2.
27. Sumimoto K, Uchida K, Mitsuyama T, et al. A proposal of a diagnostic algorithm with validation of International Consensus Diagnostic Criteria for autoimmune pancreatitis in a Japanese cohort. Pancreatology. 2013;13:230–7.
28. Kamisawa T, Takuma K, Egawa N, Tsuruta K, Sasaki T. Autoimmune pancreatitis and IgG4-related sclerosing disease. Nat Rev Gastroenterol Hepatol. 2010;7:401–9.
29. Kamisawa T, Okamoto A. Autoimmune pancreatitis: proposal of IgG4-related sclerosing disease. J Gastroenterol. 2006;41:613–25.
30. Kamisawa T, Okazaki K, Kawa S, Shimosegawa T, Tanaka M, Research Committee for Intractable Pancreatic D, Japan Pancreas S. Japanese consensus guidelines for management of autoimmune

pancreatitis: III. Treatment and prognosis of AIP. J Gastroenterol. 2010;45:471–7.
31. Ghazale A, Chari ST, Smyrk TC, Levy MJ, Topazian MD, Takahashi N, Clain JE, Pearson RK, Pelaez-Luna M, Petersen BT, Vege SS, Farnell MB. Value of serum IgG4 in the diagnosis of autoimmune pancreatitis and in distinguishing it from pancreatic cancer. Am J Gastroenterol. 2007;102:1646–53.
32. Kamisawa T, Egawa N, Nakajima H, Tsuruta K, Okamoto A, Kamata N. Clinical difficulties in the differentiation of autoimmune pancreatitis and pancreatic carcinoma. Am J Gastroenterol. 2003;98:2694–9.
33. Sahani DV, Kalva SP, Farrell J, Maher MM, Saini S, Mueller PR, Lauwers GY, Fernandez CD, Warshaw AL, Simeone JF. Autoimmune pancreatitis: imaging features. Radiology. 2004;233:345–52.
34. Bodily KD, Takahashi N, Fletcher JG, Fidler JL, Hough DM, Kawashima A, Chari ST. Autoimmune pancreatitis: pancreatic and extrapancreatic imaging findings. Am J Roentgenol. 2009;192:431–7.
35. Kamisawa T, Takuma K, Anjiki H, Egawa N, Hata T, Kurata M, Honda G, Tsuruta K, Suzuki M, Kamata N, Sasaki T. Differentiation of autoimmune pancreatitis from pancreatic cancer by diffusion-weighted MRI. Am J Gastroenterol. 2010;105:1870–5.
36. Kanno A, Ishida K, Hamada S, Fujishima F, Unno J, Kume K, Kikuta K, Hirota M, Masamune A, Satoh K, Notohara K, Shimosegawa T. Diagnosis of autoimmune pancreatitis by EUS-FNA by using a 22-gauge needle based on the International Consensus Diagnostic Criteria. Gastrointest Endosc. 2012;76:594–602.
37. Ishikawa T, Itoh A, Kawashima H, Ohno E, Matsubara H, Itoh Y, Nakamura Y, Hiramatsu T, Nakamura M, Miyahara R, Ohmiya N, Goto H, Hirooka Y. Endoscopic ultrasound-guided fine needle aspiration in the differentiation of type 1 and type 2 autoimmune pancreatitis. World J Gastroenterol. 2012;18:3883–8.

8 Clinical Features

Young Sik Woo and Kyu Taek Lee

Introduction

Autoimmune pancreatitis (AIP) is a unique type of chronic pancreatitis that has distinct pathological, histological, and clinical characteristics [1, 2]. In 1961, Sarles et al. first described a pancreatitis associated with hypergammaglobulinemia, suggesting autoimmunity as the etiology of pancreatitis [3]. The concept of autoimmune pancreatitis (AIP) was proposed by Yoshida et al. in 1995 [4]. Since then it has become recognized as a distinct entity, and many cases have been reported in Eastern countries, as well as in Western countries [5, 6].

The clinical manifestations of AIP are variable except a few common presentations. Identifying and categorizing of clinical manifestations of AIP is quite difficult because little is known about the natural history and clinical spectrum of the disease. Most reports of the clinical symptoms on AIP are based on small retrospective cohorts, case series, and case reports including the highly selected patients with advanced or unusual clinical presentations. Also, the absence of a single diagnostic test makes it difficult to assess the full spectrum of clinical symptoms associated with AIP. Recently, many AIP literatures had suggested that the entity of AIP consisted of two distinct histopathological and clinical forms of pancreatitis. Type 1 AIP refers to the subtype called lymphoplasmacytic sclerosing pancreatitis (LPSP) or granulocytic epithelial lesion (GEL)-negative AIP, whereas type 2 AIP refers to the subtype called idiopathic duct-centric pancreatitis (IDCP) or GEL-positive AIP [7–9]. This chapter will discuss about the clinical features of AIP as well as the differences and similarities between the two subtypes. The most crucial issue in clinical situation caring for patients with suspected AIP is to differentiate AIP from pancreatic cancer, because pancreatic cancer requires surgery and AIP responds dramatically to steroid treatment. So the different points in the clinical manifestation of AIP and pancreatic cancer will be reviewed.

Y.S. Woo, MD, PhD • K.T. Lee, MD, PhD (✉)
Department of Medicine, Samsung Medical Center, Sungkyunkwan University School of Medicine, Seoul, Korea
e-mail: youngsik0314.woo@samsung.com; ktcool.lee@samsung.com

Clinical Features

AIP is a heterogeneous disease with diverse clinical symptoms due to two distinct subtypes: type 1 and type 2. The two subtypes have numerous differences along with a few similarities (Table 8.1).

The relative prevalence of type 1 and type 2 AIP is different for Asia and the West. The proportion of patients with type 2 AIP is lower in Asia (3.7 %) than in both Europe (12.9 %) and North America (13.7 %) in a recent international multicenter survey [10]. Despite increasing reports on AIP, the true prevalence of AIP is unknown due to the absence of a reliable diagnostic test, the relative rarity, the under-recognition, and the underreporting. AIP prevalence was estimated to be 0.82 per 100,000 in the nationwide survey based on the diagnostic criteria of the Japanese Pancreas Society [11]. Other authors report prevalence rates of 5–6 % of all patients with a diagnosis of chronic pancreatitis in Japan and Korea [12, 13]. In North America, about 2.4 % of patients who were performed with pancreatic resection under a misdiagnosis of pancreatic cancer were found to have type 1 AIP on surgical specimens [14], and AIP resulted in 21–23 % of patients who were performed with pancreatic resection for benign conditions [15, 16].

Type 1 AIP mainly occurs in elderly males, as most patients (up to 85 %) with it are older than 50 years [2, 17, 18]. The male to female predominance is approximately 2:1 [11]. Type 2 AIP appears to affect younger patients (less than 40 years old) and may have the male predominance [7, 8].

Type 1 AIP is the pancreatic manifestation of IgG4-related disease (IgG4-RD), a multisystem disease. The variable clinical presentations can be divided into pancreatic and extrapancreatic manifestations. In addition, the pancreatic

T. Kamisawa, J.B. Chung (eds.), *Autoimmune Pancreatitis*,
DOI 10.1007/978-3-642-55086-7_8, © Springer-Verlag Berlin Heidelberg 2015

Table 8.1 Clinical profile of type 1 and type 2 AIP

	Type 1 AIP	Type 2 AIP
Synonym	Lymphoplasmacytic sclerosing pancreatitis AIP without GEL	Idiopathic duct-centric chronic pancreatitis AIP with GEL
Epidemiology	Asia > USA, Europe	Europe > USA > Asia
Age at diagnosis	Old	Young
Most common presenting complaint	Obstructive jaundice (80–90 %)	Obstructive jaundice (50–60 %)
Presenting with acute pancreatitis	(10–15 %)	(30–40 %)
Serum IgG4 level	Often elevated	Normal
Histology hallmark	Lymphoplasmacytic infiltrate, storiform fibrosis, obliterative phlebitis	Granulocytic epithelial lesion
Tissue IgG4 stain	Present	Rare
Other organ involvement	Bile duct, salivary gland, kidney, retroperitoneum	Inflammatory bowel disease
Associated with ulcerative colitis	Occasionally	Common
Steroid response	Excellent	Excellent
Recurrence	Common	Rare

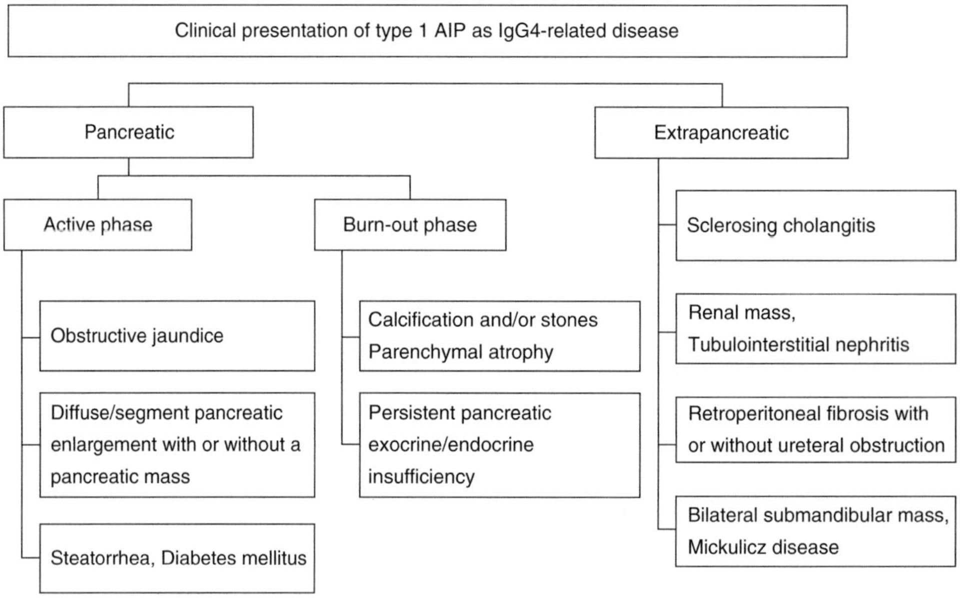

Fig. 8.1 Clinical presentation of type 1 AIP as IgG4-related disease (Adapted from Kamisawa et al. [45])

manifestation of type 1 AIP can be divided into active and late phase because of its clinical and image profile change for long times (Fig. 8.2). In the active phase of type 1 AIP, the major presentation is painless obstructive jaundice, occurring in up to 88 % of patients with a new presentation of type 1 [19, 20]. The manifestations of acute pancreatitis (abdominal pain and elevation of serum pancreatic enzymes) are more often observed in type 2 rather than type 1 [7, 21, 9]. Patients with AIP often present with mild pancreatitis that is easily cured by conservative management. It is likely to be under-recognized unless further workup is done with suspicion. According to the degree of pancreatic inflammation, it can present with a diffuse or focal pancreatic enlargement with or without a mass. The diffuse type was more common than the focal type in both groups (62.2 % in type 1 AIP and 73.3 % in type 2 AIP) [9]. In case with focal pancreatic mass, it can be clinically challenging to distinguish AIP form pancreatic cancer. Diabetes mellitus develops in up to 50 % of patients concurrently with AIP, and 8.8 % of patients developed diabetes after steroid administration as the therapy for AIP [22, 23]. Untreated or multiple-relapsed AIP may show pancreatic parenchymal atrophy and fibrosis, which in its late stages can be indistinguishable from advanced ordinary chronic pancreatitis [24]. In the late stages of disease, diabetes and steatorrhea can be caused by the failure of endocrine and exocrine function. These are discussed in more detail in subsequent chapters. In addition to the pancreatic manifestations, a characteristic feature of type 1 AIP is the extrapancreatic other organ involvement (OOI) characterized by an IgG4-positive lymphoplasmacytic infiltrate in various organs. The common involvement of other organs includes the bile duct, salivary glands, retroperitoneum, kidneys, lung, lymph nodes, and orbits. Less commonly, gallbladder and gastric involvements have been described [25–28]. OOI

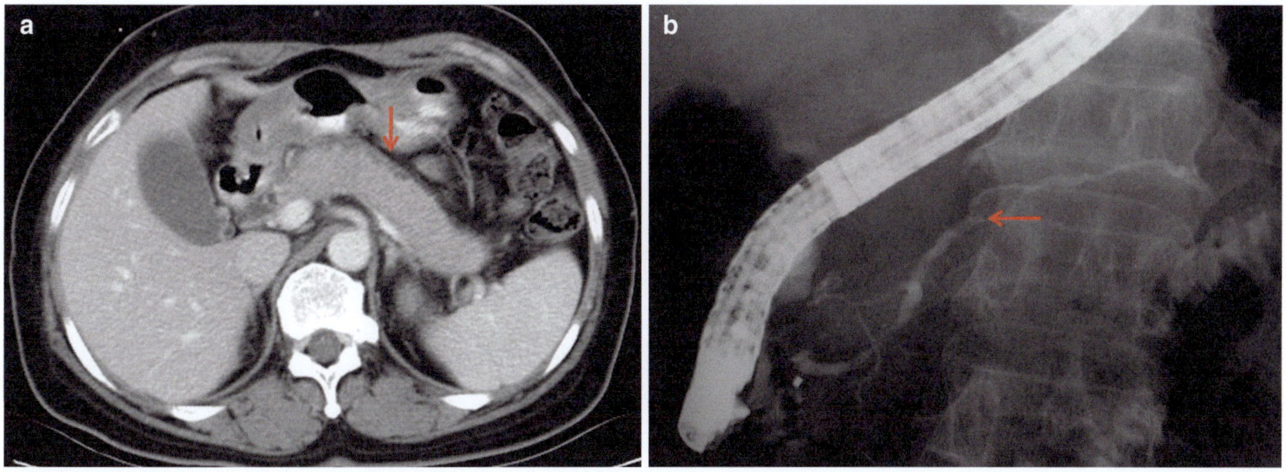

Fig. 8.2 Radiologic finding of a patient with AIP. (**a**) CT image shows diffuse enlargement with delayed enhancement and capsule-like rim (*arrow*). (**b**) ERCP shows irregular narrowing of main pancreatic duct and absence of marked upstream dilatation

may precede the diagnosis of AIP, be present concurrently, or develop metachronously over months to years after the diagnosis of AIP [25]. These extrapancreatic manifestations often provide an important clue to diagnosis.

Recent studies suggest that type 2 AIP has a clinical and histological difference from type 1 AIP and it is a distinct clinical entity. The similarities between both types are the obstructive jaundice, the diffuse pancreatic enlargement on imaging studies, and the good response to steroid therapy. However, patients with type 2 tend to be younger and are more likely to present with abdominal pain and pancreatitis than those with type 1 [8, 9]. There is an absence of elevated serum IgG4 and extrapancreatic manifestations, which are a collateral evidence of AIP to provide great clues in diagnosing AIP [8, 9, 29]. Inflammatory bowel disease is more common in type 2 than type 1 [8, 9]. Type 2 AIP has no specific serologic marker and shows minimal IgG4 immunostaining from tissues. The identifying GEL in the pancreatic tissue is the main difference from type 1 AIP and is needed for a definitive diagnosis of type 2 AIP [30]. Since occurrence is at a relatively young age and a pancreatic histology is needed for a definitive diagnosis, type 2 AIP is likely to be underrecognized. Further clinical investigation is needed to better understand the clinical profile of type 2 AIP because its clinical feature has not been defined well.

Distinguish AIP from Malignancy

The patient with AIP often presents with painless obstructive jaundice or pancreatic mass mimicking the presentation of pancreatic cancer. It is important to differentiate between these two entities due to a dismal prognosis and a narrow therapeutic window for surgical resection in pancreatic cancer. Many diagnostic criteria for AIP, such as Japanese criteria, Korean criteria, HISORt criteria, and international consensus diagnostic criteria (ICDC), have been proposed. Each of the criteria does not provide a strategy to distinguish AIP from pancreatic cancer and has strengths and weaknesses in distinguishing AIP from pancreatic cancer [31]. However, clinical feature, serology, pancreatic imaging, and steroid response may be helpful in distinguishing AIP from malignancy [32]. The jaundice in AIP sometimes fluctuates more frequently than in pancreatic cancer, whereas obstructive jaundice in pancreatic cancer typically progresses steadily. Serum IgG4 levels are frequently and significantly elevated in type 1 AIP, although it is an uncommon finding in type 2 AIP. Hamano et al. reported in 2001 that using the serum IgG4 level enabled distinguishing AIP from other pancreatic disorders with high sensitivity (95 %) and specificity (97 %) [33]. In one study, an elevation of serum IgG4 levels (>135 mg/dL) was detected in 71 % of AIP patients and 6 % of PC patients [34]. In another study, about 10 % of pancreatic cancers have elevated IgG4 levels, most being less than twice the upper limit of normal [35]. Therefore, an elevated serum IgG4 level alone cannot rule out pancreatic cancer, while this finding may be a diagnostic clue. The differential diagnosis for AIP and pancreatic malignancy usually begins with cross-sectional images. Previous studies show that diffuse enlargement with delayed enhancement, capsule-like rim, long (>1/3 the length of the main pancreatic duct) or multiple stricture, and absence of marked upstream dilatation have high specificity for AIP (Fig. 8.2) [19, 34, 36]. Furthermore, "ICDC" guidelines suggest that these findings indicate a high level of suspicion of AIP [37]. On the other hand, non-enhanced mass, upstream dilatation of the main pancreatic duct, and proximal parenchymal atrophy are highly suggestive findings for pancreatic cancer (Fig. 8.3) [19, 34, 36]. However, some AIP cases are not compatible with the typical findings of AIP. Among these

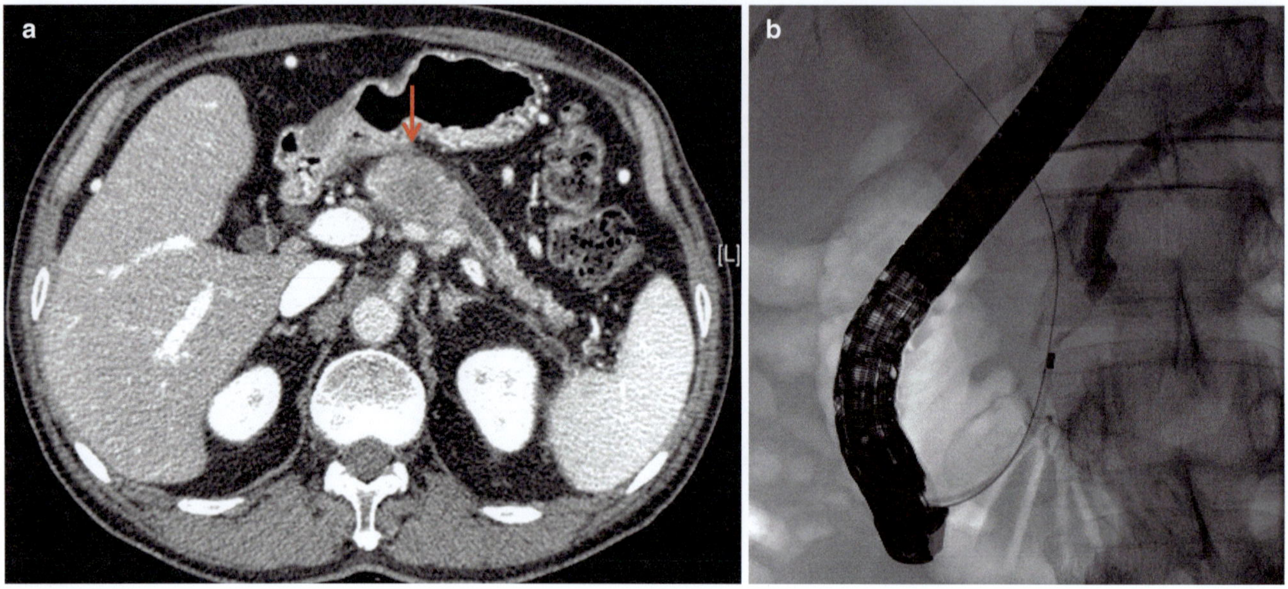

Fig. 8.3 Radiologic finding of a patient with pancreatic cancer. (**a**) CT image shows no enhancement mass (*arrow*) with upstream PD dilatation and parenchymal atrophy. (**b**) ERCP shows pancreatic duct cutoff and upstream main pancreatic duct dilatation (>5 mm)

atypical cases of AIP, focal type AIP can be difficult to differentiate from pancreatic cancer. In our series of 23 patients [38], 85.7 % (6/7) of focal-type AIP patients showed homogeneous enhancement, whereas only 3 chronic pancreatitis patients (25 %) and none of the pancreatic cancer patients showed homogeneous enhancement. None of the focal type AIP patients showed upstream duct dilatation (>5 mm) or proximal pancreatic atrophy. If a pancreatic mass has homogeneous enhancement, absence of significant upstream MPD dilatation (>5 mm), and absence of proximal pancreatic atrophy, further evaluation for AIP should be considered to avoid unnecessary surgery.

In addition, a 2-week steroid trial has been advocated as a means of differentiating the two clinical entities [39], including Korean, HISORt criteria, and ICDC. The reasons to support a 2-week steroid trial are as follows: (1) radiological improvement of AIP can occur as early as 1–2 weeks after steroid therapy [40] and (2) concern about cancer progression during the trial of steroid therapy; one study reported that complete resection was possible in all patients after the 2-week trial [39]. Improvement of clinical symptoms can be seen in pancreatic cancer patients due to the anti-inflammatory effect of steroids. The falsely elevated IgG4 in pancreatic cancer also can decrease after steroid therapy [37]. The obstructive pancreatitis associated with ductal adenocarcinoma may be relieved with steroid therapy. Therefore, the response from the steroid trial must be interpreted with an objective measurement, such as rapid (≤2 weeks) radiological resolution or marked improvement in pancreatic or extrapancreatic manifestations (Fig. 8.4). In the assessment of steroid responsiveness, relief of pancreatic ductal narrowing and/or resolution of the pancreatic mass is critical. Additionally, a steroid trial should be restricted only to suspected AIP patients who have a negative workup for cancer including EUS-FNA [41].

It is important to remember that AIP is a rare disease and thought to be much less common than pancreatic cancer. Clinical tips to help avoid misdiagnosis of pancreatic cancer as autoimmune pancreatitis are showed in Table 8.2.

Natural History and Prognosis of AIP

The natural history and long-term prognosis of AIP is unknown despite many investigation of this disease. Although types 1 and 2 AIP showed excellent response to steroid treatment, many patients develop relapse either during steroid tapering or follow-up period and steroid discontinuation. Recent studies reported that the relapses were more common in type 1 (31–50 %) than type 2 AIP (0–15.3 %) [8–10]. The location of the recurrence is predominantly in the biliary system or pancreas [10]. In a study of biliary involvement in AIP, frequent relapses occurred in proximal biliary involvement (proximal extrahepatic and intrahepatic biliary strictures) than strictures in the intrapancreatic portion of the bile duct. Continuous incomplete remission of radiological and serological abnormalities during the maintenance period can cause relapse. Relapses were more common in AIP patients with IgG4-related sclerosing cholangitis (56 % vs. 26 %), while there is controversy about whether the diffuse or focal type is an independent predictor of relapse [8, 10, 42].

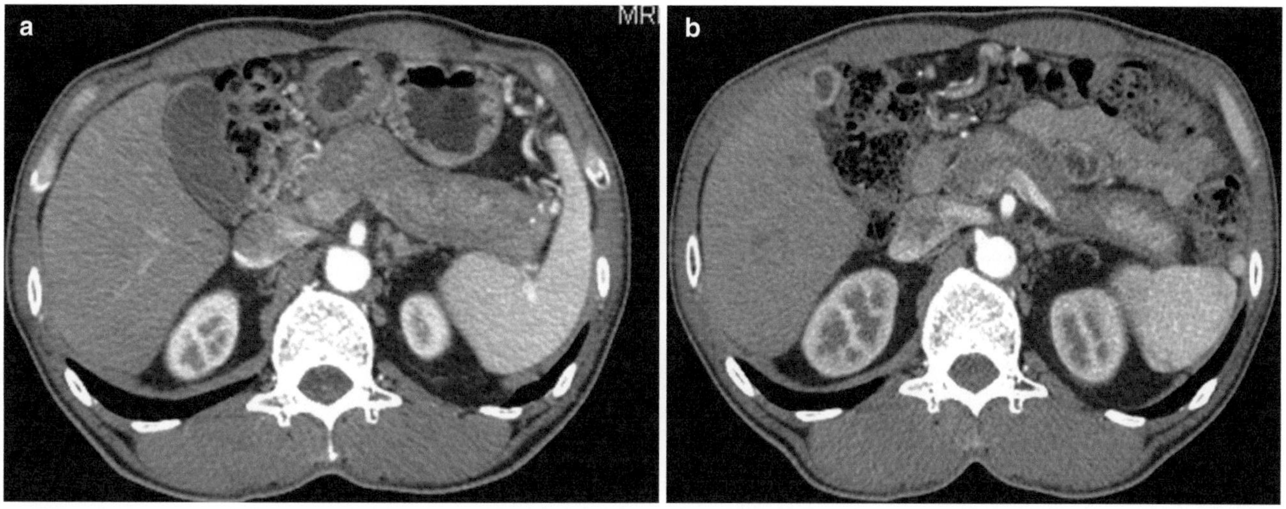

Fig. 8.4 Serial images of a patient with steroid response who was finally diagnosed with AIP. (**a**) Pretreatment: CT image shows diffuse enlargement without a discrete mass. (**b**) Posttreatment: after 2 weeks of steroid trial, the pancreatic lesion was markedly reduced

Table 8.2 Clinical tips to differentiate AIP from pancreatic cancer

1. Utilize the international consensus diagnostic criteria (ICDC) to help diagnose AIP and differentiate it from malignant disease
2. It is important to remember that AIP is a rare disease and thought to be much less common than pancreatic cancer
3. Pancreatic imaging is the basis of suspicion and diagnosis of AIP and differentiation from pancreatic cancer
4. All focal pancreatic masses should be sampled prior to initiating corticosteroids
5. An elevated serum IgG4 level alone cannot diagnose AIP or rule out pancreatic cancer. Serum IgG4 levels are elevated in 10 % of pancreatic cancer and 6 % of chronic pancreatitis
6. Elevated serum IgG4 levels can decrease in patients with pancreatic cancer who are inappropriately treated with corticosteroids
7. In the assessment of steroid responsiveness, relief of pancreatic ductal narrowing and/or resolution of the pancreatic mass is critical
8. Improvement of AIP is usually seen as early as 2 weeks after steroid therapy. If no objective response is seen within 2–4 weeks, the diagnosis is unlikely to be AIP and the resection is considered

Two major sequelae of chronic pancreatitis are pancreatic duct stone and pancreatic cancer. Patients with at least one relapse have a high prevalence of pancreatic calcification or stones. Also, multiple relapses may result in irreversible damage with fibrosis and steroid unresponsiveness [24]. For patients with AIP identified as having predictors of relapse, the treatment strategy may need to be adjusted by including higher dose or longer administration of maintenance steroid therapy or additional treatment with another immunosuppressive agent.

The life expectancy of patients with AIP has been reported to be similar to the general population. The late sequelae of AIP such as the pancreatic atrophy and pancreatic insufficiency do not seem to alter long-term survival [8].

Several cases of pancreatic cancer have been reported in patients with AIP who were suspected to have type 1. Pancreatic cancers were diagnosed synchronously with AIP or detected during the follow-up [10, 43, 44]. Because of limited date and no systematic case–control studies, further studies are needed to understand whether to increase the risk of cancer compared with the general population.

Summary

The clinical spectrum varies widely in AIP with two distinct subtypes. The AIP type 1 and type 2 have both overlapping and separate clinical features. The relative frequencies of subtypes in Asia are different from those observed in the West. The proportion of type 2 AIP is lower in East Asia than in the West. Most commonly, patients with type 1 AIP are older males presenting with painless jaundice and an elevated IgG4 level. Those with type 2 AIP tend to be younger and are likely to present with acute pancreatitis and normal IgG4 levels. Type 2 AIP is not related to the extrapancreatic disease except ulcerative colitis. Also, the differentiation of AIP from pancreatic cancer is challenging because of the presentation of AIP mimicking that of pancreatic cancer and absence of a single diagnostic test. It is important to remember several clinical tips to avoid misdiagnosis. Further clinical investigation and more experience will provide better understanding and more optimal treatment plan in AIP.

References

1. Gardner TB, Chari ST. Autoimmune pancreatitis. Gastroenterol Clin North Am. 2008;37(2):439–60.
2. Kim KP, Kim MH, Song MH, Lee SS, Seo DW, Lee SK. Autoimmune chronic pancreatitis. Am J Gastroenterol. 2004;99(8):1605–16.
3. Sarles H, Sarles JC, Muratore R, Guien C. Chronic inflammatory sclerosis of the pancreas–an autonomous pancreatic disease? Am J Dig Dis. 1961;6:688–98.
4. Yoshida K, Toki F, Takeuchi T, Watanabe S, Shiratori K, Hayashi N. Chronic pancreatitis caused by an autoimmune abnormality. Proposal of the concept of autoimmune pancreatitis. Dig Dis Sci. 1995;40(7):1561–8.
5. Finkelberg DL, Sahani D, Deshpande V, Brugge WR. Autoimmune pancreatitis. N Engl J Med. 2006;355(25):2670–6.
6. Okazaki K, Kawa S, Kamisawa T, Ito T, Inui K, Irie H, et al. Japanese clinical guidelines for autoimmune pancreatitis. Pancreas. 2009;38(8):849–66.
7. Maire F, Le Baleur Y, Rebours V, Vullierme MP, Couvelard A, Voitot H, et al. Outcome of patients with type 1 or 2 autoimmune pancreatitis. Am J Gastroenterol. 2011;106(1):151–6.
8. Sah RP, Chari ST, Pannala R, Sugumar A, Clain JE, Levy MJ, et al. Differences in clinical profile and relapse rate of type 1 versus type 2 autoimmune pancreatitis. Gastroenterology. 2010;139(1):140–8; quiz e12–3.
9. Song TJ, Kim JH, Kim MH, Jang JW, Parkdo H, Lee SS, et al. Comparison of clinical findings between histologically confirmed type 1 and type 2 autoimmune pancreatitis. J Gastroenterol Hepatol. 2012;27(4):700–8.
10. Hart PA, Kamisawa T, Brugge WR, Chung JB, Culver EL, Czako L, et al. Long-term outcomes of autoimmune pancreatitis: a multicentre, international analysis. Gut. 2013;62(12):1771–6.
11. Nishimori I, Tamakoshi A, Otsuki M. Prevalence of autoimmune pancreatitis in Japan from a nationwide survey in 2002. J Gastroenterol. 2007;42 Suppl 18:6–8.
12. Kim KP, Kim MH, Lee SS, Seo DW, Lee SK. Autoimmune pancreatitis: it may be a worldwide entity. Gastroenterology. 2004;126(4):1214.
13. Okazaki K. Autoimmune pancreatitis is increasing in Japan. Gastroenterology. 2003;125(5):1557–8.
14. Weber SM, Cubukcu-Dimopulo O, Palesty JA, Suriawinata A, Klimstra D, Brennan MF, et al. Lymphoplasmacytic sclerosing pancreatitis: inflammatory mimic of pancreatic carcinoma. J Gastrointest Surg. 2003;7(1):129–37; discussion 37–9.
15. Abraham SC, Wilentz RE, Yeo CJ, Sohn TA, Cameron JL, Boitnott JK, et al. Pancreaticoduodenectomy (Whipple resections) in patients without malignancy: are they all 'chronic pancreatitis'? Am J Surg Pathol. 2003;27(1):110–20.
16. Hardacre JM, Iacobuzio-Donahue CA, Sohn TA, Abraham SC, Yeo CJ, Lillemoe KD, et al. Results of pancreaticoduodenectomy for lymphoplasmacytic sclerosing pancreatitis. Ann Surg. 2003;237(6):853–8; discussion 8–9.
17. Chari ST, Smyrk TC, Levy MJ, Topazian MD, Takahashi N, Zhang L, et al. Diagnosis of autoimmune pancreatitis: the Mayo Clinic experience. Clin Gastroenterol Hepatol. 2006;4(8):1010–6; quiz 934.
18. Kamisawa T, Egawa N, Nakajima H, Tsuruta K, Okamoto A, Kamata N. Clinical difficulties in the differentiation of autoimmune pancreatitis and pancreatic carcinoma. Am J Gastroenterol. 2003;98(12):2694–9.
19. Chari ST, Takahashi N, Levy MJ, Smyrk TC, Clain JE, Pearson RK, et al. A diagnostic strategy to distinguish autoimmune pancreatitis from pancreatic cancer. Clin Gastroenterol Hepatol. 2009;7(10):1097–103.
20. Kamisawa T, Okamoto A. IgG4-related sclerosing disease. World J Gastroenterol (WJG). 2008;14(25):3948–55.
21. Kamisawa T, Chari ST, Giday SA, Kim MH, Chung JB, Lee KT, et al. Clinical profile of autoimmune pancreatitis and its histological subtypes: an international multicenter survey. Pancreas. 2011;40(6):809–14.
22. Nishimori I, Tamakoshi A, Kawa S, Tanaka S, Takeuchi K, Kamisawa T, et al. Influence of steroid therapy on the course of diabetes mellitus in patients with autoimmune pancreatitis: findings from a nationwide survey in Japan. Pancreas. 2006;32(3):244–8.
23. Ito T, Nakamura T, Fujimori N, Niina Y, Igarashi H, Oono T, et al. Characteristics of pancreatic diabetes in patients with autoimmune pancreatitis. J Dig Dis. 2011;12(3):210–6.
24. Takayama M, Hamano H, Ochi Y, Saegusa H, Komatsu K, Muraki T, et al. Recurrent attacks of autoimmune pancreatitis result in pancreatic stone formation. Am J Gastroenterol. 2004;99(5):932–7.
25. Stone JH, Zen Y, Deshpande V. IgG4-related disease. N Engl J Med. 2012;366(6):539–51.
26. Umehara H, Okazaki K, Masaki Y, Kawano M, Yamamoto M, Saeki T, et al. Comprehensive diagnostic criteria for IgG4-related disease (IgG4-RD), 2011. Mod Rheumatol. 2012;22(1):21–30.
27. Kamisawa T, Nakajima H, Egawa N, Hayashi Y, Funata N. Autoimmune pancreatitis can be confirmed with gastroscopy. Dig Dis Sci. 2004;49(1):155–6.
28. Leise MD, Smyrk TC, Takahashi N, Sweetser SR, Vege SS, Chari ST. IgG4-associated cholecystitis: another clue in the diagnosis of autoimmune pancreatitis. Dig Dis Sci. 2011;56(5):1290–4.
29. Pace A, Topalidis T, Blaker M, Guthoff A, de Weerth A, Lohse AW. Autoimmune pancreatitis with normal IgG4-Levels: 4 case reports and review of the literature. Zeitschrift fur Gastroenterologie. 2007;45(12):1245–51.
30. Kloppel G, Detlefsen S, Chari ST, Longnecker DS, Zamboni G. Autoimmune pancreatitis: the clinicopathological characteristics of the subtype with granulocytic epithelial lesions. J Gastroenterol. 2010;45(8):787–93.
31. Sugumar A, Chari ST. Distinguishing pancreatic cancer from autoimmune pancreatitis: a comparison of two strategies. Clin Gastroenterol Hepatol. 2009;7(11 Suppl):S59–62.
32. Kamisawa T, Takuma K, Egawa N, Tsuruta K, Sasaki T. Autoimmune pancreatitis and IgG4-related sclerosing disease. Nat Rev Gastroenterol Hepatol. 2010;7(7):401–9.
33. Hamano H, Kawa S, Horiuchi A, Unno H, Furuya N, Akamatsu T, et al. High serum IgG4 concentrations in patients with sclerosing pancreatitis. N Engl J Med. 2001;344(10):732–8.
34. Kamisawa T, Imai M, Yui Chen P, Tu Y, Egawa N, Tsuruta K, et al. Strategy for differentiating autoimmune pancreatitis from pancreatic cancer. Pancreas. 2008;37(3):e62–7.
35. Ghazale A, Chari ST, Smyrk TC, Levy MJ, Topazian MD, Takahashi N, et al. Value of serum IgG4 in the diagnosis of autoimmune pancreatitis and in distinguishing it from pancreatic cancer. Am J Gastroenterol. 2007;102(8):1646–53.
36. Shin JU, Lee JK, Kim KM, Lee KH, Lee KT, Kim YK, et al. The differentiation of autoimmune pancreatitis and pancreatic cancer using imaging findings. Hepatogastroenterology. 2013;60(125):1174–81.
37. Shimosegawa T, Chari ST, Frulloni L, Kamisawa T, Kawa S, Mino-Kenudson M, et al. International consensus diagnostic criteria for autoimmune pancreatitis: guidelines of the International Association of Pancreatology. Pancreas. 2011;40(3):352–8.
38. Chang WI, Kim BJ, Lee JK, Kang P, Lee KH, Lee KT, et al. The clinical and radiological characteristics of focal mass-forming autoimmune pancreatitis: comparison with chronic pancreatitis and pancreatic cancer. Pancreas. 2009;38(4):401–8.
39. Moon SH, Kim MH, Park DH, Hwang CY, Park SJ, Lee SS, et al. Is a 2-week steroid trial after initial negative investigation for malignancy useful in differentiating autoimmune pancreatitis from pancreatic cancer? A prospective outcome study. Gut. 2008;57(12):1704–12.

40. Kamisawa T, Egawa N, Nakajima H, Tsuruta K, Okamoto A. Morphological changes after steroid therapy in autoimmune pancreatitis. Scand J Gastroenterol. 2004;39(11):1154–8.
41. Gardner TB, Levy MJ, Takahashi N, Smyrk TC, Chari ST. Misdiagnosis of autoimmune pancreatitis: a caution to clinicians. Am J Gastroenterol. 2009;104(7):1620–3.
42. Frulloni L, Scattolini C, Falconi M, Zamboni G, Capelli P, Manfredi R, et al. Autoimmune pancreatitis: differences between the focal and diffuse forms in 87 patients. Am J Gastroenterol. 2009;104(9):2288–94.
43. Motosugi U, Ichikawa T, Yamaguchi H, Nakazawa T, Katoh R, Itakura J, et al. Small invasive ductal adenocarcinoma of the pancreas associated with lymphoplasmacytic sclerosing pancreatitis. Pathol Int. 2009;59(10):744–7.
44. Witkiewicz AK, Kennedy EP, Kennyon L, Yeo CJ, Hruban RH. Synchronous autoimmune pancreatitis and infiltrating pancreatic ductal adenocarcinoma: case report and review of the literature. Hum Pathol. 2008;39(10):1548–51.
45. Kamisawa T, Chari ST, Lerch MM, Kim MH, Gress TM, Shimosegawa T. Recent advances in autoimmune pancreatitis: type 1 and type 2. Gut. 2013;62(9):1373–80.

Serology

9

Shigeyuki Kawa, Takayuki Watanabe, and Takashi Muraki

Introduction

Serum markers associated with autoimmune pancreatitis (AIP) are roughly classified as immunoglobulins, autoantibodies, complement, and activity markers for lymphoid cells. These markers have been used for the diagnosis of AIP, differentiation of AIP from pancreatic cancer, prediction of AIP recurrence, and estimation of AIP disease activity in clinical follow-up assessments [1]. Among these markers, IgG4 is recognized to be specifically associated with AIP; thus, it is a characteristic indicator with high clinical utility [2]. Many studies have focused on the association between AIP and IgG4. However, other markers also represent useful tools in the various clinical aspects of AIP. In the following sections, we describe the clinical significance of these markers.

Diagnosis

Marker Sensitivities

Many serum markers have been assessed for their utility in diagnosing AIP, and many are included in diagnostic criteria for AIP. The first diagnostic criteria for AIP were published by the Japanese Pancreas Society (2002). Those criteria included laboratory data that demonstrated abnormally elevated levels of serum γ-globulin and/or IgG or the presence of autoantibodies [3]. After the clinical usefulness of IgG4 was discovered [2], most diagnostic criteria for AIP in Japan and other countries included only IgG4 as a diagnostic serum marker [4–10].

S. Kawa, MD, PhD (✉)
Center for Health, Safety, and Environmental Management, Shinshu University, 3-1-1 Asahi, Matsumoto 390-8621, Japan
e-mail: skawapc@shinshu-u.ac.jp

T. Watanabe, MD, PhD • T. Muraki, MD, PhD
Department of Gastroenterology, Shinshu University School of Medicine, 3-1-1 Asahi, Matsumoto 390-8621, Japan

We compared the rates of positive detection for each marker (Table 9.1) and found that IgG4 provided the best result.

Immunoglobulins

IgG4

The sera of patients with AIP exhibited a polyclonal band in the rapidly migrating fraction of gel electrophoresis that contained γ-globulins; this resulted in the finding that β–γ globulin bridging was a characteristic of AIP. Immunoprecipitation assays revealed that this polyclonal band was the result of high serum concentrations of IgG4 [2]. IgG4 is typically a minor component in IgG

Table 9.1 Rates of detection for each serum marker in autoimmune pancreatitis

Marker	Positive/total (*n*)	%
Immunoglobulins		
IgG4	80/88	90.9
IgG	59/88	67.0
IgE	33/83	39.8
IgA	7/88	8.0
IgM	4/88	4.5
Autoantibodies		
Antinuclear antibody (ANA)	39/74	52.7
Rheumatoid factor (RF)	18/67	23.9
Anti-SSA(Ro) antibody	0/56	0.0
Anti-SSB(La) antibody	0/56	0.0
Antimitochondrial antibody (AMA)	2/47	4.3
Complement components and immune complex		
C3	29/84	34.5
C4	27/84	32.1
Circulating immune complex (CIC)	68/82	82.9
Activity markers for lymphoid cells		
Soluble interleukin-2 receptor (sIL-2R)	68/81	84.0
β2 microglobulin (β2-m)	62/82	75.6

T. Kamisawa, J.B. Chung (eds.), *Autoimmune Pancreatitis*,
DOI 10.1007/978-3-642-55086-7_9, © Springer-Verlag Berlin Heidelberg 2015

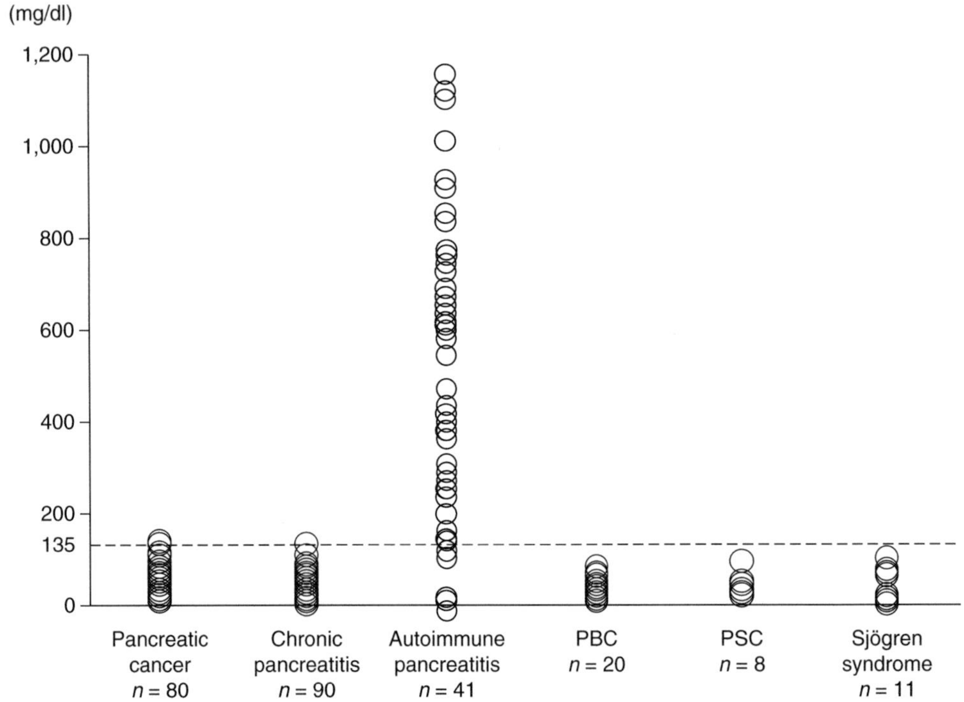

Fig. 9.1 IgG4 levels measured in patients with autoimmune pancreatitis and various other related diseases. The horizontal *dotted line* shows the maximum IgG4 level (135 mg/dl) observed in the related diseases. *PBC* primary biliary cirrhosis, *PSC* primary sclerosing cholangitis (Data are reprinted from Hamano et al. [2] with modification and from Kawa and Hamano [11] with permission from the *Journal of Gastroenterology*)

fractions; it constitutes only 3–7 % of total serum IgG. However, the serum IgG4 concentrations in patients with AIP were over tenfold higher than those in healthy subjects. In addition, we found elevated serum IgG4 concentrations in 90 % of patients with AIP, but rarely in patients with other conditions, including pancreatic cancer, chronic pancreatitis, primary biliary cirrhosis (PBC), primary sclerosing cholangitis, and Sjögren's syndrome (Fig. 9.1) [2, 11]. It has been reported that elevated serum IgG4 was found in a restricted number of conditions, including allergic disorders, parasite infestations, and pemphigus. Those results suggested that IgG4 represents a sensitive and specific marker for AIP, and it promised to be useful for the diagnosis of this disease [2]. The serum IgG4 concentration and the IgG4/IgG ratio were significantly reduced after corticosteroid therapy; this finding indicated that IgG4 might be a useful disease activity marker. Later, the clinical usefulness of IgG4 was assessed worldwide. Currently, serum IgG4 is considered a reliable marker for the diagnosis of AIP, and it has been included in various diagnostic criteria [4–10].

Patients with elevated IgG4 are considered to be in a highly active AIP disease state. Compared to patients with normal serum IgG4 levels, those with elevated IgG4 more frequently exhibit jaundice at AIP onset, diffuse pancreatic enlargement on imaging, significantly higher 18F-2-fluoro-2-deoxy-d-glucose uptake in pancreatic lesions, multiple extrapancreatic lesions, and a requirement for maintenance therapy [12, 13]. In addition, infiltration of IgG4-bearing plasma cells is a histological hallmark of AIP, and it is used in pathological diagnoses [14].

IgG

When the concept of AIP was first proposed, a high serum IgG concentration was listed as a characteristic laboratory finding [15]. Thus, IgG was considered a serological marker in the first diagnostic criteria proposed by the Japanese Pancreatic Society in 2002 [3]. However, the sensitivity and specificity of IgG are inferior for diagnosing AIP compared to IgG4. Therefore, IgG is currently used mainly as an activity marker to predict recurrence and estimate disease activity in clinical follow-ups of patients with AIP.

IgE

High serum IgE concentrations were detected in 30–40 % of patients with AIP, and the positive detection rate was also very high (86 %) [16, 17]. These findings suggested that an allergic mechanism may be contributing to the pathogenesis of AIP; thus, in some patients, AIP is complicated with an allergic response [16, 17]. However, the exact role or clinical significance of serum IgE elevation in AIP has not been fully elucidated. Although IgE does not necessarily reflect disease activity, the detection of elevated IgE might be a useful marker for the diagnosis of AIP in an inactive stage [17].

IgA and IgM

Interestingly, reduced IgA and IgM concentrations were detected in patients with AIP, in addition to increased IgG4 levels. It was reported that IgM was negatively correlated to IgG or IgG4 in patients with AIP. Moreover, the ratios of IgG:IgM and IgG:IgA in patients with AIP were significantly increased compared to those in patients with other diseases; thus, these ratios provided excellent diagnostic sensitivity and specificity in differentiating AIP from the other diseases. Those results suggested that IgG:IgM and IgG:IgA ratios may serve as novel diagnostic markers for differentiating AIP from other hepatopancreatic diseases [18].

Autoantibodies

When the concept of AIP was first proposed, serum autoantibodies, like antinuclear antibody (ANA) and rheumatoid factor (RF), were listed as a characteristic laboratory finding [15]. Thus, the presence of serum autoantibodies was considered a serological marker in the first diagnostic criteria proposed by the Japanese Pancreatic Society in 2002 [3]. To date, many autoantibodies have been studied, and below, we describe those proposed as candidates for autoantibody markers of AIP pathogenesis.

ANA and RF

ANA and RF are detectable in a wide range of autoimmune diseases, but their production may not be specifically related to those conditions. ANA and RF are typically detected in 30–50 % of AIP samples. However, this detection may represent a nonspecific, active disease state in immunological conditions [1]. After corticosteroid therapy, these autoantibodies promptly returned to undetectable levels.

Anti-SSA/Ro and Anti-SSB/La Autoantibodies and Antimitochondrial Antibody

Anti-SSA/Ro and anti-SSB/La autoantibodies are specific markers for Sjögren's syndrome. Antimitochondrial antibody (AMA) is a specific marker for PBC. These disease-specific autoantibodies are seldom detected in patients with AIP [1, 19].

Candidate Pathogenic Autoantibodies

Carbonic anhydrase II (CA II) and lactoferrin are distributed in the ductal cells of the pancreas. Both proteins have been proposed as candidate target antigens in the pathogenesis of AIP, but the presence of autoantibodies to these antigens is not sufficiently specific or sensitive for an AIP diagnosis [20, 21].

Helicobacter pylori (*H. pylori*) infections may also trigger the occurrence of AIP, possibly as a result of molecular mimicry. There is substantial structural homology between the human CA II and the *H. pylori* alpha-carbonic anhydrase; the homologous segments contain the binding motif for the HLA molecule, *DRB1*04:05*, which is closely associated with AIP [22]. Those data led to the hypothesis that the *DRB1*04:05*-restricted peptide of CA II might be presented in genetically predisposed subjects; then, when reactive T cells and autoantibodies interact with the CA II of pancreatic ductal cells, they cause injury to pancreatic tissue [23]. Similarly, selected peptides from the plasminogen-binding protein (PBP) of *H. pylori* exhibited structural homology with the ubiquitin-protein ligase E3 component, n-recognin 2 (UBR2), which is highly expressed in pancreatic acinar cells. Antibodies against the PBP peptide were detected at high levels in patients with AIP, but they were barely detectable in patients with pancreatic cancer. It seems likely that the UBR2 in pancreatic acinar cells may be targeted by an autoantibody against the PBP of *H. pylori* in patients with AIP [24].

Complement and Circulating Immune Complex

AIP is associated with reduced levels of complement in 30–40 % of cases and elevated levels of circulating immune complex (CIC; determined by C1q assay). High serum CIC levels were significantly associated with increased serum levels of IgG1, reduced levels of C4, and a tendency toward reduced levels of C3. There were no significant elevations in serum mannose-binding lectin. These results suggested that AIP was associated with high serum CIC in the active state, which then links to a complement activation system and the classical pathway, rather than the mannose-binding lectin or alternative pathways [25]. In patients with AIP, complement C3c, IgG4, and IgG were deposited in collagen IV-positive basement membranes of pancreatic ducts, bile ducts, and acini. That finding suggested that CIC-mediated destruction of ducts and acini might play a role in the pathogenesis of AIP [26]. Decreased serum complement levels have also been detected in the active stage of the IgG4-related kidney disease, tubulointerstitial nephritis [27].

Activity Markers for Lymphoid Cells

A characteristic pathological finding of AIP is abundant lymphocyte infiltration. This infiltration represents an elevation in serum markers for active lymphoid cells, such as soluble interleukin-2 receptor (sIL-2R) and β-2 microglobulin (β2-m). Thus, high elevations in serum sIL-2R and β2-m may well correlate with AIP activity [1, 28]. It is reported that the sensitivity of sIL-2R was equal to that of IgG4 and higher than that of IgG. A significant reduction in sIL-2R was associated with administration of steroid therapy; this suggested that sIL-2R may serve as an indicator of the need for maintenance therapy. Serum sIL-2R is also strongly correlated to the number of systemic lesions associated with AIP; thus, sIL-2R is thought to be a potent serological marker for assessing autoimmune activity in AIP [28].

Table 9.2 Comparison of various markers in identical sera for differentiation between autoimmune pancreatitis (AIP) and pancreatic cancer (PC)

	Sensitivity (AIP $n = 100$)	Specificity (vs. PC $n = 80$)	Accuracy (vs. PC)
IgG4	86 %	96 %	91 %
IgG	69 %	75 %	72 %
ANA	58 %	79 %	67 %
RF	23 %	94 %	54 %
IgG4 + ANA	95 %	76 %	87 %
IgG + ANA	85 %	63 %	75 %
IgG4 + IgG + ANA	95 %	63 %	81 %
IgG4 + RF	90 %	90 %	90 %
IgG + RF	78 %	73 %	76 %
IgG4 + IgG + RF	91 %	71 %	82 %
ANA + RF	69 %	60 %	78 %
IgG4 + ANA + RF	97 %	73 %	86 %
IgG + ANA + RF	91 %	61 %	78 %
IgG4 + IgG + ANA + RF	97 %	61 %	81 %

Data are reprinted from Kawa et al. [30] with permission from the *Journal of Gastroenterology*

ANA antinuclear antibody, *RF* rheumatoid factor

Differentiation from Pancreatic Cancer

Lymphoplasmacytic sclerosing pancreatitis (LPSP), which is pathologically similar to AIP, was observed in 2.5 % of patients that underwent the Whipple resection [29]. Therefore, it is necessary to differentiate AIP from pancreatic cancer. In differentiating between AIP and pancreatic cancer, IgG4 showed the best results among several markers measured in identical sera; IgG4 exhibited 86 % sensitivity, 96 % specificity, and 91 % accuracy (Table 9.2) [2, 30]. IgG4 was therefore adopted in various diagnostic criteria for AIP [4–10]. The sensitivity and specificity of IgG4 were superior to those of IgG, ANA, and RF, but the additional measurements of ANA and RF further increased the sensitivity and negative predictive value of IgG4 [30]. However, elevated serum IgG4 and numerous IgG4 bearing plasma cell infiltrations have also been found in a few patients with pancreatic cancer [31]. Thus, a high serum IgG4 concentration and numerous IgG4-positive plasma cell infiltrations in pancreatic tissue are not completely specific to AIP. These markers cannot exclude the presence of pancreatic cancer.

Estimation of AIP Activity

Prediction of Recurrence

Some patients with AIP experience recurrence during the clinical course. The recurrence rate has been estimated to vary from 30 to 50 %, but corticosteroid therapy can significantly reduce the recurrence rate [32–35]. We aimed to clarify the validity of various serum markers measured at disease onset for predicting recurrences. We found that the CIC level, determined at disease onset with the monoclonal rheumatoid method (IC-mRF), was significantly higher in the recurrence group than in the nonrecurrence group [36]. We used an IC-mRF cutoff value of 10 μg/dl to test the prediction of recurrence. The probability of recurrence was 60 % in cases where IC-mRF was >10 μg/dl, and it was 30 % in cases where IC-mRF was <10 μg/dl. We also compared the serum levels of complement components in groups with either a high or normal serum level of CIC. We found that serum C4 was significantly lower and serum C3 tended to be lower in the high-CIC group compared to levels in the normal-CIC group [25]. These results suggested that a classical pathway of complement activation system may be operating in some patients with AIP that have high serum CIC; thus, high serum CIC may predict both tissue damage and the probability of recurrence. Previous studies have shown that various factors measured at diagnosis, including diffuse pancreatic swelling, low bile duct stenosis with obstructive jaundice, IgG, CIC, sIL-2R, and complement, were highly predictive of relapse [34, 36–39].

Other studies have shown that specific HLA antigens could predict the recurrence of AIP. Furthermore, a substitution of aspartic acid at position 57 in the HLA DQβ1 was reported to affect the recurrence of AIP [40]. Another predictor of AIP recurrence is the cytotoxic T-lymphocyte antigen 4 (CTLA4) polymorphism. One study found that the +49A/A and +6230A/A polymorphic genotypes were associated with an enhanced risk of AIP recurrence [41].

In patients with AIP, extrapancreatic lesions may involve organs throughout the body and sometimes appears as recurrence lesions. Patients with AIP that had multiple extrapancreatic lesions were found to have significantly higher IgG4 levels than those with AIP, but no extrapancreatic lesion [12]. Among various extrapancreatic lesions, lachrymal and salivary gland lesions and hilar lymph adenopathy have been significantly associated with high serum IgG4 concentrations; this association suggested that patients with high serum IgG4 should be assessed for the presence of these lesions and abundant cell infiltration [12].

Follow-Up

We followed the clinical course of a 69-year-old woman that presented with two AIP recurrences. In this case, serum elevations of CIC and IgG4 were detected several months before the overt appearance of clinical recurrence. This finding indicated that CIC could represent disease activity with a sensitivity similar to that of IgG4 (Fig. 9.2) [11]. In clinical follow-ups of AIP, we currently use IgG and complement components, which are routinely measured

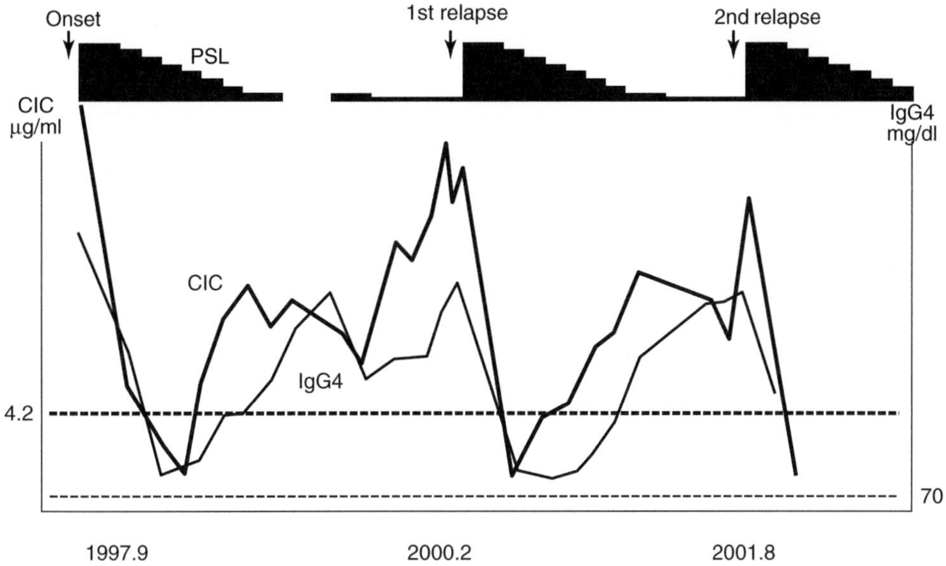

Fig. 9.2 Clinical course of autoimmune pancreatitis (AIP) in a 69-year-old female patient. After the onset of AIP and prednisolone (PSL) administration in 1997, the patient experienced two relapses in 2000 and 2001. The *black steps* indicate PSL dose reductions over time. The *horizontal dotted lines* show the typical IgG4 (light line; 70 mg/dl) and CIC (heavy line; 4.2 μg/ml) levels in healthy individuals. All three AIP occurrences were correlated with elevations in both IgG4 (*light line*) and CIC (*heavy line*). *CIC* circulating immune complex (Data are reprinted from Kawa and Hamano [11] with permission from the *Journal of Gastroenterology*)

in laboratory tests, to estimate AIP activity and predict the recurrence of AIP.

We followed two patients with AIP for 10 years each. One was a 55-year-old man with a high serum IgG4 concentration (1,135 mg/dl), and the other was a 65-year-old woman with a normal serum IgG4 concentration (42 mg/dl). The first patient experienced several recurrences, and he developed a pancreatic stone and pancreatic duct stenosis. The second patient showed no duct changes over time. These results suggested that when AIP is accompanied by normal IgG4 concentrations, it may have low activity, and it may represent a nonprogressive state [36]. Accordingly, serum IgG4 values may be useful in determining when maintenance therapy can be discontinued.

Role of IgG4

IgG4 may act in either a pathogenic or antiinflammatory role. For example, in a pathogenic role, an IgG4-type, anti-desmoglein 3 autoantibody was reported to provoke the lesions of pemphigus vulgaris [42]. Transfer of an anti-desmoglein 3 IgG4 autoantibody from a patient with pemphigus vulgaris to healthy BALB/C mice resulted in a pemphigus vulgaris-like lesion. Those studies suggested that an IgG4 autoantibody was directed against an unknown target antigen in AIP. In accordance with that hypothesis, IgG4 deposits have been detected in tissues of patients with AIP [26, 43].

In contrast, IgG4 was also found to have antiinflammatory effects against allergic reactions. IgG4 antibodies can bind to soluble antigens and block the interaction between these antigens and IgE on mast cells. This IgG4 activity resulted in the inhibition of allergic reactions.

For example, in an antiinflammatory role, it was reported that IgG4 underwent a Fab arm exchange [44]. It has been recognized that a characteristic feature of the IgG4 molecule is that it can undergo a dynamic Fab arm exchange; this exchange resulted in a Fab with bispecific activity, a loss of monospecific cross-linking activity, and a loss of the ability to form immune complexes. These findings suggested that IgG4 may primarily be an antiinflammatory agent [44].

IgG4 has been shown to act as an autoantibody against IgG, and it exhibited rheumatoid factor activity. Western blotting has shown that IgG4 from the sera of patients with AIP could bind to IgG1, IgG2, IgG3, and IgG Fc. Furthermore, IgG4 Fc, but not IgG4 Fab, was found to bind to IgG Fc; this indicated that the binding between IgG4 and IgG Fc occurred via an Fc-Fc interaction, not via rheumatoid activity [45]. The role of IgG4Fc-IgGFc is unclear, but it may have physiological and/or pathological effects. Further studies are needed to clarify this issue.

References

1. Kawa S, Hamano H, Kiyosawa K. Autoimmune pancreatitis and IgG4-related disease. In: Rose N, MacKay I, editors. The autoimmune diseases. 5th ed. St Louis: Academic Press; 2013. p. 935–49.

2. Hamano H, Kawa S, Horiuchi A, Unno H, Furuya N, Akamatsu T, et al. High serum IgG4 concentrations in patients with sclerosing pancreatitis. N Engl J Med. 2001;344(10):732–8.
3. Pearson RK, Longnecker DS, Chari ST, Smyrk TC, Okazaki K, Frulloni L, et al. Controversies in clinical pancreatology: autoimmune pancreatitis: does it exist? Pancreas. 2003;27(1):1–13.
4. Okazaki K, Kawa S, Kamisawa T, Naruse S, Tanaka S, Nishimori I, et al. Clinical diagnostic criteria of autoimmune pancreatitis: revised proposal. J Gastroenterol. 2006;41(7):626–31.
5. Otsuki M, Chung JB, Okazaki K, Kim MH, Kamisawa T, Kawa S, et al. Asian diagnostic criteria for autoimmune pancreatitis: consensus of the Japan-Korea Symposium on Autoimmune Pancreatitis. J Gastroenterol. 2008;43(6):403–8.
6. Chari ST, Smyrk TC, Levy MJ, Topazian MD, Takahashi N, Zhang L, et al. Diagnosis of autoimmune pancreatitis: the Mayo Clinic experience. Clin Gastroenterol Hepatol. 2006;4(8):1010–6; quiz 934.
7. Kim KP, Kim MH, Kim JC, Lee SS, Seo DW, Lee SK. Diagnostic criteria for autoimmune chronic pancreatitis revisited. World J Gastroenterol. 2006;12(16):2487–96.
8. Shimosegawa T, Chari ST, Frulloni L, Kamisawa T, Kawa S, Mino-Kenudson M, et al. International consensus diagnostic criteria for autoimmune pancreatitis: guidelines of the International Association of Pancreatology. Pancreas. 2011;40(3):352–8.
9. Kawa S, Fujinaga Y, Ota M, Hamano H, Bahram S. Autoimmune pancreatitis and diagnostic criteria. Curr Immunol Rev. 2011;7:144–61.
10. Maruyama M, Watanabe T, Kanai K, Oguchi T, Muraki T, Hamano H, et al. International consensus diagnostic criteria for autoimmune pancreatitis and its Japanese amendment have improved diagnostic ability over existing criteria. Gastroenterol Res Pract. 2013;2013:456965.
11. Kawa S, Hamano H. Clinical features of autoimmune pancreatitis. J Gastroenterol. 2007;42 Suppl 18:9–14.
12. Hamano H, Arakura N, Muraki T, Ozaki Y, Kiyosawa K, Kawa S. Prevalence and distribution of extrapancreatic lesions complicating autoimmune pancreatitis. J Gastroenterol. 2006;41(12): 1197–205.
13. Matsubayashi H, Sawai H, Kimura H, Yamaguchi Y, Tanaka M, Kakushima N, et al. Characteristics of autoimmune pancreatitis based on serum IgG4 level. Dig Liver Dis. 2011;43(9):731–5.
14. Hamano H, Kawa S, Ochi Y, Unno H, Shiba N, Wajiki M, et al. Hydronephrosis associated with retroperitoneal fibrosis and sclerosing pancreatitis. Lancet. 2002;359(9315):1403–4.
15. Yoshida K, Toki F, Takeuchi T, Watanabe S, Shiratori K, Hayashi N. Chronic pancreatitis caused by an autoimmune abnormality. Proposal of the concept of autoimmune pancreatitis. Dig Dis Sci. 1995;40(7):1561–8.
16. Kamisawa T, Anjiki H, Egawa N, Kubota N. Allergic manifestations in autoimmune pancreatitis. Eur J Gastroenterol Hepatol. 2009;21(10):1136–9.
17. Hirano K, Tada M, Isayama H, Kawakubo K, Yagioka H, Sasaki T, et al. Clinical analysis of high serum Ig8+E in autoimmune pancreatitis. World J Gastroenterol. 2010;16(41):5241–6.
18. Taguchi M, Kihara Y, Nagashio Y, Yamamoto M, Otsuki M, Harada M. Decreased production of immunoglobulin M and A in autoimmune pancreatitis. J Gastroenterol. 2009;44(11):1133–9.
19. Smyk DS, Rigopoulou EI, Koutsoumpas AL, Kriese S, Burroughs AK, Bogdanos DP. Autoantibodies in autoimmune pancreatitis. Int J Rheumatol. 2012;2012:940831.
20. Kino-Ohsaki J, Nishimori I, Morita M, Okazaki K, Yamamoto Y, Onishi S, et al. Serum antibodies to carbonic anhydrase I and II in patients with idiopathic chronic pancreatitis and Sjogren's syndrome. Gastroenterology. 1996;110(5):1579–86.
21. Okazaki K, Chiba T. Autoimmune related pancreatitis. Gut. 2002;51(1):1–4.
22. Kawa S, Ota M, Yoshizawa K, Horiuchi A, Hamano H, Ochi Y, et al. HLA DRB10405-DQB10401 haplotype is associated with autoimmune pancreatitis in the Japanese population. Gastroenterology. 2002;122(5):1264–9.
23. Guarneri F, Guarneri C, Benvenga S. Helicobacter pylori and autoimmune pancreatitis: role of carbonic anhydrase via molecular mimicry? J Cell Mol Med. 2005;9(3):741–4.
24. Frulloni L, Lunardi C, Simone R, Dolcino M, Scattolini C, Falconi M, et al. Identification of a novel antibody associated with autoimmune pancreatitis. N Engl J Med. 2009;361(22):2135–42.
25. Muraki T, Hamano H, Ochi Y, Komatsu K, Komiyama Y, Arakura N, et al. Autoimmune pancreatitis and complement activation system. Pancreas. 2006;32(1):16–21.
26. Detlefsen S, Brasen JH, Zamboni G, Capelli P, Kloppel G. Deposition of complement C3c, immunoglobulin (Ig)G4 and IgG at the basement membrane of pancreatic ducts and acini in autoimmune pancreatitis. Histopathology. 2010;57(6):825–35.
27. Saeki T, Nishi S, Imai N, Ito T, Yamazaki H, Kawano M, et al. Clinicopathological characteristics of patients with IgG4-related tubulointerstitial nephritis. Kidney Int. 2010;78(10):1016–23.
28. Matsubayashi H, Uesaka K, Kanemoto H, Asakura K, Kakushima N, Tanaka M, et al. Soluble IL-2 receptor, a new marker for autoimmune pancreatitis. Pancreas. 2012;41(3):493–6.
29. Abraham SC, Wilentz RE, Yeo CJ, Sohn TA, Cameron JL, Boitnott JK, et al. Pancreaticoduodenectomy (Whipple resections) in patients without malignancy: are they all 'chronic pancreatitis'? Am J Surg Pathol. 2003;27(1):110–20.
30. Kawa S, Okazaki K, Kamisawa T, Shimosegawa T, Tanaka M. Japanese consensus guidelines for management of autoimmune pancreatitis: II. Extrapancreatic lesions, differential diagnosis. J Gastroenterol. 2010;45:1264–71.
31. Ghazale A, Chari ST, Smyrk TC, Levy MJ, Topazian MD, Takahashi N, et al. Value of serum IgG4 in the diagnosis of autoimmune pancreatitis and in distinguishing it from pancreatic cancer. Am J Gastroenterol. 2007;102(8):1646–53.
32. Takayama M, Hamano H, Ochi Y, Saegusa H, Komatsu K, Muraki T, et al. Recurrent attacks of autoimmune pancreatitis result in pancreatic stone formation. Am J Gastroenterol. 2004;99(5):932–7.
33. Hirano K, Asaoka Y, Tada M, Isayama H, Sasahira N, Tsujino T, et al. No significant relation between relapse of autoimmune pancreatitis and substitution of aspartic acid at position 57 of DQbeta1. J Gastroenterol. 2009;44(7):799–800.
34. Kubota K, Watanabe S, Uchiyama T, Kato S, Sekino Y, Suzuki K, et al. Factors predictive of relapse and spontaneous remission of autoimmune pancreatitis patients treated/not treated with corticosteroids. J Gastroenterol. 2011;46(6):834–42.
35. Hart PA, Kamisawa T, Brugge WR, Chung JB, Culver EL, Czako L, et al. Long-term outcomes of autoimmune pancreatitis: a multicentre, international analysis. Gut. 2012;62(12):1771–6.
36. Kawa S, Hamano H, Ozaki Y, Ito T, Kodama R, Chou Y, et al. Long-term follow-up of autoimmune pancreatitis: characteristics of chronic disease and recurrence. Clin Gastroenterol Hepatol. 2009;7(11 Suppl):S18–22.
37. Hirano K, Tada M, Isayama H, Yagioka H, Sasaki T, Kogure H, et al. Long-term prognosis of autoimmune pancreatitis with and without corticosteroid treatment. Gut. 2007;56(12):1719–24.
38. Kim HM, Chung MJ, Chung JB. Remission and relapse of autoimmune pancreatitis: focusing on corticosteroid treatment. Pancreas. 2010;39(5):555–60.
39. Takuma K, Kamisawa T, Tabata T, Inaba Y, Egawa N, Igarashi Y. Short-term and long-term outcomes of autoimmune pancreatitis. Eur J Gastroenterol Hepatol. 2011;23(2):146–52.
40. Park do H, Kim MH, Oh HB, Kwon OJ, Choi YJ, Lee SS, et al. Substitution of aspartic acid at position 57 of the DQbeta1 affects relapse of autoimmune pancreatitis. Gastroenterology. 2008;134(2):440–6.

41. Umemura T, Ota M, Hamano H, Katsuyama Y, Muraki T, Arakura N, et al. Association of autoimmune pancreatitis with cytotoxic T-lymphocyte antigen 4 gene polymorphisms in Japanese patients. Am J Gastroenterol. 2008;103(3):588–94.
42. Rock B, Martins CR, Theofilopoulos AN, Balderas RS, Anhalt GJ, Labib RS, et al. The pathogenic effect of IgG4 autoantibodies in endemic pemphigus foliaceus (fogo selvagem). N Engl J Med. 1989;320(22):1463–9.
43. Aoki S, Nakazawa T, Ohara H, Sano H, Nakao H, Joh T, et al. Immunohistochemical study of autoimmune pancreatitis using anti-IgG4 antibody and patients' sera. Histopathology. 2005;47(2):147–58.
44. van der Neut Kolfschoten M, Schuurman J, Losen M, Bleeker WK, Martinez-Martinez P, Vermeulen E, et al. Anti-inflammatory activity of human IgG4 antibodies by dynamic Fab arm exchange. Science. 2007;317(5844):1554–7.
45. Kawa S, Kitahara K, Hamano H, Ozaki Y, Arakura N, Yoshizawa K, et al. A novel immunoglobulin-immunoglobulin interaction in autoimmunity. PLoS One. 2008;3(2):e1637.

Abdominal Ultrasonography

10

Kazuo Inui, Junji Yoshino, Hironao Miyoshi, and Satoshi Yamamoto

Introduction

Autoimmune pancreatitis (AIP) type 1 is characterized by diffuse or local enlargement of the pancreas demonstrated by imaging modalities, increased serum IgG4, and pathologic findings of abundant infiltration by IgG4-positive plasma cells, obliterative phlebitis, and storiform fibrosis [1, 2]. Pathologically, AIP type 2 shows lesions with neutrophilic infiltrates representing idiopathic duct-centric chronic pancreatitis [3]. In Japan, AIP type 1 is common, while AIP type 2 is rare, differing from frequencies in the USA and Europe. Abdominal ultrasonography (US) is the initial imaging examination performed following blood tests in patients with jaundice, exacerbation of diabetes mellitus, or abdominal pain – all common symptoms of AIP. Sometimes, AIP is detected in asymptomatic patients by mass screening programs [4]. In this section, we describe US findings in AIP type 1.

US Findings in the Pancreas

Diffusely Enlarged Type

US displays a diffusely enlarged pancreas as a hypoechoic area (Fig. 10.1) presenting a "sausage-like" appearance [5–7]. The enlarged hypoechoic area contains scattered hyperechoic spots [5, 8]. However, US cannot detect the irregular focal or diffuse narrowing of the main pancreatic duct, one of the main criteria for diagnosis of AIP by ERCP [2]. Furthermore, the diagnostic ability of US is affected by operator skill, patient condition, obesity, and excessive intestinal gas. Sometimes, US delineates a hypoechoic mass surrounding the pancreatic parenchyma (Fig. 10.2); in such cases, malignant lymphoma, pancreatic ductal adenocarcinoma, and metastatic pancreatic tumors should be distinguished from AIP using other imaging modalities.

Locally Enlarged Type

In patients with a segmentally or focally enlarged pancreas, AIP is important to differentiate from pancreatic ductal adenocarcinoma or mass-forming pancreatitis (Fig. 10.3). Wakabayashi et al. [9] reported that focal AIP is associated with clinical and radiologic features different from those of alcohol-induced mass-forming pancreatitis, but similar to those of pancreatic ductal adenocarcinoma. No dilation of the main pancreatic duct is seen in most cases of AIP, but in some patients dilation may make differential diagnosis difficult (Fig. 10.4). In AIP, US visualizes the main duct passing through the mass, which is called the "duct-penetrating

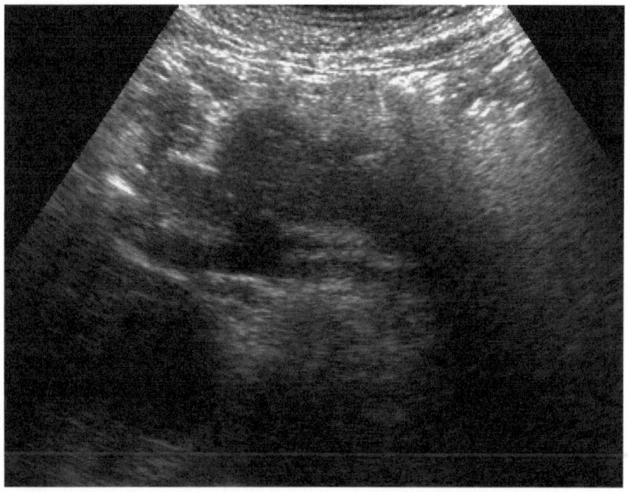

Fig. 10.1 Ultrasonography shows a diffusely enlarged pancreas as a hypoechoic area with scattered hyperechoic spots, described as a "sausage-like" appearance

K. Inui, MD, PhD (✉) • J. Yoshino, MD, PhD
H. Miyoshi, MD, PhD • S. Yamamoto, MD, PhD
Department of Gastroenterology,
Second Teaching Hospital, Fujita Health University,
3-6-10, Otobashi, Nakagawa-ku, Nagoya 454-8509, Japan
e-mail: kinui@fujita-hu.ac.jp

T. Kamisawa, J.B. Chung (eds.), *Autoimmune Pancreatitis*,
DOI 10.1007/978-3-642-55086-7_10, © Springer-Verlag Berlin Heidelberg 2015

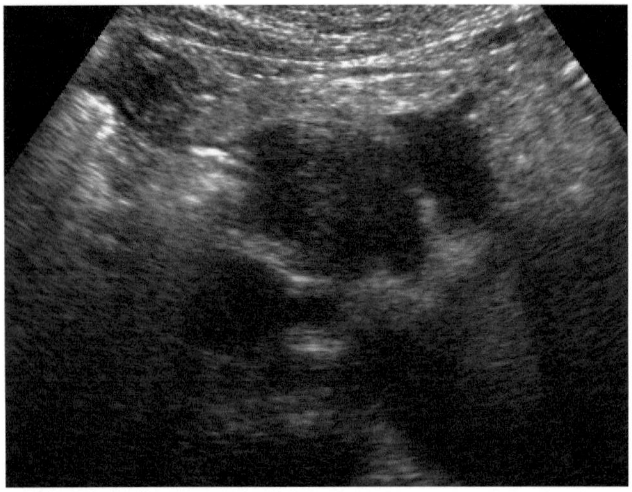

Fig. 10.2 Ultrasonography delineates multiple hypoechoic areas surrounding the pancreatic parenchyma

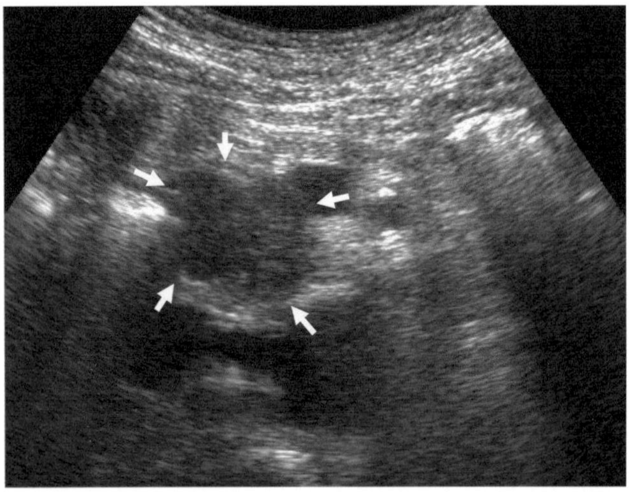

Fig. 10.3 Ultrasonography shows a hypoechoic mass (*arrows*) at the head of the pancreas. Because the internal echo is irregular, the lesion is difficult to distinguish from pancreatic ductal adenocarcinoma

sign." This sign is useful in distinguishing AIP from pancreatic ductal adenocarcinoma [10].

Contrast-Enhanced Ultrasonography for Diagnosis of AIP

Contrast-enhanced ultrasonography (CEUS) has been reported to be useful in distinguishing AIP from pancreatic ductal adenocarcinoma [6, 11–13]. In pancreatic ductal adenocarcinoma, CEUS displays enhancement only at the periphery of the mass, in associating with tumor vessels. In AIP, enhancement occurs in the entire mass, unassociated with tumor vessels. Morana et al. [6] reported that by CEUS, most inflammatory pancreatic masses showed a pattern of enhancement similar to that of normal pancreatic parenchyma ("isovascular"), while focal pancreatic tumors were hypovascular relative to surrounding parenchyma, and this criterion achieved sensitivity and accuracy in differentiating the 2 diseases of 98 and 95 %, respectively.

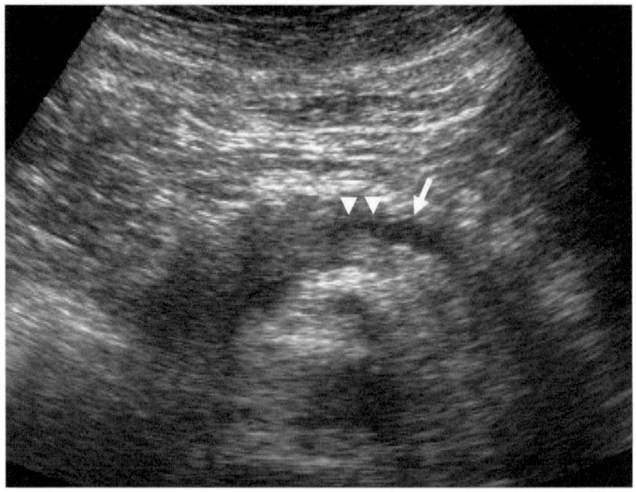

Fig. 10.4 Ultrasonography shows slight enlargement of the head of the pancreas and dilation of the main pancreatic duct (*arrow*), presenting potential difficulty in differential diagnosis. In this case, however, US displays the duct-penetrating sign (*arrowheads*)

Numata et al. [11] correlated vascularity of pancreatic lesions on CEUS with pathologic findings (fibrosis and inflammation) in 6 patients with AIP. The AIP lesions exhibited mild ($n=1$), moderate ($n=3$), or marked ($n=2$) enhancement in both early and delayed phases of the examination. A direct correlation was evident between enhancement (vascularity) and pathologic degree of inflammation, and an inverse correlation was noted between enhancement and degree of fibrosis associated with AIP. Vascularity of all 3 lesions with follow-up CEUS examinations had decreased after steroid therapy. Those authors concluded that CEUS appeared useful for evaluating both vascularity of AIP lesions and therapeutic efficacy of steroid therapy [11]. On the other hand, Miyoshi et al. [13] reported that CEUS findings in patients with AIP varied by stage of disease; areas with intense inflammation and immature fibrosis enhanced strongly, while areas with less intense inflammation and more established fibrosis enhanced weakly.

US Characteristics of the Common Bile Duct in AIP

AIP frequently complicates IgG4-related sclerosing cholangitis (IgG4-SC), in such cases. US detects thickening of the wall of the common bile duct (Fig. 10.5), and frequency of bile duct wall thickening in AIP was reported to be about 60 % [8]. A thickened bile duct wall is characterized by layered or parenchymal hypoechoic wall thickening [14, 15]. In

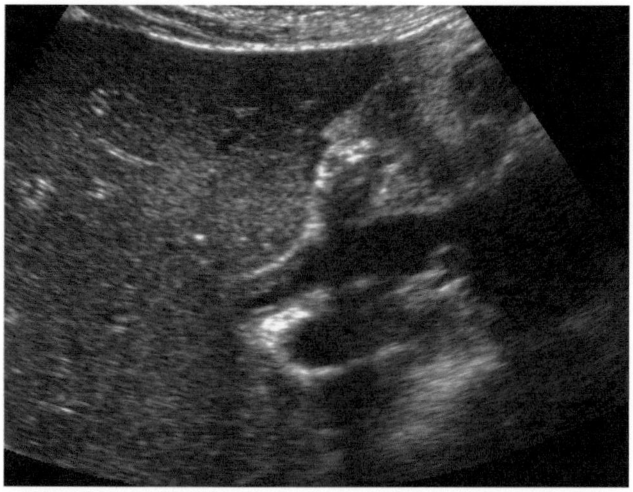

Fig. 10.5 Ultrasonography demonstrates thickening of the wall of the common bile duct (thickness, 4.7 mm). US also shows dilation of the common bile duct and a mass in the head of the pancreas

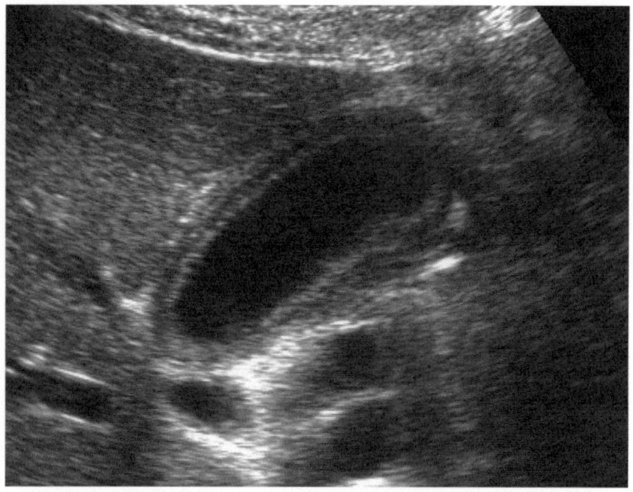

Fig. 10.6 Ultrasonography shows a thickening of the gallbladder wall (thickness, 5.4 mm). The three-layered structure of the gallbladder wall (hyperechoic-hypoechoic-hyperechoic) is wholly maintained

some cases, thickening of ducts wall beyond extrahepatic bile ducts extends to intrahepatic bile ducts. However, US cannot detect narrowing of the intrapancreatic bile duct, a feature included among the criteria for IgG4-SC [16]. Accordingly, strictures of hilar or intrahepatic bile ducts are assessed by other means in patients with AIP [16].

Duct wall thickening in AIP has been studied in detail with endoscopic ultrasonography (EUS) and intraductal ultrasonography (IDUS) [8, 17]. Although wall thickening in narrowed duct segments is not shown clearly by conventional US, EUS and IDUS depict circular, symmetric wall thickening with smooth outer and inner margins, associated with homogeneous internal echo in narrowed ducts [18, 19]. Sometimes, difficulty arises in correctly diagnosing IgG4-SC, when IDUS displays irregular wall thickening during the acute phase of disease. However, after steroid therapy, wall thickness has decreased conspicuously [20].

US Characteristics of the Gallbladder in AIP

In some patients with AIP, US detects thickening of the gallbladder wall [21]. Reported frequency of gallbladder wall thickening has ranged from 37.8 % (14/37) [22] to 52.6 % (10/19) [23]. In one of our patients, US detected diffuse thickening of the gallbladder wall, with no disruption of its structure (Fig. 10.6). US also detected thickening of the wall of the common bile duct in this patient. Kamisawa et al. [23] reported that gallbladder wall thickening was more frequent in AIP patients with extensive bile duct involvement ($P<0.01$). The same group of authors [8] described histologic findings in the thickened gallbladder wall as showing transmural lymphoplasmacytic infiltration with fibrosis, mucosal infiltration with fibrosis, or mucosal lymphoplasmacytic infiltration. Marked or moderate infiltration of the gallbladder by IgG4-positive plasma cells was detected immunohistochemically. These findings also were noted in the bile duct and the pancreas.

Conclusions

Abdominal US is effective for diagnosis of AIP. Ultrasonographic findings in AIP are a diffusely or locally enlarged pancreas with hypoechoic parenchyma. When diffusely enlarged, the pancreas is described as "sausage like." In patients with a locally enlarged pancreas or a hypoechoic mass surrounding the pancreatic parenchyma, pancreatic ductal adenocarcinoma, malignant lymphoma, and metastatic pancreatic carcinoma should be considered.

References

1. Okazaki K, Kawa S, Kamisawa T, Naruse S, Tanaka S, Nishimori I, et al. Clinical diagnostic criteria of autoimmune pancreatitis: revised proposal. J Gastroenterol. 2006;41:626–31.
2. Okazaki K, Kawa S, Kamisawa T, Shimosegawa T, Tanaka M, Research Committee for Intractable Pancreatic Disease and Japan Pancreas Society. Japanese consensus guidelines for management of autoimmune pancreatitis: I. Concept and diagnosis of autoimmune pancreatitis. J Gastroenterol. 2010;45:249–65.
3. Shimosegawa T, Chari ST, Frulloni L, Kamisawa T, Kawa S, Mino-Kenudson M, et al. International consensus diagnostic criteria for autoimmune pancreatitis: guidelines of the International Association of Pancreatology. Pancreas. 2011;40:352–8.
4. Yoda Y, Kobayashi K, Enomoto N. Study of category classification in abdominal ultrasonographic mass screening. J Gastroenterol Mass Surv. 2006;44:12–20 (In Japanese with English abstract).
5. Irie H, Ito T. US, CT and MRI findings of autoimmune pancreatitis based on "Clinical diagnostic criteria of autoimmune pancreatitis 2006". Suizo. 2007;22:629–33 (In Japanese with English abstract).

6. Morana G, Tapparelli M, Faccioli N, D'Onofrio M, Pozzi Mucelli R. Autoimmune pancreatitis: instrumental diagnosis. JOP. 2005;6(1 Suppl):102–7.
7. Ito T, Nakano I, Koyanagi S, Miyahara T, Migita Y, Ogoshi K, et al. Autoimmune pancreatitis as a new clinical entity. Three cases of autoimmune pancreatitis with effective steroid therapy. Dig Dis Sci. 1997;42:1458–68.
8. Kamisawa T, Egawa N, Nakajima H, Tsuruta K, Okamoto A, Kamata N, et al. Comparison of radiological and histological findings in autoimmune pancreatitis. Hepatogastroenterol. 2006; 53:953–6.
9. Wakabayashi T, Kawaura Y, Satomura Y, Watanabe H, Motoo Y, Okai T, et al. Clinical and imaging features of autoimmune pancreatitis with focal pancreatic swelling or mass formation: comparison with so-called tumor-forming pancreatitis and pancreatic carcinoma. Am J Gastroenterol. 2003;98:2679–87.
10. Muraki T, Ozaki Y, Hamano H, Niikura N, Ochi Y, Kawa S, et al. Ultrasonographic diagnosis of autoimmune pancreatitis. Tan to Sui. 2005;26:711–6 (In Japanese without English abstract).
11. Nagase M, Furuse J, Ishii H, Yoshino M. Evaluation of contrast enhancement patterns in pancreatic tumors by coded harmonic sonographic imaging with a microbubble contrast agent. J Ultrasound Med. 2003;22:789–95.
12. Numata K, Ozawa Y, Kobayashi N, Kubota T, Akinori N, Nakatani Y, et al. Contrast-enhanced sonography of autoimmune pancreatitis: comparison with pathologic findings. J Ultrasound Med. 2004;23:199–206.
13. Miyoshi H, Inui K, Yoshino J, Okushima K, Hattori M, Yamamto T. Usefulness of contrast-enhanced ultrasonography in autoimmune pancreatitis. Suizo. 2010;25:117–24 (In Japanese with English abstract).
14. Hyodo N, Hyodo T. Ultrasonographic evaluation in patients with autoimmune-related pancreatitis. J Gastroenterol. 2003;38:1155–61.
15. Honjo H, Takeuchi K, Nagashima N, Yamamoto T, Yamamoto T, Sakurai N, et al. Biliary duct lesions associated with autoimmune pancreatitis. Tan to Sui. 2001;22:581–7 (In Japanese without English abstract).
16. Ohara T, Okazaki K, Tsubouchi H, Inui K, Kawa S, Kamisawa T, et al. Clinical diagnostic criteria of IgG4-related sclerosing cholangitis 2012. J Helpatobiliary Pancreat Sci. 2012;9:536–42.
17. Hasebe O, Arakura N, Imai Y, Yokosawa S, Tokoo M, Goto A, et al. The findings of ERC and IDUS in autoimmune pancreatitis. J Gastroenterol Imaging. 2002;4:41–8.
18. Nakazawa T, Ando T, Hayashi K, Naitoh I, Ohara H, Joh T. Diagnostic procedures for IgG4-related sclerosing cholangitis. J Hepatobiliary Pancreat Sci. 2011;18:127–36.
19. Kubota K, Kato S, Uchiyama T, Watanabe S, Nozaki Y, Fujita K, et al. Discrimination between sclerosing cholangitis-associated autoimmune pancreatitis and primary sclerosing cholangitis, cancer using intraductal ultrasonography. Dig Endosc. 2011;23:10–6.
20. Inui K, Yoshino J, Miyoshi H. Differential diagnosis and treatment of biliary strictures. Clin Gastroenterol Hepatol. 2009;7:S79–83.
21. Kamisawa T, Tu Y, Nakajima H, Egawa N, Tsuruta K, Okamoto A, Horiguchi S. Sclerosing cholecystitis associated with autoimmune pancreatitis. World J Gastroenterol. 2006;12:3736–9.
22. Koyama R, Imamura T, Okuda C, Sakamoto N, Honjo H, Takeuchi K. Ultrasonograhic imaging of bile duct lesions in autoimmune pancreatitis. Pancreas. 2008;37:259–64.
23. Kamisawa T, Takuma K, Anjiki H, Egawa N, Kurata M, Honda G, et al. Biliary lesions associated with autoimmune pancreatitis. Hepatogastroenterol. 2009;56:1190–3.

Imaging Findings: CT and MRI with MRCP

11

Min Jung Park, Young Eun Chung, and Mi-Suk Park

Introduction

Autoimmune pancreatitis has a wide range of possible imaging features, and there are overlaps in appearance with other pancreatic diseases. However, in the diagnosis of autoimmune pancreatitis, imaging findings are important components of diagnostic criteria and should be considered in conjunction with the clinical, serologic, and pathological findings. Imaging methods employed in the diagnosis and treatment response evaluation of autoimmune pancreatitis include computed tomography (CT), magnetic resonance imaging (MRI), transabdominal ultrasonography (US), endoscopic retrograde cholangiopancreatography (ERCP), and endoscopic ultrasonography (EUS) [1–4]. Here we focus on typical and atypical findings of autoimmune pancreatitis in CT, MRI, and MRCP and the differential points with other diseases.

Pancreas

Typical Findings

The most important imaging feature of autoimmune pancreatitis is pancreatic enlargement with loss of the lobular architecture often termed "sausage-shaped pancreas" (seen in 40–60 % of cases) [2–6], which is typical when diffuse, and atypical when focal or segmental enlargement according to the International Consensus Diagnostic Criteria [7]. These findings are well delineated on cross-sectional imaging studies, CT (Fig. 11.1) and MRI (Fig. 11.2), the most commonly used modalities due to their availability, reproducibility, and noninvasive nature.

On CT or MRI, autoimmune pancreatitis enhances less than normal pancreas in the pancreatic phase (or arterial phase) and then demonstrates delayed enhancement in the portal venous and equilibrium phase in over 90 % of cases [2, 7–9]. This delayed enhancement pattern of autoimmune pancreatitis is one of the most important imaging features and useful in differentiating from other diseases, which will be discussed afterward in this chapter. On MRI, the pancreas appears moderately hyperintense on T2-weighted images and hypointense on T1-weighted images in autoimmune pancreatitis patients (Fig. 11.2).

Hypoattenuating or hypointense capsule-like rim surrounding the pancreas is a supplementary finding of autoimmune pancreatitis seen in 12–40 % of cases on CT and MRI [2, 6, 10] (Fig. 11.2). The rim reflects intense inflammatory infiltration and fibrosis of the peripancreatic tissue [8, 10]. On MRI, the rim appears hypointense on T1- and T2-weighted images and delayed enhancement. Peripancreatic fat stranding, which is a common feature in other causes of pancreatitis, is usually minimal in autoimmune pancreatitis [6] (Fig. 11.2). Regional lymphadenopathy and involution of the pancreatic tail can occur in patients with autoimmune pancreatitis [1, 5].

Another imaging hallmark of autoimmune pancreatitis is an irregular luminal narrowing of the main pancreatic duct, of which MRCP is the modality of choice [11, 12] (Fig. 11.2). Typically, there is long (>1/3 of the main pancreatic duct) or multiple strictures in the main pancreatic duct without marked upstream dilatation. And segmental or focal narrowing of the main pancreatic duct without marked upstream dilatation in atypical cases [7]. However, ERCP is necessary if there is any symptomatic biliary obstruction [11, 12].

Of the two known forms of autoimmune pancreatitis, type 1 (lymphoplasmacytic sclerosing pancreatitis) is associated with IgG4-related disease and tends to develop in middle-aged and elderly men (mean age, 59–68 years) with a male-to-female ratio of 4–7.5:1 [13, 14]. The prevalence rate is 2–11 % among patients with chronic pancreatitis [15]. On the other hand, autoimmune pancreatitis type 2 is seen in a younger population in comparison with patients with autoimmune pancreatitis type 1, which lacks elevated IgG4 levels. However, there was no imaging feature of the pancreas

M.J. Park, MD (✉) • Y.E. Chung, MD • M.-S. Park, MD
Department of Radiology and Research Institute of Radiological Science, Yonsei University College of Medicine, Seoul, Korea
e-mail: mindungs@yuhs.ac; RADPMS@yuhs.ac

T. Kamisawa, J.B. Chung (eds.), *Autoimmune Pancreatitis*,
DOI 10.1007/978-3-642-55086-7_11, © Springer-Verlag Berlin Heidelberg 2015

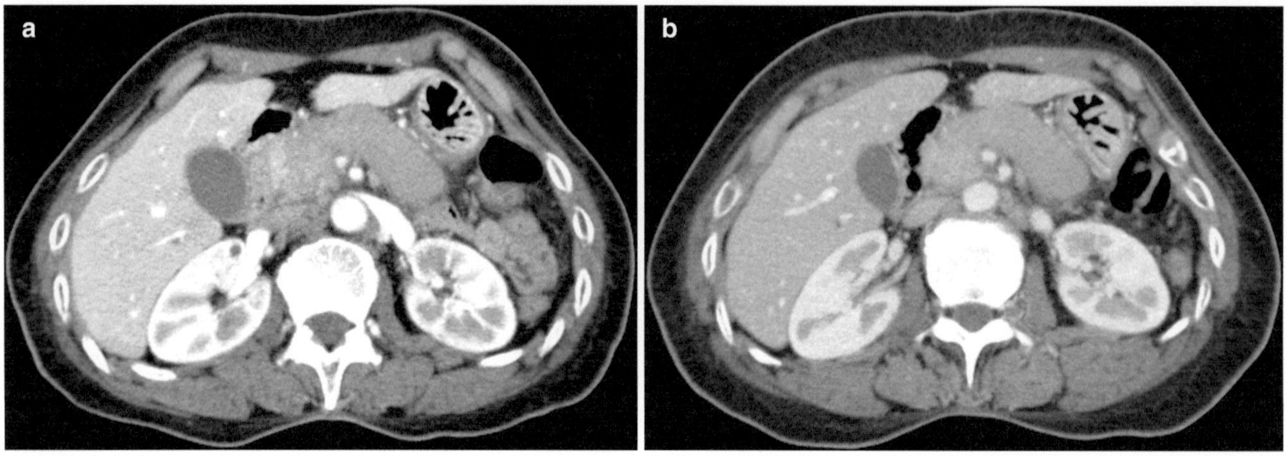

Fig. 11.1 A 59-year-old woman with typical imaging features of autoimmune pancreatitis in the pancreatic (**a**) and portal venous phase images (**b**) of CT showing mild diffuse enlargement of the pancreas with loss of the lobular architecture ("sausage-shaped pancreas"), hypoattenuation in the pancreatic phase and hyperattenuation on the portal venous phase ("delayed enhancement"). Note that the pancreas enhances less than the normal pancreas in the pancreatic phase (**a**) and then exhibits delayed enhancement in the portal venous phase (**b**). Also note the paucity of peripancreatic stranding

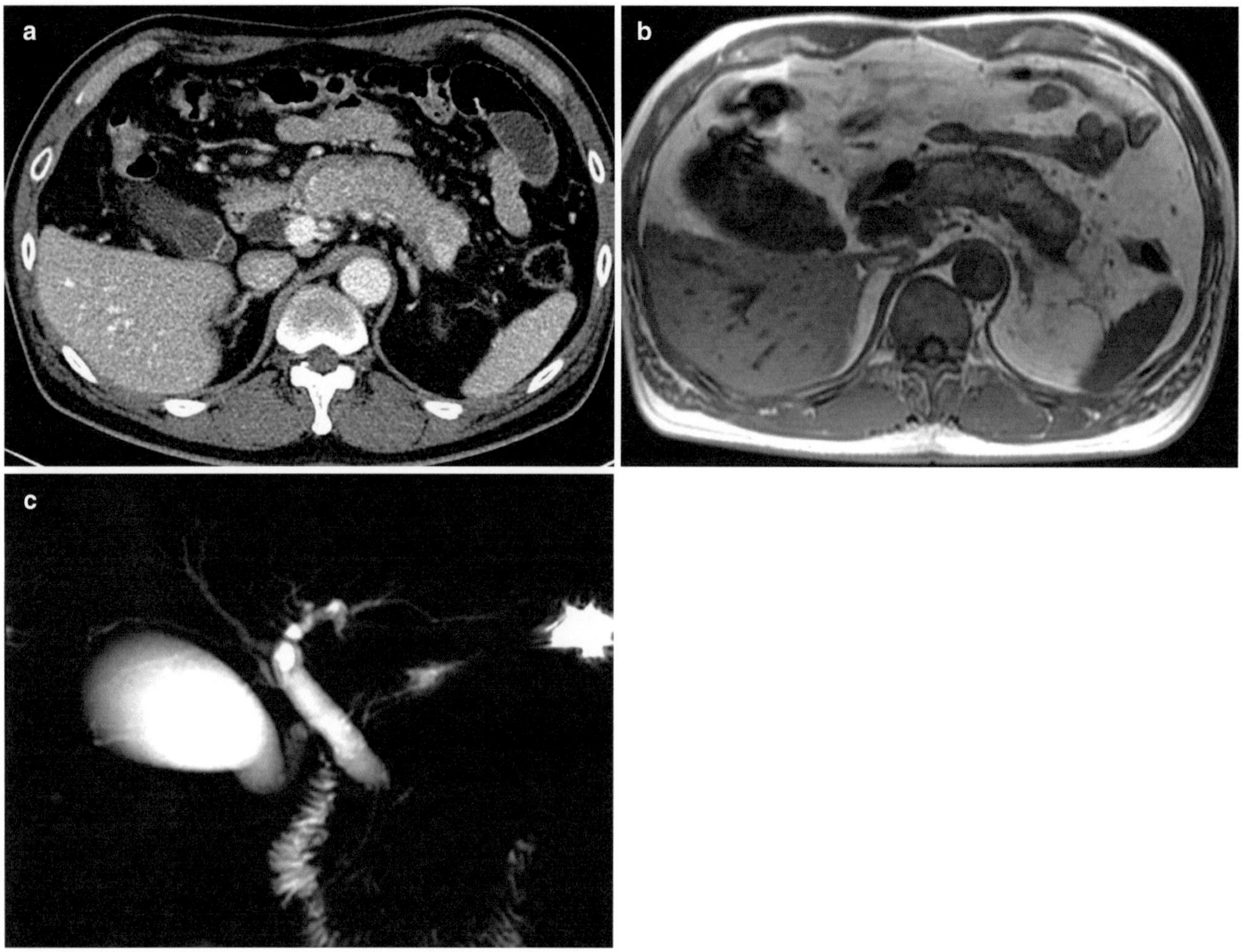

Fig. 11.2 A 56-year-old man with typical imaging features of autoimmune pancreatitis. (**a**) Axial portal venous phase CT image shows mild diffuse enlargement of the pancreas with hypoattenuating capsule-like rim surrounding the pancreas. (**b**) Axial T2-weighted MR image shows diffuse enlargement of the pancreas appearing as moderate hyperintensity with hypointense capsule-like rim around the pancreas. (**c**) MRCP image shows diffuse irregular luminal narrowing of the main pancreatic duct

reported to differentiate the two types of autoimmune pancreatitis. And the two types may be definitively distinguished only by histopathologic assessment [14].

Atypical Findings and Differential Diagnosis

Autoimmune pancreatitis sometimes exhibits atypical imaging features, which makes the diagnosis difficult. Therefore, the diagnosis of autoimmune pancreatitis requires a combination of clinical, laboratory, imaging, and histologic findings.

The most important atypical imaging finding in autoimmune pancreatitis is focal pancreatic mass-like lesion in 30–40 % of cases, resulting from localized involvement of autoimmune pancreatitis seen commonly in the pancreatic head [1] (Fig. 11.3). The focal form of autoimmune pancreatitis may simulate pancreatic ductal adenocarcinoma, and there are ancillary imaging features helpful in distinguishing the two diseases; prominent lymphadenopathy, vascular occlusion, abrupt narrowing of the pancreatic duct, and marked atrophy of the pancreas distal to the mass increase the possibility of pancreatic carcinoma rather than autoimmune pancreatitis. The pancreatic duct penetrating through the mass-like lesion, known as "duct-penetrating sign," is considered to be helpful for differentiating focal form of autoimmune pancreatitis from pancreatic cancer even though the finding has low specificity as up to 50 % [16] (Figs. 11.3 and 11.4). Although both autoimmune pancreatitis and pancreatic carcinoma show restricted diffusion (Fig. 11.3), diffusion-weighted MRI has been reported to be helpful in differentiation between autoimmune pancreatitis and pancreatic carcinoma [17, 18]. In a series of Kamisawa et al., the apparent diffusion coefficient (ADC) values were lower in patients with autoimmune pancreatitis than in those

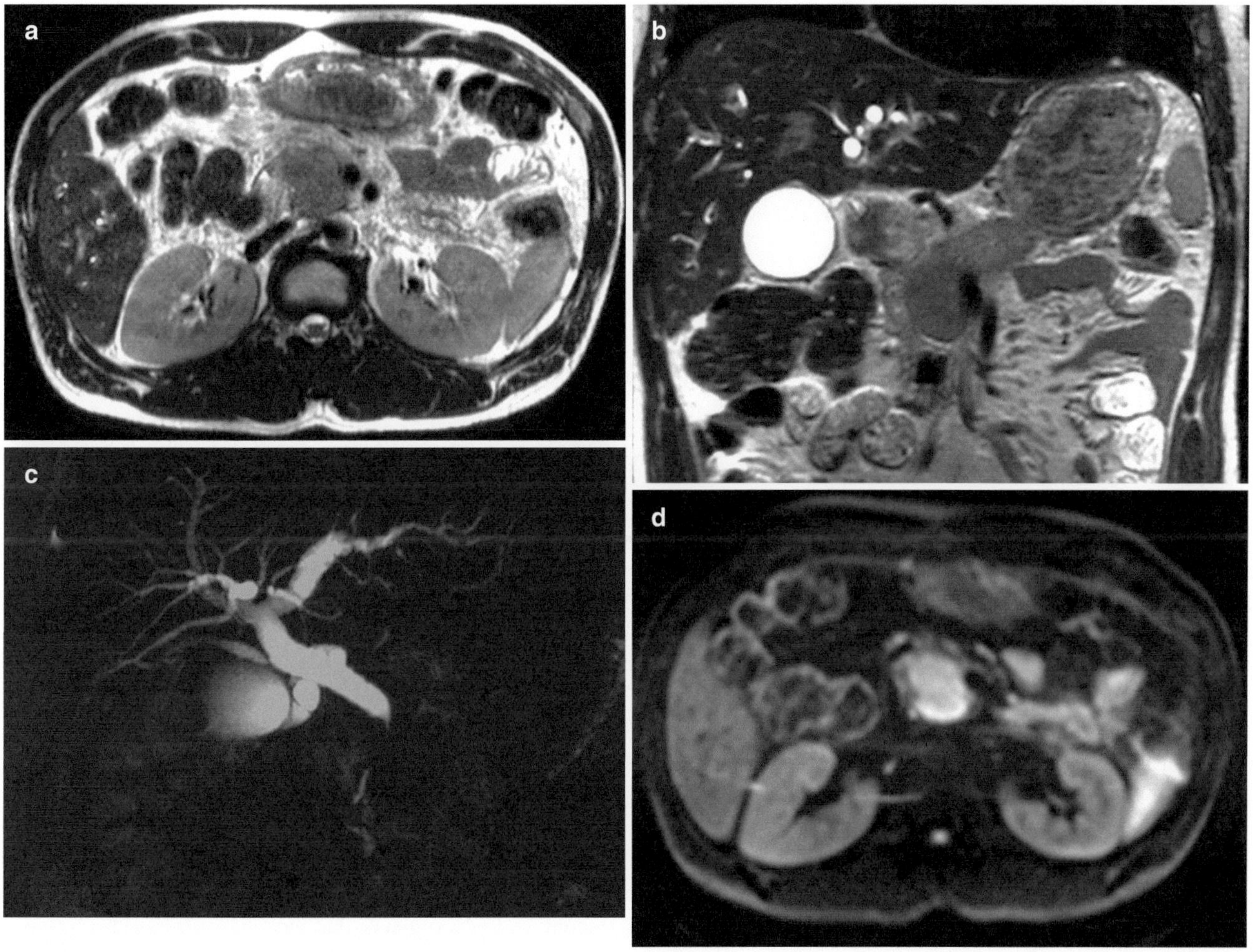

Fig. 11.3 A 56-year-old man with focal autoimmune pancreatitis. A round mass in the pancreas head appearing as moderate hyperintense lesion on (**a**) axial and (**b**) coronal T2-weighted MR images. (**c**) On MRCP image, the distal common bile duct shows segmental narrowing at level of the mass-like lesion in the pancreas head, but patency was preserved ("duct-penetrating sign"). (**d**) Diffusion-weighted image obtained at b value of 400 s/mm^2 and (**e**) apparent diffusion coefficient map show restricted diffusion of the mass-like lesion in the pancreas head. After steroid treatment, the mass-like lesion in the pancreas head and distal CBD narrowing disappeared on (**f**) axial CT and (**g**) ERCP images

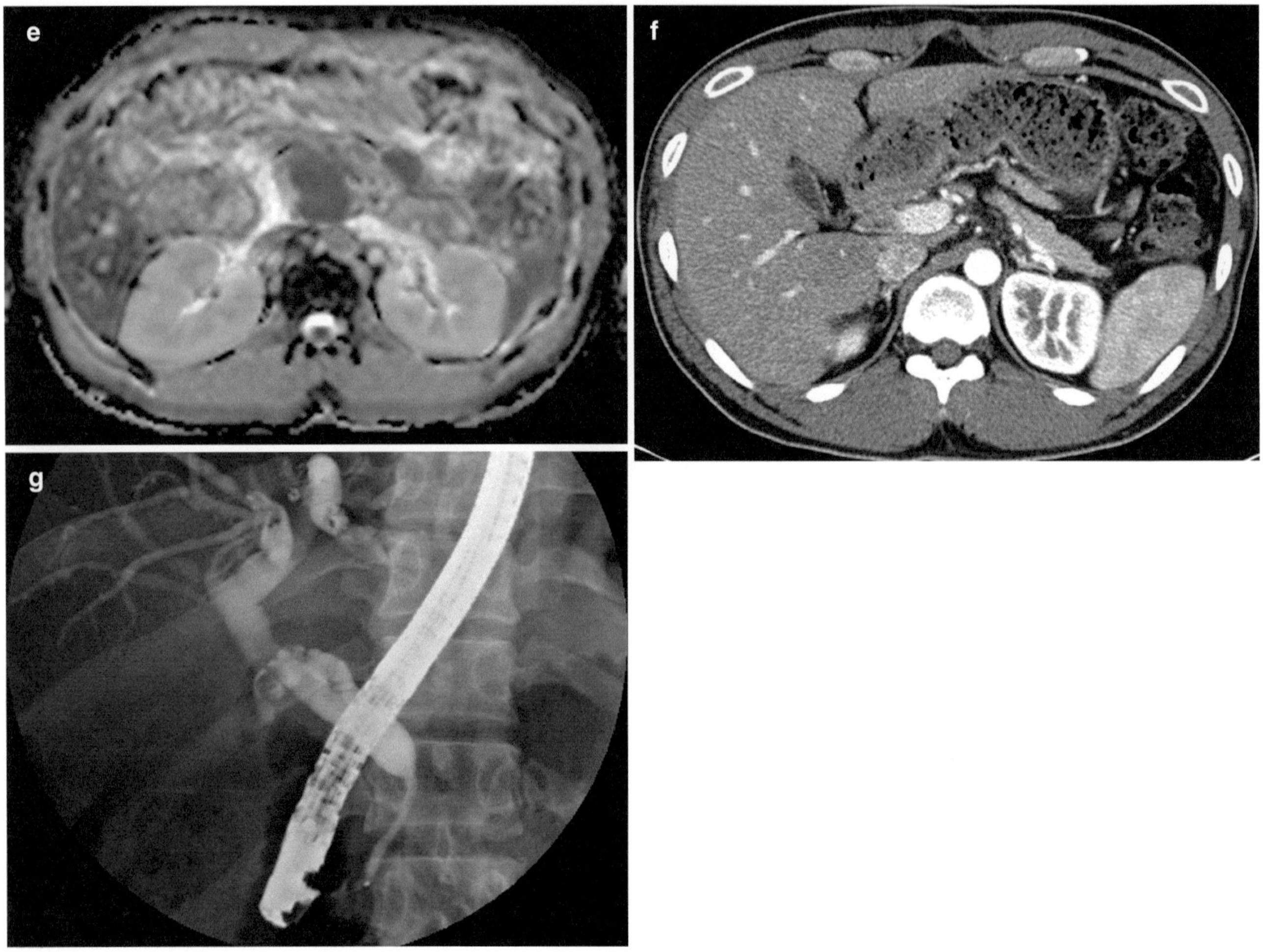

Fig. 11.3 (continued)

with pancreatic carcinoma. A possible ADC cutoff value ($1.075 \times 10–3$ mm^2/s) can be used in distinguishing between the two entities [18]. Histological confirmation, however, remains for a diagnosis for many cases of focal autoimmune pancreatitis for differentiation from pancreatic carcinoma. Moreover, although rare in prevalence, pancreatic carcinoma may occur concurrently or during follow-up for autoimmune pancreatitis, even after histological confirmation of the diagnosis [19, 20].

Diffuse autoimmune pancreatitis must be differentiated from other causes of pancreatitis or diffuse pancreatic infiltration. Features that favor autoimmune pancreatitis over acute pancreatitis include the presence of a peripancreatic halo or capsule-like rim, minimal or no peripancreatic fat stranding, and the absence of peripancreatic necrosis [5, 21]. The presence of causative factors, such as gallstones, in addition to imaging features of acute pancreatitis, such as peripancreatic fat stranding and fluid collections, and necrosis of the pancreas or peripancreatic tissue reduce the likelihood of autoimmune pancreatitis (Fig. 11.5) Pseudocyst is a rare finding of autoimmune pancreatitis [5, 22], but often combined in patients with alcohol-induced pancreatitis [23].

Another differential diagnosis of autoimmune pancreatitis is lymphoma. Multiple and widespread lymphadenopathy and diffuse pancreatic infiltration would suggest lymphoma. Also, the delayed enhancement pattern of autoimmune pancreatitis is useful in differentiating from lymphoma and ductal adenocarcinoma, which exhibit lower degree of contrast enhancement compared to that of autoimmune pancreatitis in both of the pancreatic and portal venous phases [8, 9, 24].

Imaging Features After Treatment

Recent evidence suggests that most patients have been found to have significant symptomatic improvement after treatment with corticosteroids, and this is usually accompanied by radiological resolution [3, 25, 26] (Fig. 11.3). However, the resolution of radiological features is dependent upon the degree of fibrosis, and inflammatory change is more likely to resolve quickly. Therefore, a long-standing fibrotic disease

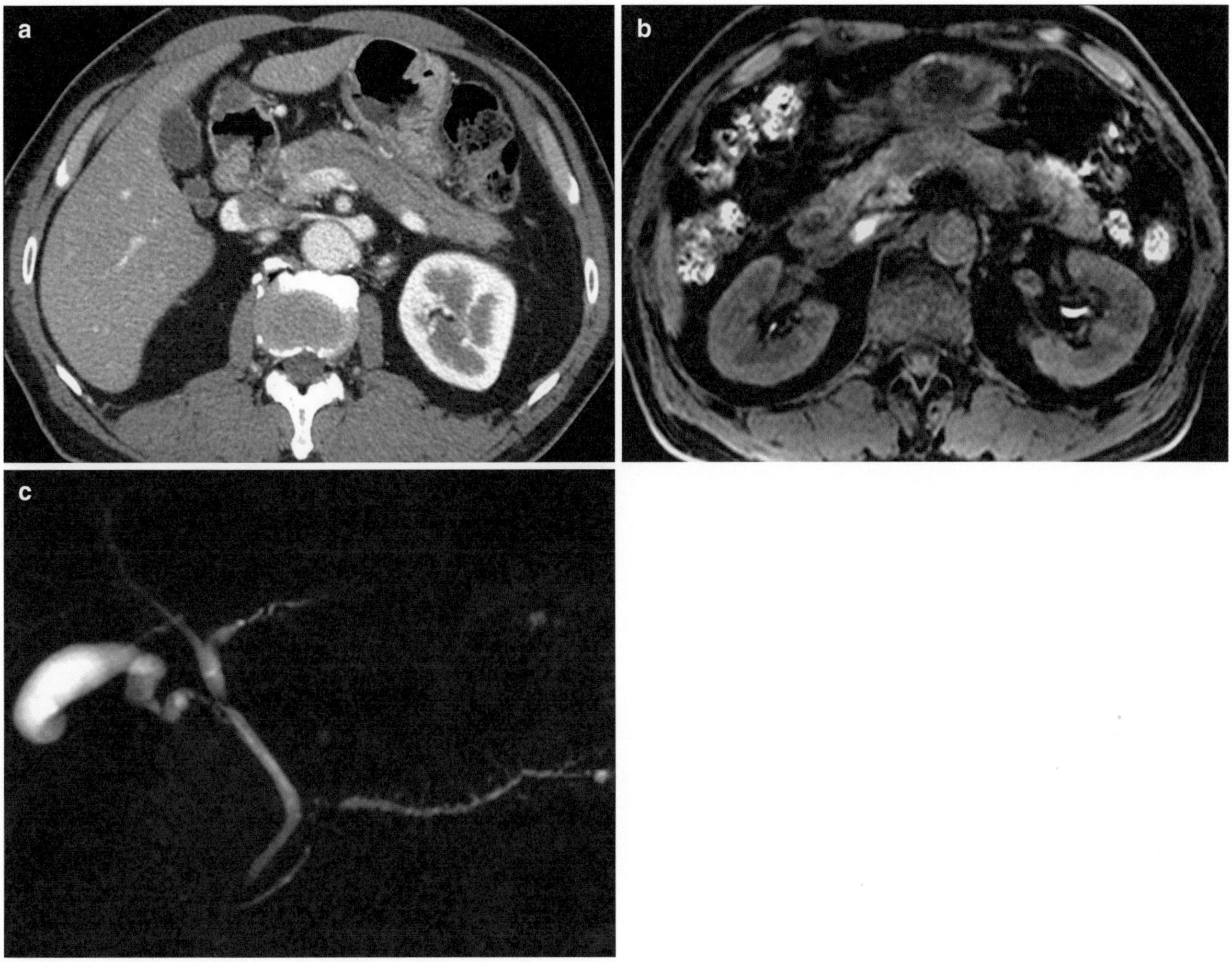

Fig. 11.4 A 64-year-old man with pancreatic ductal adenocarcinoma. (**a**) On axial contrast-enhanced CT image, mild dilatation of the main pancreatic duct and cutoff at body portion was observed without any visible mass lesion. Further evaluation was performed under the suspicion of isoattenuating pancreatic cancer. (**b**) On axial precontrast T1-weighted MR image, it shows hypointense mass at the portion of duct cutoff. (**c**) MRCP image also shows abrupt termination of the main pancreatic duct (*arrow*) at the level of mass. Duct-penetrating sign is negative here, which suggests pancreatic carcinoma

may not change appearance with treatment, and extrapancreatic manifestations may resolve at a different rate from the pancreatic findings [27].

Bile Duct and Gallbladder

Biliary involvement is the most common extrapancreatic manifestation of autoimmune pancreatitis seen in up to 67–96 % cases, especially in type 1 autoimmune pancreatitis, which is a multisystem fibro-inflammatory disorder and called as IgG4-related disease [3, 16, 28–30]. This condition has been termed IgG4-related sclerosing cholangitis. It can occur without pancreatic findings, and the distal common bile duct is the most common site of biliary involvement.

On contrast-enhanced CT and MRI, the affected segments of the bile duct show mural thickening with enhancement, luminal narrowing, and stenosis (Fig. 11.6). In addition to CT and MRI, MRCP is helpful for a precise assessment of the location and extent of biliary involvement, especially when there are multifocal involvement in both the intra- and extrahepatic bile ducts.

There are some overlaps in the imaging features of IgG4-related sclerosing cholangitis and cholangiocarcinoma [21] and primary sclerosing cholangitis in 10–35 % of cases [31]. On MRCP, primary sclerosing cholangitis shows multifocal, short segmental, band-like strictures. A beaded appearance with alternating strictures and normal or slightly dilated segments, a pruned-tree appearance with decreased in number of visible peripherally located intrahepatic ducts, and diverticulum-like lesions involving the intra- or extrahepatic bile ducts are characteristic findings [28] (Fig. 11.7). In IgG4-related sclerosing cholangitis, stricture typically affects a long segment and is continuous

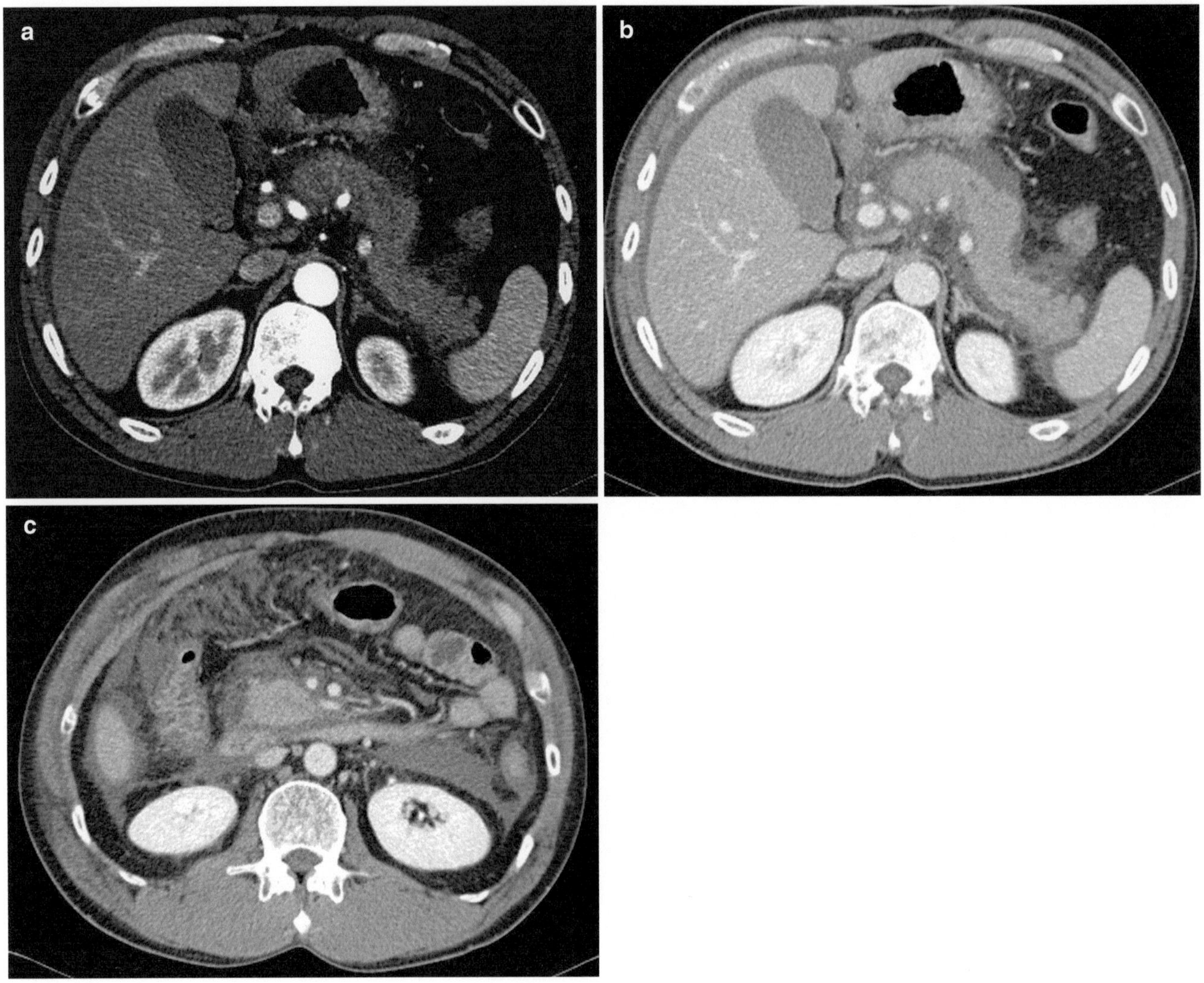

Fig. 11.5 A 42-year-old man with acute alcoholic pancreatitis. (**a**) The arterial phase and (**b–c**) portal venous phase images of axial contrast-enhanced CT show extensive peripancreatic fat stranding (*arrows*) and peripancreatic fluid collection in addition to diffuse enlargement of the pancreas. These imaging features point toward acute pancreatitis rather than autoimmune pancreatitis

with prestenotic dilatation. And isolated stricture of the distal common bile duct is common unlike multifocal involvement in primary sclerosing cholangitis [28]. In a series of Kim et al., multifocal stricture and/or wall thickening of intrahepatic bile duct stricture and pruned-tree appearance were more frequent on MRCP in primary sclerosing cholangitis than in IgG4-related sclerosing cholangitis patients [32]. In their series, on CT and MRI, the bile duct wall was thicker (5.1 mm vs. 3.1 mm and 4.3 mm vs. 3.0 mm, respectively) in IgG4-related sclerosing cholangitis than in primary sclerosing cholangitis patients.

When present, soft tissue around the bile ducts in IgG4-related sclerosing cholangitis tends to be larger in extent compared to that in primary sclerosing cholangitis. Periductal soft tissue mass is rarely seen, but can mimic cholangiocarcinoma [31]. In the differentiation of IgG4-related sclerosing cholangitis and cholangiocarcinoma, IgG4-related sclerosing cholangitis was reported to have more frequently intrapancreatic common bile duct involvement, concentric wall thickening, smooth outer margin of the thickened wall, and lower degrees of wall thickening, upstream dilatation, and contrast enhancement of the bile duct compared to common bile duct cancer in a series of Kim et al. [33]. Also in their study, IgG4-related sclerosing cholangitis appeared to have more frequently smooth margin, gradual and symmetric narrowing, multifocal involvement, and hourglass appearance of the bile duct than common bile duct cancer on ERCP and MRCP.

Gallbladder involvement can also occur in up to 25 % of patients with IgG4-related autoimmune pancreatitis with concurrent sclerosing cholangitis and manifest as diffuse thickening of the gallbladder wall [31]. In contrast to the nonspecific imaging appearance of acalculous diffuse cholecystitis of other causes, IgG4-related cholecystitis shows predominant extramural involvement and subserosal inflammatory nodules.

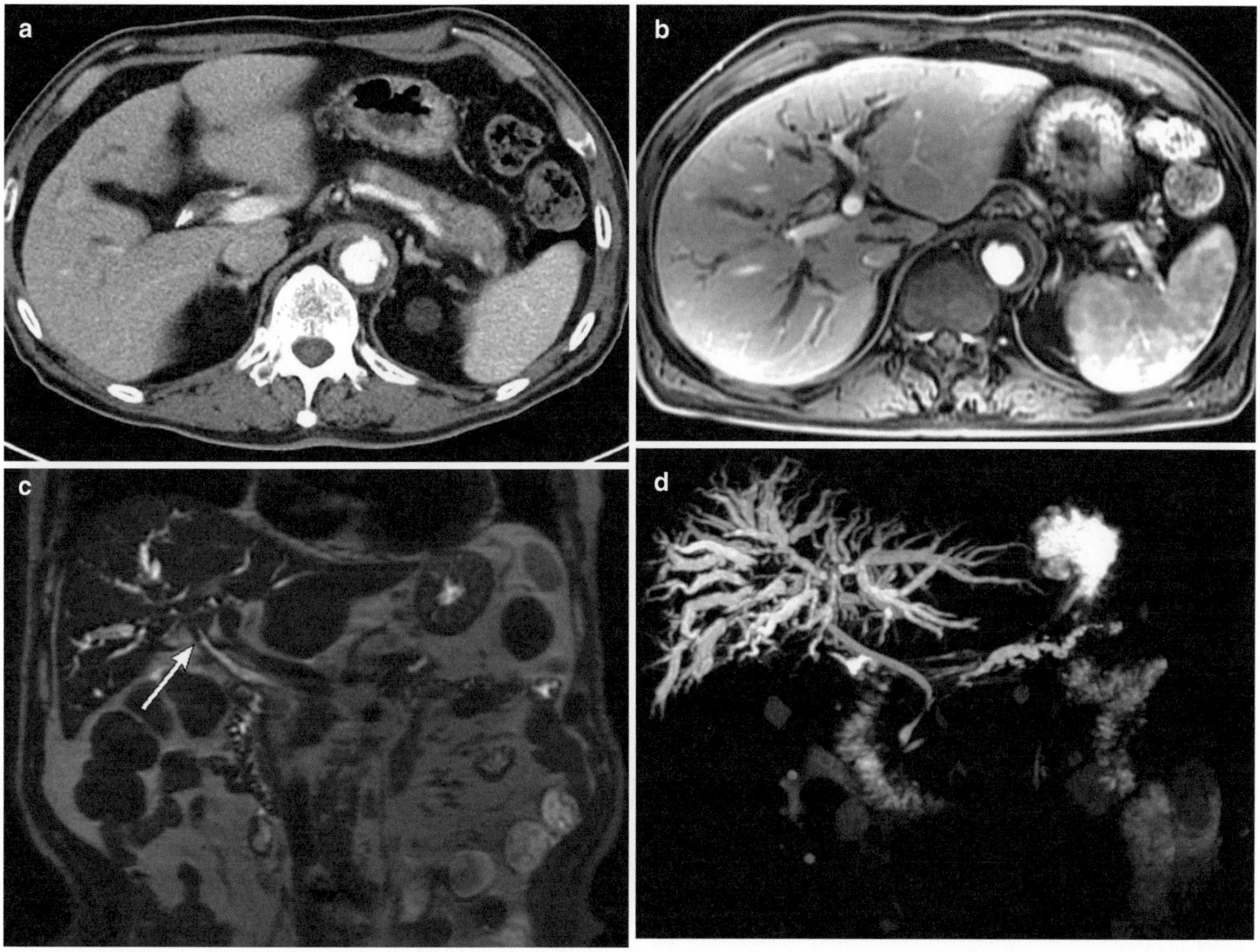

Fig. 11.6 A 71-year-old man presented with diffuse biliary dilatation. (**a**) On axial CT image, the pancreas shows mild enlargement with hypoattenuating capsule-like rim around the pancreas. (**b**) On axial contrast-enhanced T1-weighted image and (**c**) coronal T2-weighted MR image, long segmental luminal narrowing and wall thickening of the hilar duct (*arrow*) was noted at the hepatic hilum. (**d**) On MRCP, multifocal stenosis and dilatation of IHD and irregular stricture and dilatation of the main pancreatic duct

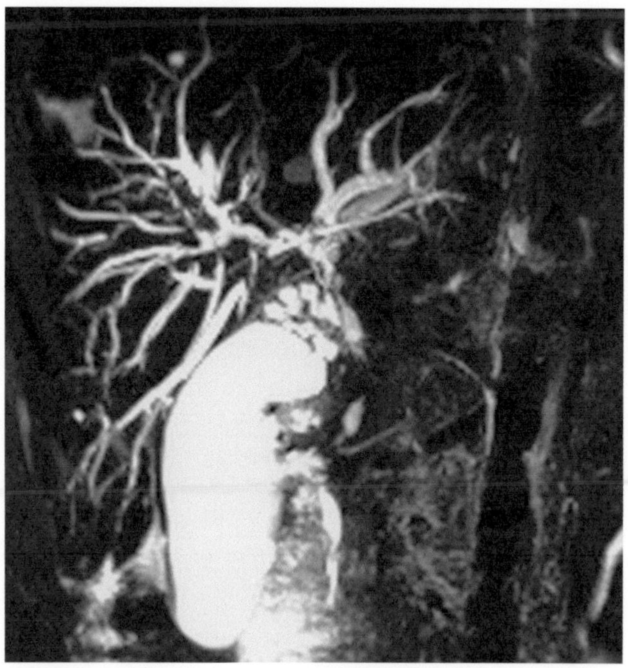

Fig. 11.7 A 41-year-old man with primary sclerosing cholangitis. MRCP image demonstrates beaded and prune-tree appearance of the intra- and extrahepatic bile ducts

References

1. Finkelberg DL, Sahani D, Deshpande V, Brugge WR. Autoimmune pancreatitis. N Engl J Med. 2006;355(25):2670–6.
2. Suzuki K, Itoh S, Nagasaka T, Ogawa H, Ota T, Naganawa S. CT findings in autoimmune pancreatitis: assessment using multiphase contrast-enhanced multisection CT. Clin Radiol. 2010;65(9):735–43.
3. Sahani DV, Kalva SP, Farrell J, et al. Autoimmune pancreatitis: imaging features. Radiology. 2004;233(2):345–52.
4. Okazaki K, Kawa S, Kamisawa T, et al. Japanese consensus guidelines for management of autoimmune pancreatitis: I. Concept and diagnosis of autoimmune pancreatitis. J Gastroenterol. 2010;45(3):249–65.
5. Shanbhogue AK, Fasih N, Surabhi VR, Doherty GP, Shanbhogue DK, Sethi SK. A clinical and radiologic review of uncommon types and causes of pancreatitis. Radiographics. 2009;29(4):1003–26.
6. Kawamoto S, Siegelman SS, Hruban RH, Fishman EK. Lymphoplasmacytic sclerosing pancreatitis (autoimmune pancreatitis): evaluation with multidetector CT. Radiographics. 2008;28(1):157–70.
7. Shimosegawa T, Chari ST, Frulloni L, et al. International consensus diagnostic criteria for autoimmune pancreatitis: guidelines of the International Association of Pancreatology. Pancreas. 2011;40(3):352–8.
8. Takahashi N, Fletcher JG, Hough DM, et al. Autoimmune pancreatitis: differentiation from pancreatic carcinoma and normal pancreas on the basis of enhancement characteristics at dual-phase CT. AJR Am J Roentgenol. 2009;193(2):479–84.
9. Ishigami K, Tajima T, Nishie A, et al. MRI findings of pancreatic lymphoma and autoimmune pancreatitis: a comparative study. Eur J Radiol. 2010;74(3):e22–8.
10. Kwak SW, Kim S, Lee JW, et al. Evaluation of unusual causes of pancreatitis: role of cross-sectional imaging. Eur J Radiol. 2009;71(2):296–312.
11. Kamisawa T, Tu Y, Egawa N, et al. Can MRCP replace ERCP for the diagnosis of autoimmune pancreatitis? Abdom Imaging. 2009;34(3):381–4.
12. Park SH, Kim MH, Kim SY, et al. Magnetic resonance cholangiopancreatography for the diagnostic evaluation of autoimmune pancreatitis. Pancreas. 2010;39(8):1191–8.
13. Kamisawa T, Yoshiike M, Egawa N, et al. Chronic pancreatitis in the elderly in Japan. Pancreatology. 2004;4(3–4):223–7; discussion 227–8.
14. Zhang L, Chari S, Smyrk TC, et al. Autoimmune pancreatitis (AIP) type 1 and type 2: an international consensus study on histopathologic diagnostic criteria. Pancreas. 2011;40(8):1172–9.
15. Divatia M, Kim SA, Ro JY. IgG4-related sclerosing disease, an emerging entity: a review of a multi-system disease. Yonsei Med J. 2012;53(1):15–34.
16. Kim JH, Kim MH, Byun JH, et al. Diagnostic strategy for differentiating autoimmune pancreatitis from pancreatic cancer: is an endoscopic retrograde pancreatography essential? Pancreas. 2012;41: 639–647
17. Taniguchi T, Kobayashi H, Nishikawa K, et al. Diffusion-weighted magnetic resonance imaging in autoimmune pancreatitis. Jpn J Radiol. 2009;27(3):138–42.
18. Kamisawa T, Takuma K, Anjiki H, et al. Differentiation of autoimmune pancreatitis from pancreatic cancer by diffusion-weighted MRI. Am J Gastroenterol. 2010;105(8):1870–5.
19. Loos M, Esposito I, Hedderich DM, et al. Autoimmune pancreatitis complicated by carcinoma of the pancreatobiliary system: a case report and review of the literature. Pancreas. 2011;40(1):151–4.
20. Takuma K, Kamisawa T, Tabata T, Inaba Y, Egawa N, Igarashi Y. Short-term and long-term outcomes of autoimmune pancreatitis. Eur J Gastroenterol Hepatol. 2011;23(2):146–52.
21. Vlachou PA, Khalili K, Jang HJ, Fischer S, Hirschfield GM, Kim TK. IgG4-related sclerosing disease: autoimmune pancreatitis and extrapancreatic manifestations. Radiographics. 2011;31(5):1379–402.
22. Welsch T, Kleeff J, Esposito I, Buchler MW, Friess H. Autoimmune pancreatitis associated with a large pancreatic pseudocyst. World J Gastroenterol. 2006;12(36):5904–6.
23. Gouyon B, Levy P, Ruszniewski P, et al. Predictive factors in the outcome of pseudocysts complicating alcoholic chronic pancreatitis. Gut. 1997;41(6):821–5.
24. Miller FH, Rini NJ, Keppke AL. MRI of adenocarcinoma of the pancreas. AJR Am J Roentgenol. 2006;187(4):W365–74.
25. Church NI, Pereira SP, Deheragoda MG, et al. Autoimmune pancreatitis: clinical and radiological features and objective response to steroid therapy in a UK series. Am J Gastroenterol. 2007;102(11):2417–25.
26. Ghazale A, Chari ST, Zhang L, et al. Immunoglobulin G4-associated cholangitis: clinical profile and response to therapy. Gastroenterology. 2008;134(3):706–15.
27. Sohn JH, Byun JH, Yoon SE, et al. Abdominal extrapancreatic lesions associated with autoimmune pancreatitis: radiological findings and changes after therapy. Eur J Radiol. 2008;67(3):497–507.
28. Nakazawa T, Ohara H, Sano H, et al. Cholangiography can discriminate sclerosing cholangitis with autoimmune pancreatitis from primary sclerosing cholangitis. Gastrointest Endosc. 2004;60(6):937–44.
29. Nishino T, Toki F, Oyama H, et al. Biliary tract involvement in autoimmune pancreatitis. Pancreas. 2005;30(1):76–82.
30. Kamisawa T, Egawa N, Nakajima H, Tsuruta K, Okamoto A. Extrapancreatic lesions in autoimmune pancreatitis. J Clin Gastroenterol. 2005;39(10):904–7.
31. Bodily KD, Takahashi N, Fletcher JG, et al. Autoimmune pancreatitis: pancreatic and extrapancreatic imaging findings. AJR Am J Roentgenol. 2009;192(2):431–7.
32. Kim JH, Byun JH, Kim SY, et al. Sclerosing cholangitis with autoimmune pancreatitis versus primary sclerosing cholangitis: comparison on endoscopic retrograde cholangiography, MR cholangiography, CT, and MRI. Acta Radiol. 2013;54(6):601–7.
33. Kim JH, Byun JH, Lee SJ, et al. Differential diagnosis of sclerosing cholangitis with autoimmune pancreatitis and periductal infiltrating cancer in the common bile duct at dynamic CT, endoscopic retrograde cholangiography and MR cholangiography. Eur Radiol. 2012;22(11):2502–13.

Endoscopy: ERCP and EUS

12

Tae Jun Song and Myung-Hwan Kim

Introduction

The diagnosis of autoimmune pancreatitis (AIP) still may be challenging. Major pancreatic resections continue to be performed for this benign disease, although surgeries for AIP have been dwindling as clinical experience increases. Until now, imaging of the pancreas and biliary tree with endoscopic retrograde cholangiopancreatography (ERCP) and endoscopic ultrasound (EUS) plays an important role in the diagnosis of AIP.

An international consensus diagnostic criteria and algorithms (ICDC) for AIP has been recently proposed, based on a consensus of expert opinion, to nonsurgically diagnose AIP and to avoid misdiagnosis of pancreatobiliary malignancies as AIP [1]. According to the ICDC, endoscopic evaluations including ERCP and EUS play a key role for the diagnosis of AIP and for the differentiation of AIP from pancreatic cancer. ERCP also plays a role in the relief of obstructive jaundice and also in the assessment of steroid responsiveness.

ERCP

Endoscopic Retrograde Pancreatography

The typical pancreatographic appearance of AIP has been reported as a diffusely attenuated duct with irregular wall (Fig. 12.1) [2–4]. An international multicenter study on ERP of AIP has identified 4 specific ERP features of AIP being useful in the differential diagnosis between AIP and pancreatic cancer: (1) a long (>1/3 the length of the pancreatic duct) stricture, (2) lack of upstream dilatation from the stricture (>5 mm) (Fig. 12.2), (3) multiple strictures, and (4) side branches arising from the stricture site [3]. Interestingly, the ability to diagnose AIP based on ERP features alone could be improved by awareness of these key features. In a recent study, the typical pancreatographic abnormalities seen in type 1 AIP also were seen in type 2 AIP with similar frequencies [5]. Particularly type 2 AIP benefits the most from diagnostic ERP because patients with type 2 AIP typically have normal levels of serum IgG4 and no OOI [6].

There has been substantial disparity between the Asian and the HISORt criteria in the use of ERP to diagnose AIP [7, 8]. The former mandates the use of an ERP to diagnose AIP, whereas the latter does not. According to a recent study, in which patients with AIP were divided into two subgroups according to CT features (typical vs. atypical), little incremental benefit was obtained from additional ERP in patients with typical CT features for AIP (diffuse pancreatic enlargement ± rim with homogeneous enhancement) [9]. On the other hand, in patients with atypical CT features (segmental/focal enlargement, marked dilatation/cutoff of the main pancreatic duct, or pancreatic mass), additional ERP could increase the sensitivity and specificity in distinguishing AIP from pancreatic cancer. In the clinical setting of suspected AIP, therefore, the use of ERP may be tailored depending on CT features. Actually, when initial CT fea-

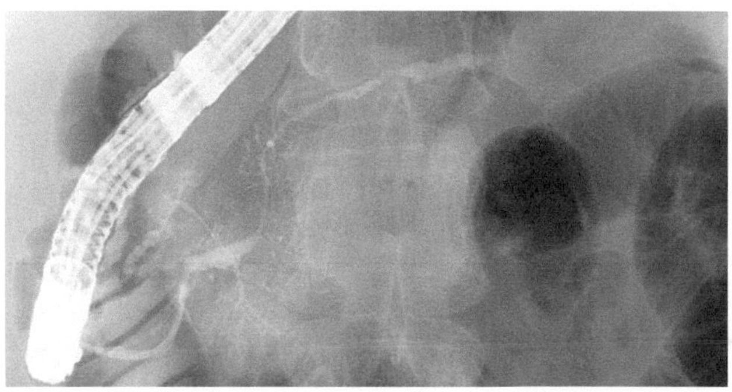

Fig. 12.1 Endoscopic retrograde pancreatography demonstrates a diffuse irregular narrowing of the main pancreatic duct in autoimmune pancreatitis

T.J. Song, MD, PhD • M.-H. Kim, MD, PhD (✉)
Department of Internal Medicine, Asan Medical Center, University of Ulsan College of Medicine, Asanbyeongwon-Gil 86, Songpa-Gu, Seoul 138-736, South Korea
e-mail: mhkim@amc.seoul.kr

T. Kamisawa, J.B. Chung (eds.), *Autoimmune Pancreatitis*,
DOI 10.1007/978-3-642-55086-7_12, © Springer-Verlag Berlin Heidelberg 2015

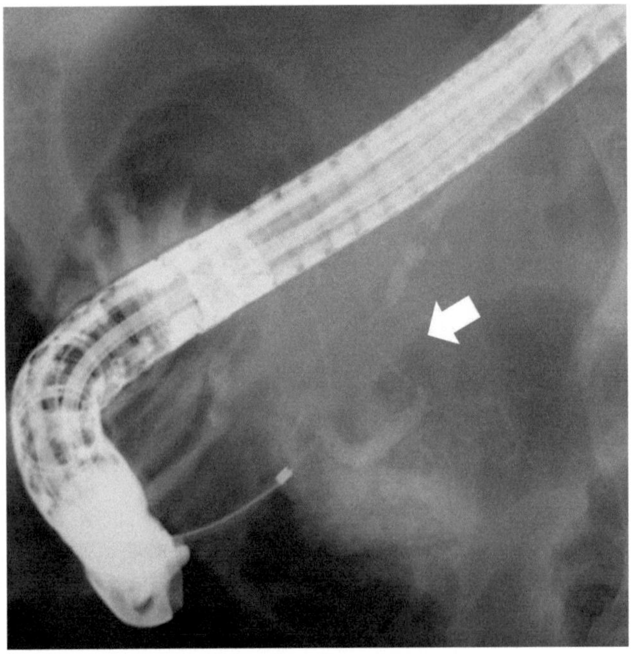

Fig. 12.2 Endoscopic retrograde pancreatography demonstrates a focal narrowing of the main pancreatic duct (*arrow*) at the pancreatic head in autoimmune pancreatitis. The upstream dilatation of the main pancreatic duct is mild (<5 mm)

tures are typical for AIP, the ICDC do not use ERP at all for differentiating AIP from pancreatic cancer. According to the ICDC, ERP is not usually used in cases with typical CT features and is only recommended in patients with atypical CT features or when there is no collateral evidence to support the diagnosis [1].

Many western endoscopists do not use ERP in patients with obstructive jaundice for fear of post-ERCP pancreatitis [1]. In the previous studies, however, there was no post-ERCP pancreatitis in patients with AIP [4, 5, 9]. One plausible explanation is that AIP is a unique form of chronic pancreatitis and that post-ERCP pancreatitis is rare in patients with chronic pancreatitis [10]. This may reflect a protective effect of chronic pancreatitis against post-ERCP pancreatitis due to fibrosis and decreased enzymatic activity.

Endoscopic Retrograde Cholangiography

AIP frequently accompanies the common bile duct (CBD) and the proximal bile duct involvement [11–13]. Biliary involvement of AIP or IgG4-related systemic disease is referred to as IgG4-SC and presents radiographically as bile duct strictures with ductal wall thickening [14, 15]. ERCP can reveal strictures of the biliary tree as well as the pancreatic duct. The most common feature of endoscopic retrograde cholangiography (ERC) is intrapancreatic CBD stricture, but proximal (hilar/intrahepatic) bile duct strictures may also be observed [11, 13]. IgG4-SC should be differentiated from primary sclerosing cholangitis (PSC), cholangiocarcinoma, and pancreatic cancer. Differential diagnosis depends on the location and characteristics of the biliary stricture. In cases with isolated intrapancreatic CBD strictures, differential diagnosis includes distal CBD cancer and pancreatic cancer [11, 16]. On the other hand, hilar cholangiocarcinoma and PSC should be differentiated in cases with intrahepatic/hilar bile duct strictures. Intrahepatic/hilar bile duct strictures can be an important clue for distinguishing AIP from pancreatic cancer [15, 17–19]. An international multicenter study reported that proximal bile duct strictures were detected in 20–79 % of AIP patients, whereas pancreatic cancer did not accompany proximal bile duct strictures [20].

Characteristic features of ERC may allow discrimination of IgG4-SC from PSC. Typical cholangiographic features for PSC include short annular or band-like strictures, diverticulum-like outpouching, and beaded or pruned-tree appearance, whereas these features are rarely observed in IgG4-SC [19, 21]. On the other hand, IgG4-SC has longer stricture and more prestenotic dilatation [15].

Characteristic cholangiographic features of IgG4-SC being useful in differential diagnosis from hilar cholangiocarcinoma are the following: symmetric (concentric) wall thickening, thickening of the bile duct wall (>1 mm) in a nonstenotic bile duct on ERC, smooth luminal surface and preservation of wall layer structure, multifocal strictures (skipped lesions), and mild proximal duct dilatation despite a long stricture [22]. Several clinical and radiological features other than cholangiography can also be helpful in differential diagnosis [11, 19]. The coexistence of pancreatic lesions (e.g., pancreatic enlargement) and OOI (e.g., salivary gland, kidney, or retroperitoneum) can further support the diagnosis of IgG4-SC [22].

Endobiliary biopsy for bile duct stricture may be helpful to exclude malignancy [19]. Endobiliary biopsy can be performed easily during endoscopic biliary drainage for obstructive jaundice [23]. Although the biopsy specimen is usually too small to observe the full spectrum of lymphoplasmacytic sclerosing histology, IgG4 immunostaining may provide further histologic support for the diagnosis of AIP/IgG4-SC. The sensitivity and specificity for IgG4 immunostaining of endobiliary biopsy specimens in the differential diagnosis between AIP/IgG4-SC and malignancy were 18–88 % and 9–100 %, respectively [11, 19, 24, 25]. Endobiliary biopsy for diagnosing AIP/IgG4-SC is included in the ICDC [1].

Duodenal Papillary Biopsy for IgG4 Immunostaining

Anatomically, the major duodenal papilla corresponds to the junction of the common bile duct and the main pancreatic duct and is often involved in AIP [26]. Kamisawa et al. first reported that positive IgG4 immunostaining in papillary biopsies was specific for AIP [27]. The sensitivity and specificity of positive IgG4 immunostaining of the major duodenal papilla were 52–80 % and 89–100 %, respectively [24, 27–29]. Significant adverse events such as bleeding or pancreatitis have not been reported during/after endoscopic biopsy of the major duodenal papilla. Positive IgG4 immunostaining of the major duodenal papilla occurs regardless of serum IgG4 level [29, 30]. Duodenal papillary biopsy with IgG4 immunostaining may, therefore, be attractive especially when AIP is clinically suspected, whereas serum IgG4 levels are normal or pancreatic core biopsy is not available [22].

The ICDC also recommend endoscopic biopsy of the major duodenal papilla at the time of ERCP [1]. In the ICDC, the presence of marked lymphoplasmacytic infiltrate and abundant IgG4-positive cells seen in duodenal papillary biopsy specimen is currently classified as level 2 OOI in diagnosing type 1 AIP.

Endoscopic Ultrasound

EUS is used to verify the presence or absence of a pancreatic mass. EUS is superior to multidetector CT for the diagnosis of small pancreatic neoplasms [31]. The negative predictive value of a normal EUS exam for pancreatic tumor detection is nearly 100 % [32]. EUS examination and EUS-FNA is highly recommended for patients who have atypical features of AIP because (1) EUS has excellent negative predictive value and can detect a small pancreatic cancer not visible on CT, and (2) EUS-FNA is the most reliable tool for excluding pancreatic cancer and avoiding unnecessary pancreatic surgery [22, 32]. For the diagnosis of pancreatic cancer, EUS-guided trucut biopsy (EUS-TCB) may not offer advantages over EUS-FNA; however, EUS-TCB should be considered when details of tissue architecture and immunostaining are required to establish a specific diagnosis [33]. EUS elastography and contrast-enhanced harmonic EUS may provide information complementary to conventional EUS imaging [22].

Conventional EUS Imaging

Although the role of EUS in the diagnosis of pancreatic cancer is well established, there is lack of evidence in the definite diagnosis of AIP. It is unclear if EUS imaging alone can reliably suggest definite diagnosis of AIP and differentiating between AIP and pancreatic cancer, since there are no pathognomonic findings suggestive of AIP on EUS. The lack of pathognomonic features and diverse spectrum of EUS imaging features limits the utility of EUS imaging alone

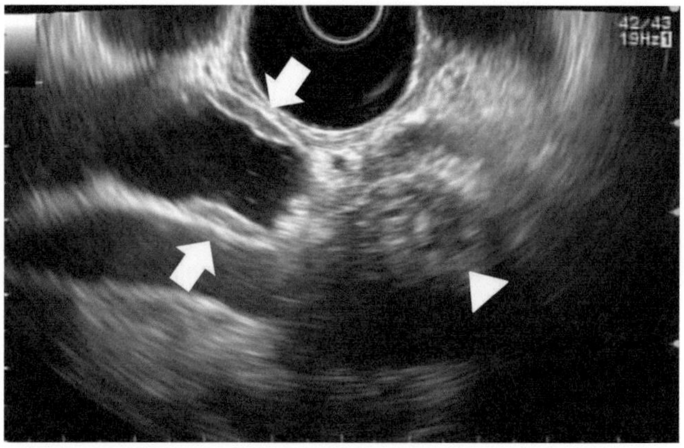

Fig. 12.3 EUS demonstrates an enlargement of pancreas head (*arrowhead*) and a wall thickening of dilated bile duct (*arrow*) in autoimmune pancreatitis

[34]. The reported EUS finding for AIP is diffuse hypoechoic pancreatic enlargement, sometimes with coarse hyperechoic inclusions, and a mass lesion mimicking pancreatic cancer may be observed [16, 34, 35]. In AIP, on EUS, ductal wall thickening commonly spreads continuously from intrapancreatic CBD to the suprapancreatic middle bile duct (Fig. 12.3). In contrast, on EUS finding of patients with pancreatic head cancer, bile duct wall thickening is observed only at the intrapancreatic area. Hoki et al. reported that the findings of diffuse hypoechoic areas, diffuse enlargement, bile duct wall thickening, and peripancreatic hypoechoic margins are more frequent in AIP than in pancreatic cancer [36]. On the other hand, a focal hypoechoic area and focal enlargement are significantly more common in pancreatic cancer.

EUS-FNA and Core Biopsy

Real-time EUS can guide cytology/biopsy, allowing distinction of benign from malignant lesions for the pancreatic mass [22]. The EUS-guided fine-needle aspiration (FNA) provides sensitivity of about 80–90 %, specificity of about 95–100 %, and accuracy of about 90–95 % in the differential diagnosis between benign pancreatic disease and pancreatic cancer [34, 37, 38]. Although diagnostic sensitivity of EUS-FNA for pancreatic cancer is very high, some of the difficulty may exist in cases with well-differentiated carcinoma, those with extensive necrosis, and those with a background of chronic pancreatitis [39–41]. We should remember that a negative result of cytology/biopsy is not a guarantee of benign disease; hence repeat EUS-FNA or short-term follow-up imaging to assess steroids responsiveness is necessary [8, 23]. Actually, AIP is much less common than pancreatobiliary malignancies such as pancreatic cancer or cholangiocarcinoma. It should be emphasized that repeat EUS-FNA is warranted in patients with high suspicion of pancreatobiliary malignancies despite negative results at initial EUS-FNA [39]. If the steroid responsiveness is negative or equivocal, a definitive diagnosis always should be pursued by surgical exploration or resection. In the ICDC, negative work-up for pancreatobiliary malignancies is a prerequisite for a steroids trial [1].

For the histological diagnosis of AIP, EUS-guided trucut biopsy (TCB) is necessary. The primary role of EUS-FNA in a diagnosis of AIP may be to exclude malignancy rather than to provide definitive histological evidence for AIP [42]. While EUS-FNA with a small caliber (22/25 gauge) provides only cytological samples, a TCB needle (19 gauge) can acquire larger tissue specimen preserving tissue architecture and can permit a nonsurgical diagnosis of AIP [34, 43, 44]. For establishing a diagnosis of pancreatic cancer, EUS-TCB does not offer advantage over EUS-FNA; however, EUS-TCB should be considered when details of tissue architecture and immunostaining are required to establish a specific diagnosis [5, 34, 43]. EUS-TCB is particularly useful for diagnosing type 2 AIP patients who are seronegative and lack of OOI [22]. Until now, EUS-TCB is only available in a few specialized tertiary-care centers and is often not technically feasible according to a location of mass/enlargement in the pancreas [1, 34, 45]. However, EUS-TCB is expected to become more widespread with the availability of newly developed core biopsy needles with enhanced flexibility and improved tissue acquisition [44]. Newly developed core biopsy needles can access all areas in the pancreas. This may attain two goals of histologic examination in one sitting with the use of the same needle: exclusion of pancreatic cancer and histological diagnosis of AIP.

EUS Elastography/Contrast-Enhanced Harmonic EUS

To overcome the limitations related to conventional EUS imaging, endosonographers have used several techniques including the characterization of tumor vascularization and estimation of elasticity distribution in normal and pathologic areas in the pancreas [46]. These imaging techniques can make EUS less operator dependent and improve the diagnostic yield of EUS-guided tissue sampling by selecting the most suspicious area of a tumor.

Elastography noninvasively gather informations about the relative hardness of the examined lesions compared with the surrounding tissues [47–49]. The premise is that malignant tumors are of harder consistency than benign ones. In a study by Dietrich et al., elastographic imaging of pancreatic cancer showed a markedly firmer area confined to the site of the low-echoic mass area, while in AIP cases, the hard area was not restricted to the mass lesion (Fig. 12.4).

Contrast-enhanced EUS use contrast agents to provide perfusion imaging [46, 50]. The contrast agent creates microbubbles and enhances the Doppler signal. Therefore, it can enable the depiction of microvessels and give imaging of vascularization. Contrast-enhanced EUS may increase the diagnostic accuracy in distinguishing AIP from pancreatic cancer by characterization of microvasculature inside the organ. According to a recent study on contrast-enhanced EUS, the lesions of AIP typically appeared as hypervascularization, whereas hypoechoic tumors caused by pancreatic cancer appeared as hypovascular masses (Fig. 12.5) [50, 51].

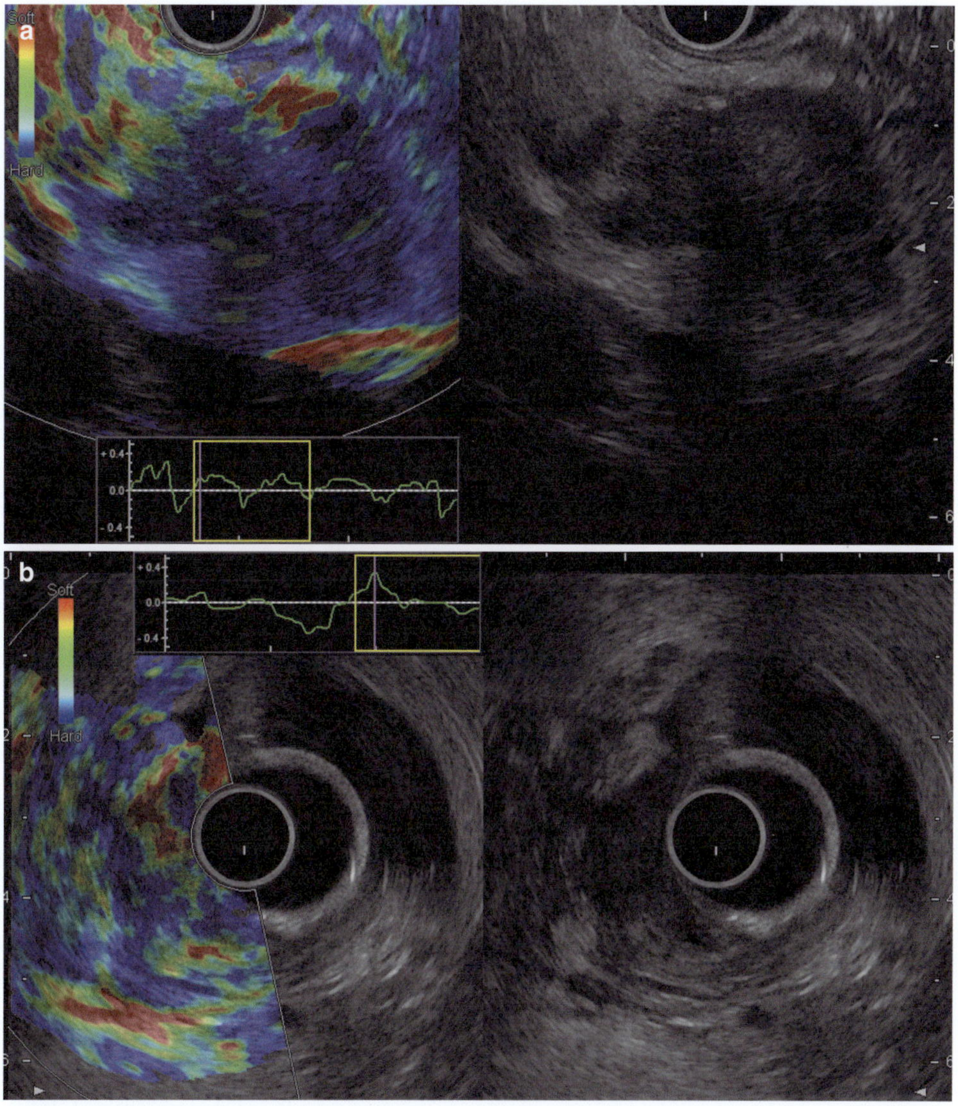

Fig. 12.4 (**a**) EUS elastography demonstrates the very hard area (*blue*) with soft spots (*yellow*) inside the tumor, which proved to be irregularly dilated cancer ducts surrounded cancerous fibrous tissue in pancreatic cancer. (**b**) EUS elastography in autoimmune pancreatitis demonstrates the random color signals apparently different from those of pancreatic cancer

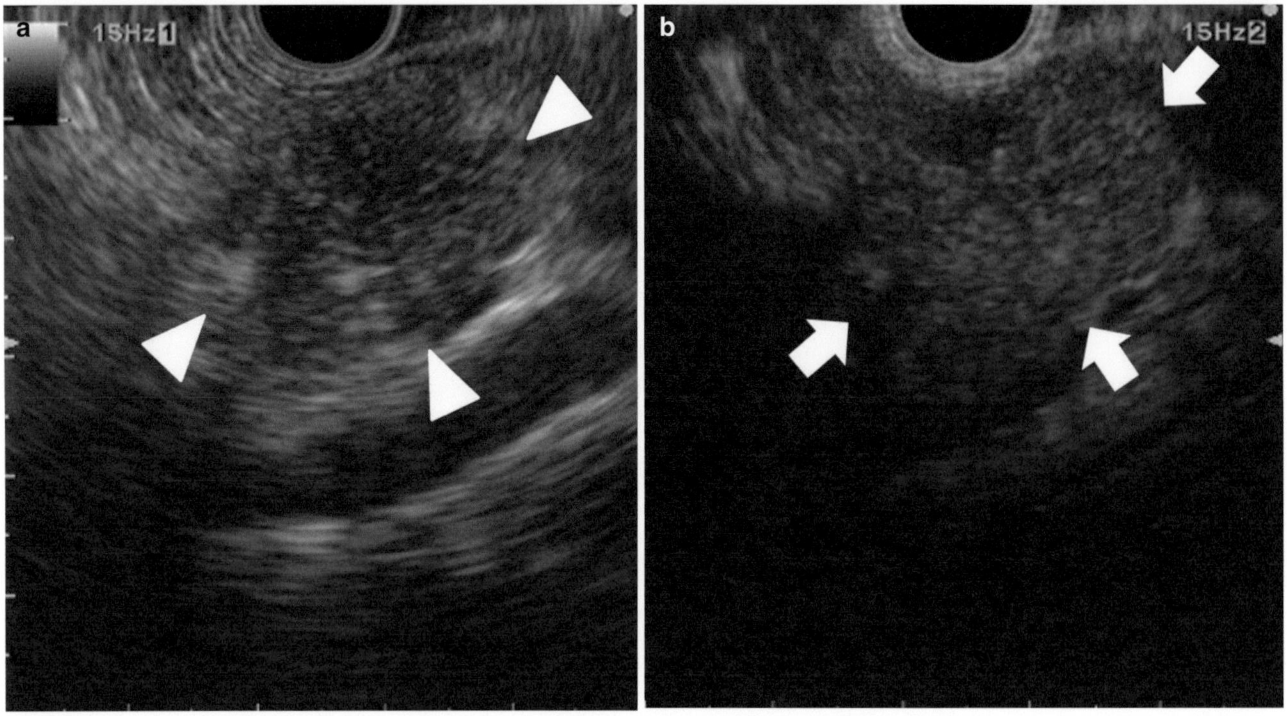

Fig. 12.5 (**a**) EUS demonstrates a low-echoic mass (*arrowheads*) at the pancreas body. (**b**) Contrast-enhanced harmonic EUS demonstrates a homogeneous iso-enhancement in the mass in autoimmune pancreatitis

Conclusion

Diverse endoscopic techniques are being used for the purpose of diagnosis and differential diagnosis between AIP and pancreatobiliary malignancies. Both ERCP and EUS are the key procedures of endoscopic evaluation for AIP. Some ERCP and EUS findings can be particularly useful for differentiating from pancreatic cancer in those with atypical CT features of AIP. The endoscopists are necessary to be fully aware of the advantages, disadvantages, strengths, and limitations of the various endoscopic tests and to use these tools properly. The role of ERCP and EUS in the initial evaluation and diagnosis of patients with suspected AIP continues to evolve.

Acknowledgment The authors are grateful to Dr. Yoshiki Hirooka (Nagoya University, Japan) for providing beautiful figures of EUS elastography and to Dr. Masayuki Kitano (Kinki University, Japan) for providing beautiful figures of contrast-enhanced EUS.

References

1. Shimosegawa T, Chari ST, Frulloni L, et al. International consensus diagnostic criteria for autoimmune pancreatitis: guidelines of the International Association of Pancreatology. Pancreas. 2011;40:352–8.
2. Kim KP, Kim MH, Song MH, et al. Autoimmune chronic pancreatitis. Am J Gastroenterol. 2004;99:1605–16.
3. Sugumar A, Levy MJ, Kamisawa T, et al. Endoscopic retrograde pancreatography criteria to diagnose autoimmune pancreatitis: an international multicentre study. Gut. 2011;60:666–70.
4. Horiuchi A, Kawa S, Hamano H, et al. ERCP features in 27 patients with autoimmune pancreatitis. Gastrointest Endosc. 2002;55:494–9.
5. Song TJ, Kim JH, Kim MH, et al. Comparison of clinical findings between histologically confirmed type 1 and type 2 autoimmune pancreatitis. J Gastroenterol Hepatol. 2012;27:700–8.
6. Lerch MM, Mayerle J. The benefits of diagnostic ERCP in autoimmune pancreatitis. Gut. 2011;60:565–6.
7. Otsuki M, Chung JB, Okazaki K, et al. Asian diagnostic criteria for autoimmune pancreatitis: consensus of the Japan-Korea Symposium on Autoimmune Pancreatitis. J Gastroenterol. 2008;43:403–8.
8. Chari ST, Takahashi N, Levy MJ, et al. A diagnostic strategy to distinguish autoimmune pancreatitis from pancreatic cancer. Clin Gastroenterol Hepatol. 2009;7:1097–103.
9. Kim JH, Kim MH, Byun JH, et al. Diagnostic strategy for differentiating autoimmune pancreatitis from pancreatic cancer: is an endoscopic retrograde pancreatography essential? Pancreas. 2012;41:639–47.
10. Freeman ML, DiSario JA, Nelson DB, et al. Risk factors for post-ERCP pancreatitis: a prospective, multicenter study. Gastrointest Endosc. 2001;54:425–34.
11. Ghazale A, Chari ST, Zhang L, et al. Immunoglobulin G4-associated cholangitis: clinical profile and response to therapy. Gastroenterology. 2008;134:706–15.
12. Kamisawa T, Kim MH, Liao WC, et al. Clinical characteristics of 327 Asian patients with autoimmune pancreatitis based on Asian diagnostic criteria. Pancreas. 2011;40:200–5.
13. Nishino T, Toki F, Oyama H, et al. Biliary tract involvement in autoimmune pancreatitis. Pancreas. 2005;30:76–82.
14. Nakazawa T, Ohara H, Sano H, et al. Schematic classification of sclerosing cholangitis with autoimmune pancreatitis by cholangiography. Pancreas. 2006;32:229.

15. Nakazawa T, Naitoh I, Hayashi K, et al. Diagnostic criteria for IgG4-related sclerosing cholangitis based on cholangiographic classification. J Gastroenterol. 2012;47:79–87.
16. Kawa S, Okazaki K, Kamisawa T, et al. Japanese consensus guidelines for management of autoimmune pancreatitis: II. Extrapancreatic lesions, differential diagnosis. J Gastroenterol. 2010;45:355–69.
17. Nishino T, Oyama H, Toki F, et al. Differentiation between autoimmune pancreatitis and pancreatic carcinoma based on endoscopic retrograde cholangiopancreatography findings. J Gastroenterol. 2010;45:988–96.
18. Chari ST, Smyrk TC, Levy MJ, et al. Diagnosis of autoimmune pancreatitis: the Mayo Clinic experience. Clinical Gastroenterol Hepatol. 2006;4:1010–6; quiz 934.
19. Oh HC, Kim MH, Lee KT, et al. Clinical clues to suspicion of IgG4-associated sclerosing cholangitis disguised as primary sclerosing cholangitis or hilar cholangiocarcinoma. J Gastroenterol Hepatol. 2010;25:1831–7.
20. Kamisawa T, Chari ST, Giday SA, et al. Clinical profile of autoimmune pancreatitis and its histological subtypes: an international multicenter survey. Pancreas. 2011;40:809–14.
21. Nakazawa T, Ohara H, Sano H, et al. Cholangiography can discriminate sclerosing cholangitis with autoimmune pancreatitis from primary sclerosing cholangitis. Gastrointest Endosc. 2004;60:937–44.
22. Moon SH, Kim MH. The role of endoscopy in the diagnosis of autoimmune pancreatitis. Gastrointest Endosc. 2012;76:645–56.
23. Moon SH, Kim MH, Park DH, et al. Is a 2-week steroid trial after initial negative investigation for malignancy useful in differentiating autoimmune pancreatitis from pancreatic cancer? A prospective outcome study. Gut. 2008;57:1704–12.
24. Kawakami H, Zen Y, Kuwatani M, et al. IgG4-related sclerosing cholangitis and autoimmune pancreatitis: histological assessment of biopsies from Vater's ampulla and the bile duct. J Gastroenterol Hepatol. 2010;25:1648–55.
25. Naitoh I, Nakazawa T, Ohara H, et al. Endoscopic transpapillary intraductal ultrasonography and biopsy in the diagnosis of IgG4-related sclerosing cholangitis. J Gastroenterol. 2009;44:1147–55.
26. Kim MH, Moon SH, Kamisawa T. Major duodenal papilla in autoimmune pancreatitis. Dig Surg. 2010;27:110–4.
27. Kamisawa T, Tu Y, Egawa N, et al. A new diagnostic endoscopic tool for autoimmune pancreatitis. Gastrointest Endosc. 2008;68:358–61.
28. Kubota K, Kato S, Akiyama T, et al. Differentiating sclerosing cholangitis caused by autoimmune pancreatitis and primary sclerosing cholangitis according to endoscopic duodenal papillary features. Gastrointest Endosc. 2008;68:1204–8.
29. Moon SH, Kim MH, Park do H, et al. IgG4 immunostaining of duodenal papillary biopsy specimens may be useful for supporting a diagnosis of autoimmune pancreatitis. Gastrointest Endosc. 2010;71:960–6.
30. Deheragoda MG, Church NI, Rodriguez-Justo M, et al. The use of immunoglobulin g4 immunostaining in diagnosing pancreatic and extrapancreatic involvement in autoimmune pancreatitis. Clin Gastroenterol Hepatol. 2007;5:1229–34.
31. DeWitt J, Devereaux B, Chriswell M, et al. Comparison of endoscopic ultrasonography and multidetector computed tomography for detecting and staging pancreatic cancer. Ann Intern Med. 2004;141:753–63.
32. Klapman JB, Chang KJ, Lee JG, et al. Negative predictive value of endoscopic ultrasound in a large series of patients with a clinical suspicion of pancreatic cancer. Am J Gastroenterol. 2005;100:2658–61.
33. Polkowski M, Larghi A, Weynand B, et al. Learning, techniques, and complications of endoscopic ultrasound (EUS)-guided sampling in gastroenterology: European Society of Gastrointestinal Endoscopy (ESGE) Technical Guideline. Endoscopy. 2012;44:190–206.
34. Levy MJ, Wiersema MJ, Chari ST. Chronic pancreatitis: focal pancreatitis or cancer? Is there a role for FNA/biopsy? Autoimmune pancreatitis. Endoscopy. 2006;38 Suppl 1:S30–5.
35. Farrell JJ, Garber J, Sahani D, et al. EUS findings in patients with autoimmune pancreatitis. Gastrointest Endosc. 2004;60:927–36.
36. Hoki N, Mizuno N, Sawaki A, et al. Diagnosis of autoimmune pancreatitis using endoscopic ultrasonography. J Gastroenterol. 2009;44:154–9.
37. Zhang MM, Yang H, Jin ZD, et al. Differential diagnosis of pancreatic cancer from normal tissue with digital imaging processing and pattern recognition based on a support vector machine of EUS images. Gastrointest Endosc. 2010;72:978–85.
38. Wiersema MJ, Vilmann P, Giovannini M, et al. Endosonography-guided fine-needle aspiration biopsy: diagnostic accuracy and complication assessment. Gastroenterology. 1997;112:1087–95.
39. Eloubeidi MA, Varadarajulu S, Desai S, et al. Value of repeat endoscopic ultrasound-guided fine needle aspiration for suspected pancreatic cancer. J Gastroenterol Hepatol. 2008;23:567–70.
40. Fritscher-Ravens A, Brand L, Knofel WT, et al. Comparison of endoscopic ultrasound-guided fine needle aspiration for focal pancreatic lesions in patients with normal parenchyma and chronic pancreatitis. Am J Gastroenterol. 2002;97:2768–75.
41. Varadarajulu S, Tamhane A, Eloubeidi MA. Yield of EUS-guided FNA of pancreatic masses in the presence or the absence of chronic pancreatitis. Gastrointest Endosc. 2005;62:728–36; quiz 51, 53.
42. Finkelberg DL, Sahani D, Deshpande V, et al. Autoimmune pancreatitis. N Engl J Med. 2006;355:2670–6.
43. Mizuno N, Bhatia V, Hosoda W, et al. Histological diagnosis of autoimmune pancreatitis using EUS-guided trucut biopsy: a comparison study with EUS-FNA. J Gastroenterol. 2009;44:742–50.
44. Iglesias-Garcia J, Poley JW, Larghi A, et al. Feasibility and yield of a new EUS histology needle: results from a multicenter, pooled, cohort study. Gastrointest Endosc. 2011;73:1189–96.
45. Levy MJ. Endoscopic ultrasound-guided trucut biopsy of the pancreas: prospects and problems. Pancreatology. 2007;7:163–6.
46. Fusaroli P, Saftoiu A, Mancino MG, et al. Techniques of image enhancement in EUS (with videos). Gastrointest Endosc. 2011;74:645–55.
47. Hirooka Y, Itoh A, Kawashima H, et al. Diagnosis of pancreatic disorders using contrast-enhanced endoscopic ultrasonography and endoscopic elastography. Clin Gastroenterology Hepatol. 2009;7:S63–7.
48. Dietrich CF, Hirche TO, Ott M, et al. Real-time tissue elastography in the diagnosis of autoimmune pancreatitis. Endoscopy. 2009;41:718–20.
49. Janssen J, Schlorer E, Greiner L. EUS elastography of the pancreas: feasibility and pattern description of the normal pancreas, chronic pancreatitis, and focal pancreatic lesions. Gastrointest Endosc. 2007;65:971–8.
50. Hocke M, Ignee A, Dietrich CF. Contrast-enhanced endoscopic ultrasound in the diagnosis of autoimmune pancreatitis. Endoscopy. 2011;43:163–5.
51. Hocke M, Ignee A, Dietrich CF. Three-dimensional contrast-enhanced endoscopic ultrasound for the diagnosis of autoimmune pancreatitis. Endoscopy. 2011;43(Suppl 2 UCTN):E381–2.

13 A Role of PET/CT in the Diagnosis of Autoimmune Pancreatitis

Nobumasa Mizuno and Kenji Yamao

Introduction

Autoimmune pancreatitis (AIP) is a special entity of chronic pancreatitis of presumed autoimmune etiology that is associated with characteristic clinical, histological, and morphological findings [1, 2]. Over the last decade, significant progress has been made in understanding this disease, including identification of two distinct histological subtypes with different clinical phenotypes (termed type 1 and type 2 AIP), incorporation of seemingly unrelated diseases within the spectrum of IgG4-related disease [2–4]. Despite advances, many questions remain unanswered. Among the remaining questions, distinguishing AIP from pancreatic cancer is still challenging. AIP mimics pancreatic cancer in terms of clinical features, such as advanced age, painless jaundice, weight loss, new-onset diabetes mellitus, and the presence of a mass lesion of the pancreas [1, 5].

Positron-emission tomography (PET) is a functional imaging modality that has shown promise in tumor depiction, but it is unable to provide detailed, high-spatial-resolution images [6]. PET/CT combines the functional information of PET with the detailed anatomic information of CT [7]. To date, several studies have been conducted to assess the utility of PET or PET/CT in the diagnosis of AIP. In this chapter, we review the clinical impact of PET and PET/CT in the diagnosis of AIP, especially in its differentiation from pancreatic cancer.

Positron-Emission Tomography (PET)

^{18}F-fluorodeoxyglucose positron-emission tomography (FDG-PET), a functional and molecular imaging modality, is widely used for the diagnosis of pancreatic cancer [7]. Integrated PET/CT scanners produce both PET and CT images of the entire body in one setting.

Malignant lesions generally show avid FDG uptake, whereas most benign lesions are characterized by normal or minimally increased FDG accumulation. In distinguishing mass-forming pancreatitis from pancreatic cancer, several studies have shown that PET is better for characterizing tissue than contrast material-enhanced CT [7]. PET or PET/CT imaging findings in patients with AIP have been explored in a small number of studies. In these studies, FDG uptake was increased in patients with AIP [5, 8, 9]. The accumulation of FDG in inflammatory diseases is based on high uptake in activated granulocytes. Transport of FDG across the cellular membrane is mediated by the glucose transporter (GLUT) proteins, which are also present in a higher amount on the cell membranes of inflammatory and infectious cells.

Pancreatic Imaging of PET

Pancreatic cancer is the most important disease to distinguish from AIP, and we review the pancreatic imaging with PET. Ozaki et al. reported that the prevalence and manner of FDG accumulation in the pancreatic lesions were significantly different between autoimmune pancreatitis and pancreatic cancer [9]. In their study, FDG uptake was found in all 15 patients with autoimmune pancreatitis, whereas it was found in 19 of 26 patients (73.1 %) with pancreatic cancer. A Korean group reported the similar result [5]. ^{18}F-FDG uptake by the pancreas was found in all (17/17) patients with autoimmune pancreatitis and in 82 % (124/151) of patients with pancreatic cancer. Overall, the frequency of FDG uptake did not differ between the two conditions. However, diffusely increased FDG uptake by the pancreas may be a characteristic PET/CT finding of AIP. Lee et al. reported that diffuse FDG uptake by the pancreas was significantly more frequent in patients with autoimmune pancreatitis than in pancreatic cancer (53 % vs. 3 %, $p<0.001$) [5]. In their study, there

N. Mizuno, MD, PhD (✉) • K. Yamao, MD, PhD
Department of Gastroenterology, Aichi Cancer Center Hospital, 1-1 Kanokoden, Chikusa-ku, Nagoya 464-8681, Japan
e-mail: nobumasa@aichi-cc.jp

T. Kamisawa, J.B. Chung (eds.), *Autoimmune Pancreatitis*,
DOI 10.1007/978-3-642-55086-7_13,

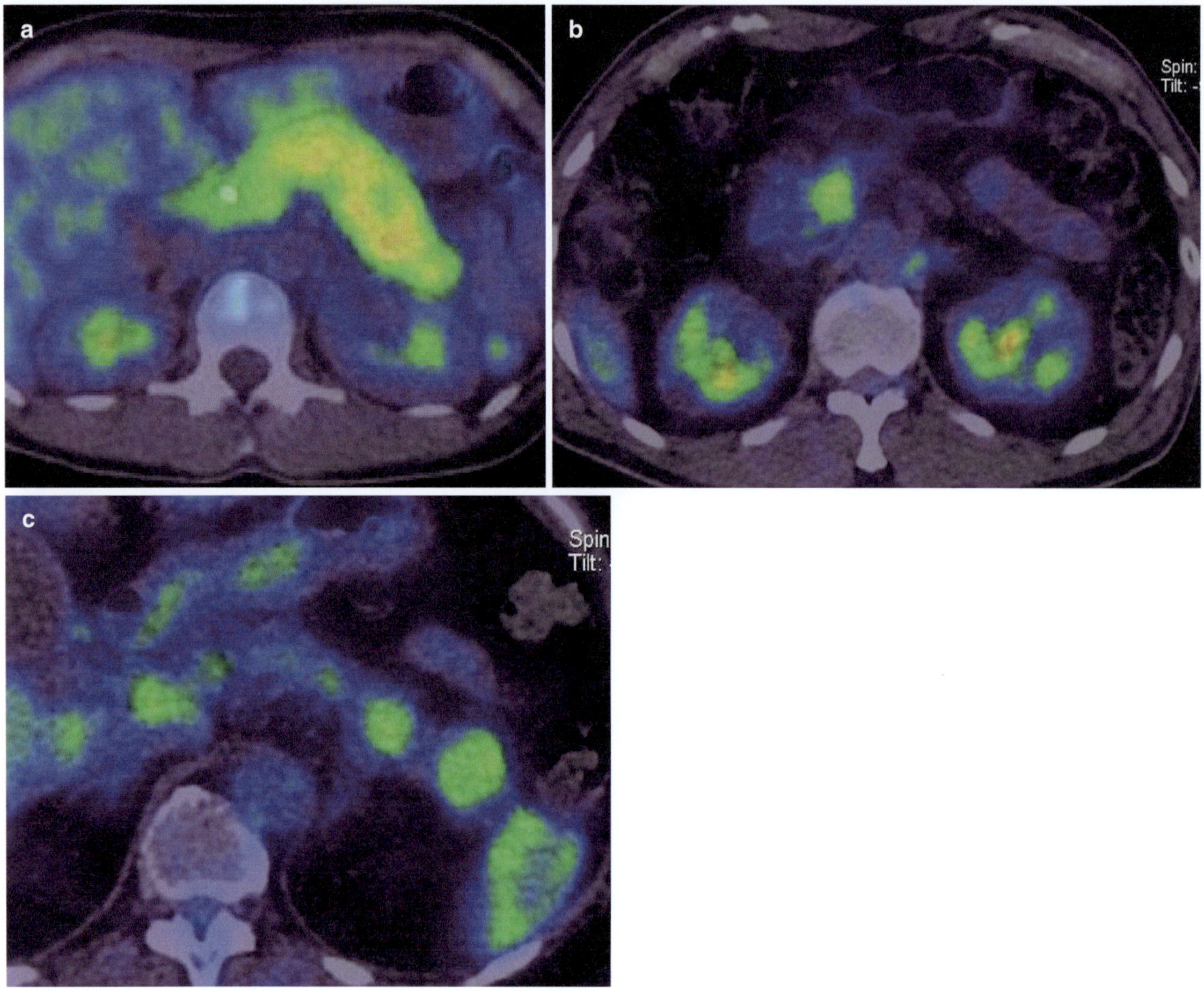

Fig. 13.1 FDG uptake pattern of the pancreas. (**a**) Diffuse uptake; (**b**) solitary uptake; and (**c**) multifocal uptake

Table 13.1 FDG uptake pattern in the pancreas

	AIP	Pancreatic cancer	
Diffuse	12 (50 %)	3 (12 %)	$P<0.001$
Solitary	9 (36 %)	21 (88 %)	
Multifocal	3 (14 %)	0(0 %)	

was no significant difference between AIP and pancreatic cancer in terms of SUV_{max} and segmental distribution. On the other hand, heterogeneous FDG accumulation in the pancreas may be helpful in distinguishing AIP from pancreatic cancer [9]. In our study, diffuse FDG uptake was more likely in AIP than in pancreatic cancer, but diffuse FDG uptake was found in patients with pancreatic cancer (unpublished data Fig. 13.1 and Table 13.1). Thus, careful attention is necessary when evaluating the FDG uptake pattern in the pancreas to discriminate AIP from pancreatic cancer.

Other Organ Involvement

The presence of extrapancreatic lesions, in other words, other organ involvement (OOI), is categorized as one of the cardinal features of type 1 AIP in the International Consensus Diagnostic Criteria for Autoimmune Pancreatitis (ICDC) [2, 3, 10, 11]. OOI is also part of the manifestation of IgG4-related systemic disease. OOI may be diagnosed by histological evaluation of tissue, by imaging (proximal bile duct stricture, retroperitoneal fibrosis), or by clinical examination (salivary gland enlargement). Concomitant extrapancreatic FDG uptake by other organs, such as the salivary glands and bile duct, has been shown to be indicative of systemic disease [5, 7, 8]. Lee et al. reported that abnormal FDG uptake by extrapancreatic lesions was found in 12 of the 17 patients (70 %). The salivary gland was the most frequent site of FDG uptake, followed by the retroperitoneal space, kidneys, thyroid, hilar lymph nodes,

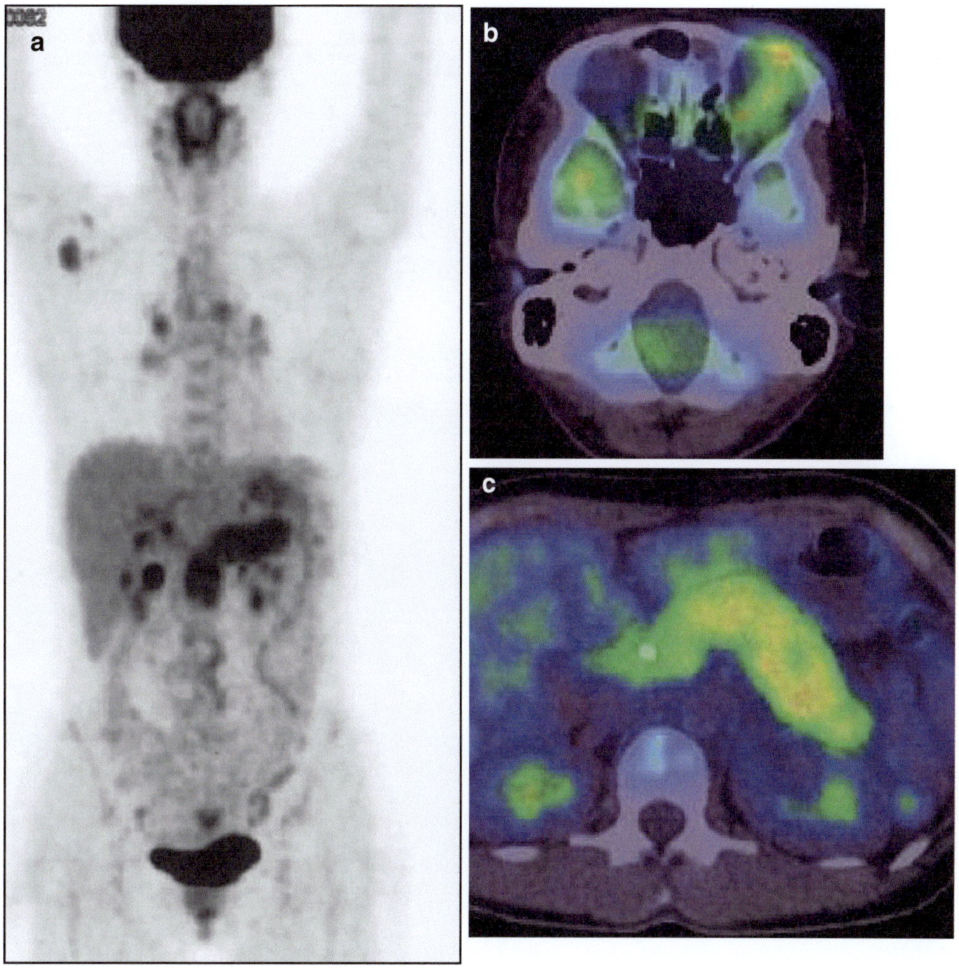

Fig. 13.2 FDG uptake in the intra- and extrapancreatic lesions. (**a**) FDG uptake in the pancreas and axillary and mediastinal lymph nodes; (**b**) FDG uptake in the left lacrimal gland; and (**c**) diffuse FDG uptake in the pancreas

bile ducts, and lungs [5]. The diagnostic impact of PET for OOI was evaluated in some studies. Ozaki et al. compared PET findings between AIP and pancreatic cancer [9]. Hilar lymph node involvement was significantly more frequent in patients with AIP than in those with pancreatic cancer; however, there was no significant difference in lacrimal gland, salivary gland, biliary duct, and retroperitoneal space involvement. The prevalence of OOI differs across studies, because PET/CT findings in patients with AIP have been explored in only a small number of studies. In any case, extrapancreatic FDG uptake concomitant with pancreatic uptake may support a diagnosis of AIP (Fig. 13.2).

Response to Steroids

In some cases, it is difficult to distinguish AIP from pancreatic cancer even after a negative workup for pancreatic cancer. In cases of AIP, steroids would result in a definitive improvement of imaging abnormalities, including biliary strictures and pancreatic enlargement. Steroids are indicated under the following circumstances: (1) patients with typical imaging findings who have appropriate collateral findings of AIP or (2) patients without typical imaging findings who have a negative workup for cancer and have appropriate collateral evidence of AIP [12]. The recommended duration of steroid therapy is 2 weeks based on the study by Moon et al., the only study which has examined this issue [2, 13]. Response to steroid therapy was assessed using morphologic imaging modalities such as CT, ERP, and/or MRCP in their study. FDG-PET is a functional imaging modality that reflects the severity of inflammation and regression of inflammation after steroid therapy. We evaluated changes in FDG uptake before and after steroid therapy in 6 patients with AIP and in 3 patients with pancreatic cancer [14]. Changes in FDG uptake in pancreatic and extrapancreatic lesions were estimated semiquantitatively and visually within 1 week. FDG uptake was dramatically decreased within a week in most cases of AIP (5/6) (Table 13.2 and Fig. 13.3), whereas FDG uptake was unchanged or increased in cases of pancreatic cancer (Fig. 13.4). Our study indicates that FDG-PET may allow a more rapid (within 1 week) and objective assessment of the response to steroids, as compared with morphological imaging modalities.

Table 13.2 Changes of SUVmax before and after steroid therapy

	Age/gender	Pre SUV_{max}	Post SUV_{max}	Interval (days)	Changes in SUV_{max} (%)
AIP-1	66/M	9.46	4.27	43	−54.7
AIP-2	43/M	9.41	4.29	2	−54.4
AIP-3	74/M	5.24	3.08	7	−41.2
AIP-4	55/F	8.95	7.25	4	−19.0
AIP-5	41/F	10.50	3.26	3	−68.9
AIP-6	75/M	5.07	5.49	4	8.30
PC-1	62/F	2.80	7.88	5	181
PC-2	76/M	9.11	8.70	3	−4.50
PC-3	59/M	5.10	5.97	4	17.1

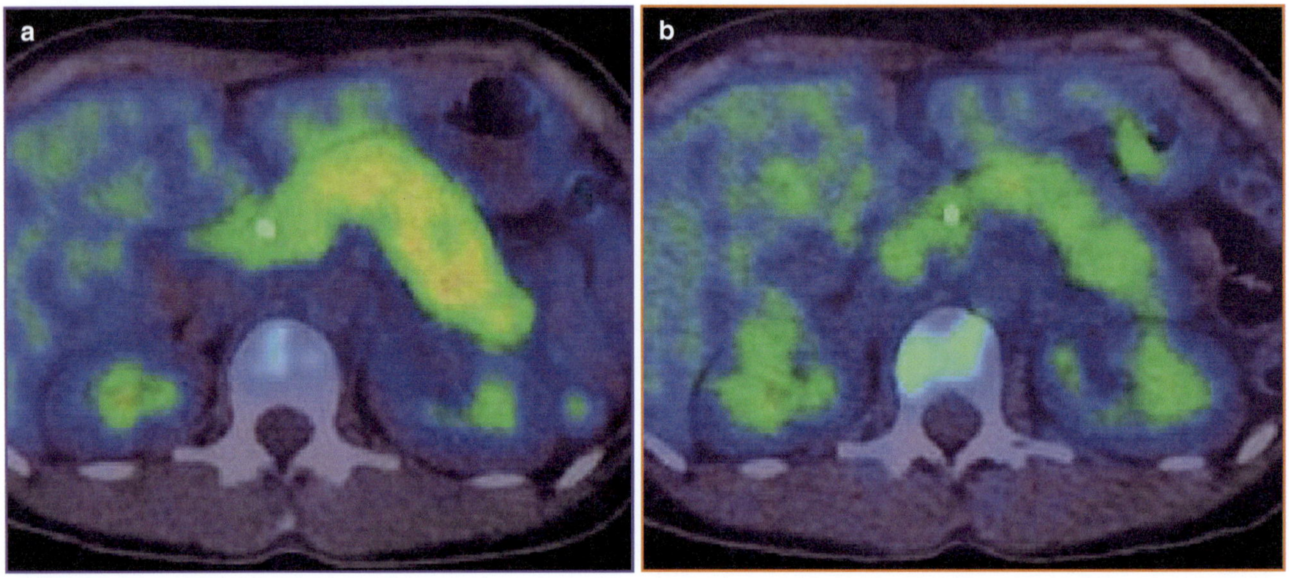

Fig. 13.3 Change in FDG uptake before and after steroid therapy in patients with AIP. (**a**) Before steroid and (**b**) after steroid

PET/CT Findings of AIP by Subtypes

The ICDC defines two distinct subtypes of AIP, type 1 and type 2 AIP [2]. Type 1 AIP is regarded as part of the IgG4-RD spectrum. Lymphoplasmacytic sclerosing pancreatitis (LPSP) is a pathological feature of type I AIP; it is characterized by infiltration of tissues with IgG4-positive plasma cells, fibrosis with subsequent irregular narrowing of the main pancreatic duct, and obliterative phlebitis. Serum IgG4 is increased in most patients with type 1 AIP. On the other hand, neutrophilic infiltration within the lumen and epithelium of interlobular ducts is a characteristic pathological feature of type 2 AIP. Type 2 AIP patients are less likely to show elevated serum IgG4 levels and IgG4-related extrapancreatic sclerosing lesions. This concept of two subtypes of AIP has been established recently [1, 2, 15]. In addition, the definitive diagnosis of type 2 AIP requires pancreatic histology provided by surgical resection or core biopsy. Therefore, most reports focused on PET or PET/CT findings of AIP regardless of its distinct subtype.

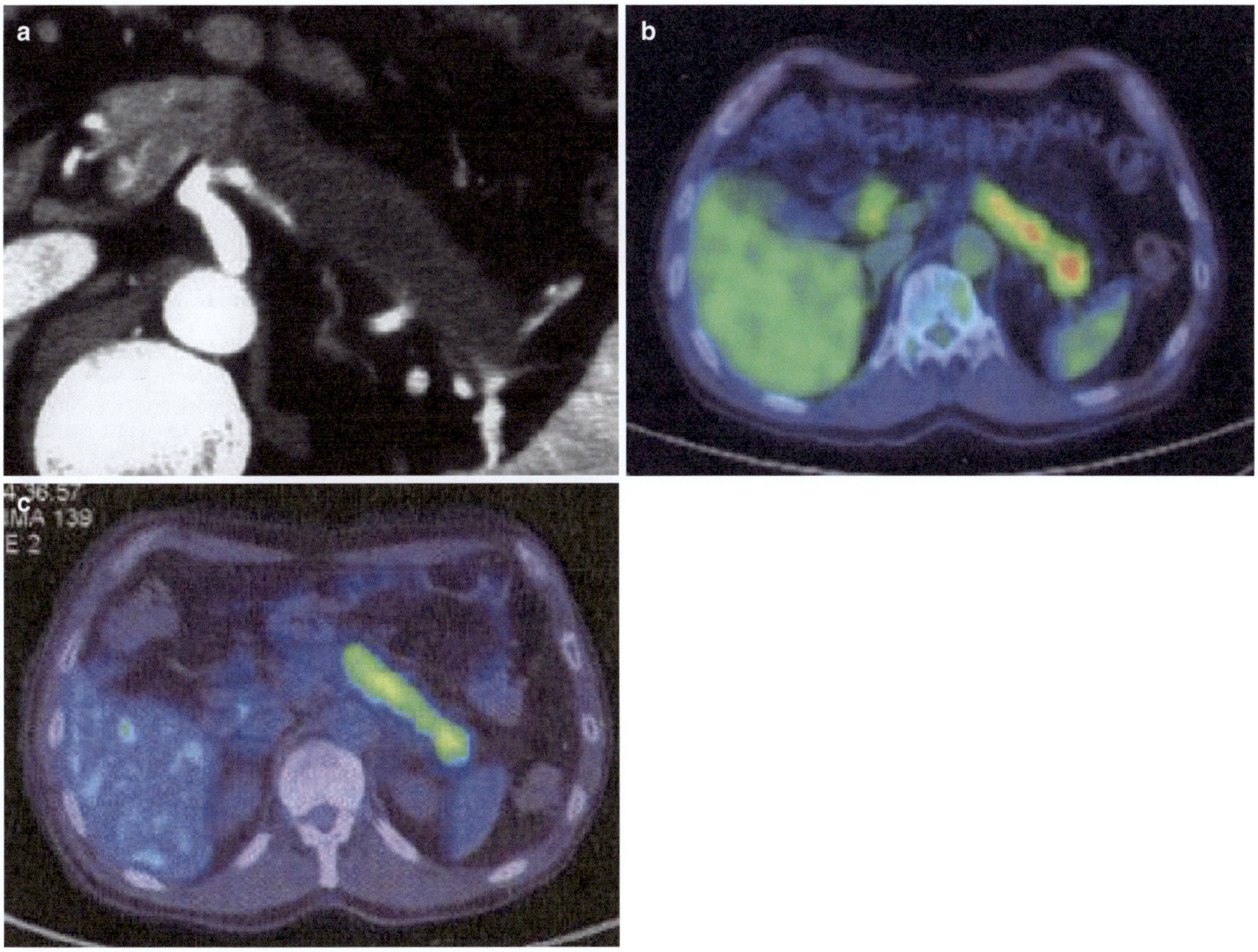

Fig. 13.4 Change in FDG uptake before and after steroid therapy in patients with pancreatic cancer (PC-3 in Table 13.2). (**a**) FDG-PET scan before steroid therapy; (**b**) enhanced CT before steroid therapy; and (**c**) FDG-PET scan after steroid therapy

Summary

The diagnosis of AIP remains challenging, especially with respect to distinguishing it from pancreatic cancer. Although endoscopic ultrasonography-guided fine-needle aspiration (EUS-FNA) is a useful modality for the discrimination of pancreatic cancer from AIP [16, 17], EUS-FNA sometimes results in an inconclusive outcome. When faced with a diagnostic dilemma between AIP and pancreatic cancer, the intra- and/or extrapancreatic FDG uptake pattern and/or response to steroids may help to solve this clinical problem. A trial with a large sample size that takes into account the subtype of AIP is necessary to clarify the clinical impact of PET/CT in the diagnosis of AIP.

References

1. Kamisawa T, Chari ST, Lerch MM, Kim MH, Gress TM, Shimosegawa T. Recent advances in autoimmune pancreatitis: type 1 and type 2. Gut. 2013;62:1373–80.
2. Shimosegawa T, Chari ST, Frulloni L, Kamisawa T, Kawa S, Mino-Kenudson M, Kim MH, Kloppel G, Lerch MM, Lohr M, Notohara K, Okazaki K, Schneider A, Zhang L. International consensus diagnostic criteria for autoimmune pancreatitis: guidelines of the International Association of Pancreatology. Pancreas. 2011;40:352–8.
3. Okazaki K, Uchida K, Ikeura T, Takaoka M. Current concept and diagnosis of IgG4-related disease in the hepato-bilio-pancreatic system. J Gastroenterol. 2013;48:303–14.
4. Chari ST, Kloeppel G, Zhang L, Notohara K, Lerch MM, Shimosegawa T. Histopathologic and clinical subtypes of autoimmune pancreatitis: the Honolulu consensus document. Pancreas. 2010;39:549–54.
5. Lee TY, Kim MH, Park do H, Seo DW, Lee SK, Kim JS, Lee KT. Utility of 18F-FDG PET/CT for differentiation of autoimmune pancreatitis with atypical pancreatic imaging findings from pancreatic cancer. AJR Am J Roentgenol. 2009;193:343–8.
6. Glaudemans AW, De Vries EF, Galli F, Dierckx RA, Slart RH, Signore A. The use of (18)F-FDG-PET/CT for diagnosis and treatment monitoring of inflammatory and infectious diseases. Clin Dev Immunol. 2013;2013, 623036.
7. Sahani DV, Bonaffini PA, Catalano OA, Guimaraes AR, Blake MA. State-of-the-art PET/CT of the pancreas: current role and emerging indications. Radiographics. 2012;32:1133–58; discussion 1158–60.

8. Kamisawa T, Takum K, Anjiki H, Egawa N, Kurata M, Honda G, Tsuruta K. FDG-PET/CT findings of autoimmune pancreatitis. Hepatogastroenterology. 2010;57:447–50.
9. Ozaki Y, Oguchi K, Hamano H, Arakura N, Muraki T, Kiyosawa K, Momose M, Kadoya M, Miyata K, Aizawa T, Kawa S. Differentiation of autoimmune pancreatitis from suspected pancreatic cancer by fluorine-18 fluorodeoxyglucose positron emission tomography. J Gastroenterol. 2008;43:144–51.
10. Umehara H, Okazaki K, Masaki Y, Kawano M, Yamamoto M, Saeki T, Matsui S, Sumida T, Mimori T, Tanaka Y, Tsubota K, Yoshino T, Kawa S, Suzuki R, Takegami T, Tomosugi N, Kurose N, Ishigaki Y, Azumi A, Kojima M, Nakamura S, Inoue D. A novel clinical entity, IgG4-related disease (IgG4RD): general concept and details. Mod Rheumatol. 2012;22:1–14.
11. Stone JH, Zen Y, Deshpande V. IgG4-related disease. N Engl J Med. 2012;366:539–51.
12. Chari ST, Takahashi N, Levy MJ, Smyrk TC, Clain JE, Pearson RK, Petersen BT, Topazian MA, Vege SS. A diagnostic strategy to distinguish autoimmune pancreatitis from pancreatic cancer. Clin Gastroenterol Hepatol. 2009;7:1097–103.
13. Moon SH, Kim MH, Park DH, Hwang CY, Park SJ, Lee SS, Seo DW, Lee SK. Is a 2-week steroid trial after initial negative investigation for malignancy useful in differentiating autoimmune pancreatitis from pancreatic cancer? A prospective outcome study. Gut. 2008;57:1704–12.
14. Shigekawa M, Yamao K, Sawaki A, Hara K, Takagi T, Bhatia V, Nishio M, Tamaki T, El-Amin H, Sayed Zel A, Mizuno N. Is (18) F-fluorodeoxyglucose positron emission tomography meaningful for estimating the efficacy of corticosteroid therapy in patients with autoimmune pancreatitis? J Hepatobiliary Pancreat Sci. 2010;17:269–74.
15. Sah RP, Chari ST, Pannala R, Sugumar A, Clain JE, Levy MJ, Pearson RK, Smyrk TC, Petersen BT, Topazian MD, Takahashi N, Farnell MB, Vege SS. Differences in clinical profile and relapse rate of type 1 versus type 2 autoimmune pancreatitis. Gastroenterology. 2010;139:140–8.
16. Ogura T, Yamao K, Sawaki A, Mizuno N, Hara K, Hijioka S, Niwa Y, Tajika M, Kondo S, Shimizu Y, Bhatia V, Higuchi K, Hosoda W, Yatabe Y. Clinical impact of K-ras mutation analysis in EUS-guided FNA specimens from pancreatic masses. Gastrointest Endosc. 2012;75:769–74.
17. Mizuno N, Bhatia V, Hosoda W, Sawaki A, Hoki N, Hara K, Takagi T, Ko SB, Yatabe Y, Goto H, Yamao K. Histological diagnosis of autoimmune pancreatitis using EUS-guided trucut biopsy: a comparison study with EUS-FNA. J Gastroenterol. 2009; 44:742–50.

Tissue Acquisition for Histologic Diagnosis

14

Ji Kon Ryu

Introduction

Autoimmune pancreatitis (AIP) is recognized as a distinct clinical entity, and it is also identified as a chronic inflammatory process of the pancreas in which the autoimmune mechanism is involved. The diagnosis of AIP is clinically challenging because it is a rare disease, which closely mimics more common pancreaticobiliary malignancies in its presentation such as obstructive jaundice and pancreatic mass. Type 1 AIP has dense periductal lymphoplasmacytic infiltrate with storiform fibrosis and obliterative phlebitis, whereas type 2 is distinguished from type 1 by granulocyte epithelial lesion, less prominent lymphoplasmacytic infiltrate, and less prominent storiform fibrosis [1]. The international consensus diagnostic criteria (ICDC) for AIP were developed based on the agreement of an international panel of experts and ICDC include both type 1 and 2 AIP [2].

The histological criteria of type 1 AIP are categorized as level 1, if more than three of the four criteria are met (lymphoplasmacytic infiltrate without granulocytic infiltration, obliterative phlebitis, storiform fibrosis, and >10 IgG4-positive plasma cells per HPF). If at least two of the criteria are met, the findings are categorized as level 2. Level 1 histological criterion for type 2 AIP is the presence of granulocytic epithelial lesions and the absence or scant presence of IgG4-positive cells. Level 2 histological criteria for type 2 AIP are the presence of granulocytic epithelial lesions with lymphoplasmacytic acinar infiltrate and the absence or scant presence of IgG4-positive cells. Therefore, adequate tissue acquisition is very important for a definite diagnosis of AIP.

J.K. Ryu, MD, PhD
Division of Gastroenterology, Department of Internal Medicine, Seoul National University College of Medicine, Seoul, Korea
e-mail: jkryu@snu.ac.kr

Indication for Tissue Acquisition

Although histopathological features are considered as the gold standard for a diagnosis of AIP, adequate tissue acquisition for a diagnosis of AIP is clinically difficult without surgical resection. So, we should know the indication of tissue acquisition. Because the most important decision for the differential diagnosis of pancreatic mass is to differentiate AIP from pancreatic cancer, endoscopic ultrasound-guided fine-needle aspiration (EUS-FNA) is usually performed to exclude the pancreatic cancer. However, a histological diagnosis of AIP using the small samples obtained by EUS-FNA is somewhat difficult. Another problem is that some AIP cases are difficult to distinguish as type 1 or type 2 AIP with small samples because these cases show less intense lymphoplasmacytic infiltration but more fibrosis, venulitis without obliterative phlebitis, and scattered neutrophils are present but granulocytic epithelial lesions are not.

Type 1 AIP can be diagnosed frequently without histological analysis. According to ICDC diagnostic algorithm, a diagnosis of type 1 AIP is possible with additional one non-ductal level 1/2 criteria if the pancreatic parenchymal image is typical. Non-ductal level 1/2 criteria include serology and other organ involvement. However, if the pancreatic parenchymal image is indeterminate or atypical, work-up for cancer is recommended. If there are two or more level 1 criteria such as ductal imaging, serology (IgG4, >2X upper limit of normal value), and other organ involvement, a definite diagnosis is possible without histology. Therefore, tissue acquisition should be done in all cases if there is no enough evidence of AIP. Of course, for the exact diagnosis of type 2 AIP, histology is always necessary because serum IgG4 level is normal and there is no other organ involvement except inflammatory bowel disease in type 2 AIP.

T. Kamisawa, J.B. Chung (eds.), *Autoimmune Pancreatitis*,
DOI 10.1007/978-3-642-55086-7_14, © Springer-Verlag Berlin Heidelberg 2015

Method of Tissue Acquisition

Percutaneous transabdominal ultrasonography-guided pancreatic tissue acquisition was a standard method before the era of EUS-FNA. The success rate and diagnostic yield are known to be higher in EUS-FNA for the diagnosis of pancreatic cancer. In addition, the problem of percutaneous approach is the high risk of cancer seeding. Micames et al. reported that the risk of peritoneal seeding was significantly lower with EUS-FNA (2.2 %) than with ultrasound-guided transabdominal FNA (16.3 %) [3]. Therefore, EUS-FNA is the standard method for the histologic diagnosis of possible pancreatic cancer, and percutaneous approach should not be done in patients with potentially resectable pancreatic cancer. Although EUS-FNA is sufficient to diagnose the pancreatic cancer, EUS-guided core biopsy is essential to obtain specimens of adequate size that preserves tissue architecture and permits an exact histological diagnosis of AIP. Usually, the primary role of EUS-FNA of the pancreas in patients with suspected AIP may be to exclude malignancy rather than to provide definitive evidence for a diagnosis of AIP. We should keep in mind that a negative biopsy/cytology is not a guarantee of non-malignancy. So, a short-term follow-up imaging to assess corticosteroid responsiveness is needed. If the patient does not respond to a diagnostic corticosteroid trial, a definitive diagnosis should always be pursued by core biopsy or resection. The ICDC suggest that negative work-up for pancreatobiliary malignancies is a prerequisite for a corticosteroid trial [2]. It should be emphasized that repeated EUS-FNA is warranted in patients with continued suspicion of pancreatobiliary malignancies despite indeterminate or negative findings at initial EUS-FNA. We should be aware that AIP is much less common than pancreatic cancer or cholangiocarcinoma.

In 2009, Detlefsen S et al. reported the role of core biopsy samples for the diagnosis of AIP [4]. The core needle biopsy specimens could be able to recognize AIP in 22 of 29 (76 %) specimens. In that study, most of core biopsy samples were obtained by percutaneous methods. However, another study concluded that percutaneous needle biopsy of pancreas was not satisfactory for the diagnosis of AIP even after IgG4-immunostaining because diagnostic sensitivity was only 47 % among 15 core biopsy samples [5]. Whereas FNA with a small caliber (22 or 25 gauge) provides material only for cytological review, a 19-gauge trucut biopsy (TCB) needle (Cook Endoscopy Inc, Winston-Salem, NC) acquires larger tissue samples to allow a histological diagnosis of AIP by preserving tissue architecture. Levy et al. reported the results of their retrospective study using EUS-TCB in patients with AIP [6]. The specimens obtained were adequate for histologic analysis in all 14 AIP patients and revealed diagnostic findings or abundant IgG4-positive plasma cells in 57 % of the patients (8 of 14). Mizuno et al. performed both EUS-TCB and EUS-FNA with a 22-gauge needle in 11 patients who were given a final diagnosis of AIP [7]. They reported that pancreatic specimens obtained by EUS-TCB showed full-spectrum lymphoplasmacytic sclerosing pancreatitis in 50 % (4 of 8) of the patients and probable lymphoplasmacytic sclerosing pancreatitis in another 4 patients (50 %, 4 of 8). However, EUS-FNA result showed that three out of eight patients with AI had full-spectrum lymphosplasmacytic sclerosing pancreatitis. One was reported as normal and 4 cases were inconclusive.

The complication rates of EUS-FNA for pancreatic mass were reported to be 0–2 % [8]. The complication rate of EUS-TCB is comparable to that of EUS-FNA. Although a TCB needle obtains the specimen on the tissue tray after cutting the tissue with only one sliding movement of the outer sheath, the FNA needle suctions the specimen inside of the needle after multiple movements of the needle inside the lesion. Theoretically, these differences in the specimen collection method might cause more distortions in the FNA specimen than that obtained by a TCB needle. However, the EUS-TCB has a technical limitation with regard to needle manipulation in the duodenum and in the approach to the pancreatic head because a puncture from the duodenum to the head of the pancreas usually requires an angulated scope position, endoscopic tip angulation, and the use of an elevator function, which makes the passage of the TCB needle difficult. So, overall diagnostic accuracy of EUS- trucut biopsy is known to be 50–72 % (Table 14.1). In addition, EUS-TCB is available in only a few specialized tertiary-care centers. Iwashita T et al. evaluated the samples collected by EUS-FNA with a conventional 19-gauge needle by histologic analysis, to look for features of AIP from 44 patients who were diagnosed with AIP [9]. EUS-FNA was performed successfully in all patients using a 19-gauge needle for the pancreatic lesions. However, 19 patients (43 %) were diagnosed with AIP based on histologic analysis.

In order to overcome the limitation of the 19-gauge needle, a EUS-guided fine-needle biopsy (EUS-FNB) device (Echotip Procore; Wilson Cook Medical Inc., Winston-Salem, North Carolina, USA) was developed. In a randomized trial, diagnostic sufficiency, technical performance, and safety profiles of the 22-gauge biopsy needle were comparable to those of the conventional 22-gauge aspiration needle for sampling of pancreatic mass [12]. In another prospective comparison study, the correct diagnosis rate of EUS-FNB was higher than that of EUS-FNA in the pancreatic mass group (86.8 % vs. 75 %, $P=0.046$) [13]. Larghi et al. reported the prospective result of EUS-FNB in 61 patients with pancreatic masses [14]. EUS-FNB was technically feasible in 98 % of patients with a solid pancreatic mass. A suitable sample for histological evaluation was obtained in 88.5 % of the cases after only one single needle pass. However, no article was published on the yield of

Table 14.1 Diagnostic yields of pancreatic biopsies in patients with AIP

Author (year)	Nation	Number	Technique	Diagnostic yield
Levy (2006) [6]	United States	14	EUS-trucut	Diagnostic 57 % (8/14) Suggestive 29 % (4/14) Inconclusive 14 % (2/14)
Hirano (2009) [5]	Japan	15	Percutaneous	Diagnostic 47 % (7/15) Suggestive 20 % (3/15) Inconclusive 33 % (5/15)
Mizuno (2009) [7]	Japan	8	EUS-trucut	Diagnostic 50 % (4/8) Suggestive 50 % (4/8) Inconclusive 0 % (0/8)
Detlefsen (2009) [4]	Germany Denmark	26	Percutaneous Intraoperative EUS-trucut	Diagnostic 81 % (21/26) Suggestive 19 % (5/26) Inconclusive 0 % (0/26)
Iwashita (2012) [9]	Japan	44	EUS-FNA (19G)[a]	Diagnostic 43 % (19/44) Suggestive 43 % (19/44) Inconclusive 7 % (3/44) Analysis impossible 7 % (3/44)
Song (2012) [10]	Korea	54	Percutaneous EUS-trucut	Diagnostic 72 % (39/54) Suggestive 0 % (0/54) Inconclusive 28 % (15/54
Fujii (2013) [11]	United States	7	EUS-trucut	Diagnostic 72 % (5/7) Suggestive 14 % (1/7) Inconclusive 14 % (1/7)

[a]EUS-guided tissue acquisition by using a conventional 19-gauge needle

EUS-FNB using the new needle for AIP diagnosis. Further studies are required to assess the diagnostic performance of EUS-FNB and comparison study between EUS-TCB and EUS-FNB for the better histologic diagnosis of AIP is necessary.

Summary

Type 1 AIP can be diagnosed frequently without histological analysis if image is typical and there are additional criteria. However, if the pancreatic parenchymal image is indeterminate or atypical, work-up for cancer is recommended. Therefore, tissue acquisition should be done in all cases if there is no enough evidence of AIP. Even if percutaneous transabdominal ultrasonography-guided pancreatic tissue acquisition was a standard method before the era of EUS-FNA, nowadays EUS-guided tissue acquisition is recommended because diagnostic yield is high and the risk of peritoneal seeding is low if the mass has possibility of pancreatic cancer. Theoretically, EUS-TCB seems to be a better method for obtaining core tissue; however, there are some technical limitations and diagnostic yield that are not satisfactory till now. The better needle should be developed to obtain the core tissue without technical limitation, and further studies are required to find the ideal and standard tissue acquisition method.

References

1. Zhang L, Chari S, Smyrk TC, et al. Autoimmune pancreatitis type 1 and type 2: an international consensus study on histopathologic diagnostic criteria. Pancreas. 2011;40:1172–9.
2. Shimosegawa T, Chari ST, Frulloni L, et al. International consensus diagnostic criteria for autoimmune pancreatitis: guidelines of the International Association of Pancreatology. Pancreas. 2011;40:352–8.
3. Micames C, Jowell PS, White R, et al. Lower frequency of peritoneal carcinomatosis in patients with pancreatic cancer diagnosed by EUS-guided FNA vs. percutaneous FNA. Gastrointest Endosc. 2003;58:690–5.
4. Detlefsen S, Mohr Drewes A, Vyberg M, et al. Diagnosis of autoimmune pancreatitis by core needle biopsy: application of six microscopic criteria. Virchows Arch. 2009;454:531–9.
5. Hirano K, Fukushima N, Tada M, et al. Diagnostic utility of biopsy specimens for autoimmune pancreatitis. J Gastroenterol. 2009;44:765–73.
6. Levy MJ, Wiersema MJ, Chari ST. Chronic pancreatitis: focal pancreatitis or cancer? Is there a role for FNA/biopsy? Autoimmune pancreatitis. Endoscopy. 2006;38 Suppl 1:S30–5.
7. Mizuno N, Bhatia V, Hosoda W, et al. Histological diagnosis of autoimmune pancreatitis using EUS-guided trucut biopsy: a comparison study with EUS-FNA. J Gastroenterol. 2009;44:742–50.
8. Yoshinaga S, Suzuki H, Oda I, Saito Y. Role of endoscopic ultrasound-guided fine needle aspiration (EUS-FNA) for diagnosis of solid pancreatic masses. Dig Endosc. 2011;23 Suppl 1:29–33.
9. Iwashita T, Yasuda I, Doi S, et al. Use of samples from endoscopic, ultrasound-guided, 19-gauge, fine-needle aspiration in diagnosis of autoimmune pancreatitis. Clin Gastroenterol Hepatol. 2012;10:316–22.

10. Song TJ, Kim JH, Kim MH, et al. A comparison of clinical findings between histologically confirmed type 1 and type 2 autoimmune pancreatitis. J Gastroenterol Hepatol. 2012;27:700–8.
11. Fujii LL, Chari ST, El-Youssef M, Takahashi N, Topazian MD, Zhang L, Levy MJ. Pediatric pancreatic EUS-guided trucut biopsy for evaluation of autoimmune pancreatitis. Gastrointest Endosc. 2013;77:824–8.
12. Bang JY, Hebert-Magee S, Trevino J, et al. Randomized trial comparing the 22-gauge aspiration and 22-gauge biopsy needles for EUS-guided sampling of solid pancreatic mass lesions. Gastrointest Endosc. 2012;76:321–7.
13. Hucl T, Wee E, Anuradha S, Gupta R, Ramchandani M, Rakesh K, et al. Feasibility and efficiency of a new 22G core needle: a prospective comparison study. Endoscopy. 2013;45:792–8.
14. Larghi A, Iglesias-Garcia J, Poley JW, et al. Feasibility and yield of a novel 22-gauge histology EUS needle in patients with pancreatic masses: a multicenter prospective cohort study. Surg Endosc. 2013;27:3733–8.

Part III

Other Organ Involvements

IgG4-Related Sclerosing Cholangitis 15

Takahiro Nakazawa, Itaru Naitoh, and Hirotaka Ohara

Introduction

We begin this chapter with an introduction to our original cholangiographic classification to help readers easily understand this chapter and the concept of IgG4-SC [1].

Cholangiographic Classification

IgG4-SC displays various cholangiographic features similar to those of pancreatic cancer (PCa), PSC, and CC. The characteristic features of IgG4-SC can be classified into 4 types based on the stricture regions revealed by cholangiography and differential diagnosis (Fig. 15.1) [1]. Type 1 IgG4-SC displays stenosis only in the lower part of the common bile duct and thus should be differentiated from chronic pancreatitis, PCa, and CC. Type 2 IgG4-SC, in which stenosis is diffusely distributed throughout the intrahepatic and extrahepatic bile ducts, should be differentiated from PSC and is further subdivided into 2 subtypes: type 2a, characterized with narrowing of the intrahepatic bile ducts with prestenotic dilation, and type 2b, characterized by the narrowing of the intrahepatic bile ducts without prestenotic dilation and reduced bile duct branches, which is caused by marked lymphocytic and plasmacyte infiltrations into the peripheral bile ducts. Type 3 IgG4-SC is characterized by stenosis in the hilar hepatic lesions and the lower part of the common bile duct. Type 4 IgG4-SC presents with strictures of the bile duct only in the hilar hepatic lesions. The cholangiographic findings of types 3 and 4 IgG4-SC should be discriminated from those of CC.

T. Nakazawa, MD, PhD (✉) • I. Naitoh, MD, PhD
Department of Gastroenterology and Metabolism,
Nagoya City University Graduate School of Medical Sciences,
1 Kawasumi, Mizuho-cho, Mizuho-ku, Nagoya 467-8601, Japan
e-mail: tnakazaw@med.nagoya-cu.ac.jp

H. Ohara, MD, PhD
Department of Community-Based Medical Education,
Nagoya City University Graduate School of Medical Sciences,
Nagoya, Japan

Frequency of Association with AIP and IgG4-SC

The Frequency of Associated IgG4-SC with AIP

IgG4-SC is one of the frequently associated diseases with AIP. In one study, 59 (95 %) of 62 patients with IgG4-SC had associated AIP, with high prevalence [2]. Ghazale et al. [3] reported that an incidence rate of AIP association was 92 % in 53 patients with IgG4-SC, which was a comparatively large sample.

These two series included all types of IgG4-SC [2, 3]. The frequency of occurrence of IgG4-SC depends on the definition of IgG4-SC being considered. Inclusion of type 1 IgG4-SC into the IgG4-SC category has been disputed. Some researchers claim that the stricture of the lower common bile duct, which is observed in type 1 IgG4-SC, is caused by compression due to AIP [4]. This claim is based on the fact that type 1 IgG4-SC was not found in some cases of focal-type AIP with only body and tail involvement. However, we believe that type 1 IgG4-SC should be classified as one of the IgG4-SC types because of the following reasons. First, pathological examination of the bile duct wall obtained from surgically resected samples showed abundant IgG4-positive plasma cell infiltration, storiform fibrosis, and obstructive phlebitis, which are characteristics of IgG4-SC-associated inflammation [5]. In addition, some cases showed inflammation of only the bile duct wall and not of the pancreas. Second, the results of an intraductal ultrasonography (IDUS) study showed continuous thickening of the bile duct wall from the intrapancreatic to the extrapancreatic bile duct [6]. In fact, it is difficult to identify which is the major factor contributing to the thickening of the bile duct wall—inflammation of the bile duct or compression due to AIP.

Therefore, understanding statistical data is essential for determining the frequency of occurrence of IgG4-SC. The frequency of IgG4-SC occurrence also changes depending on whether type 1 IgG4-SC is included in the IgG4-SC classification.

T. Kamisawa, J.B. Chung (eds.), *Autoimmune Pancreatitis*,
DOI 10.1007/978-3-642-55086-7_15, © Springer-Verlag Berlin Heidelberg 2015

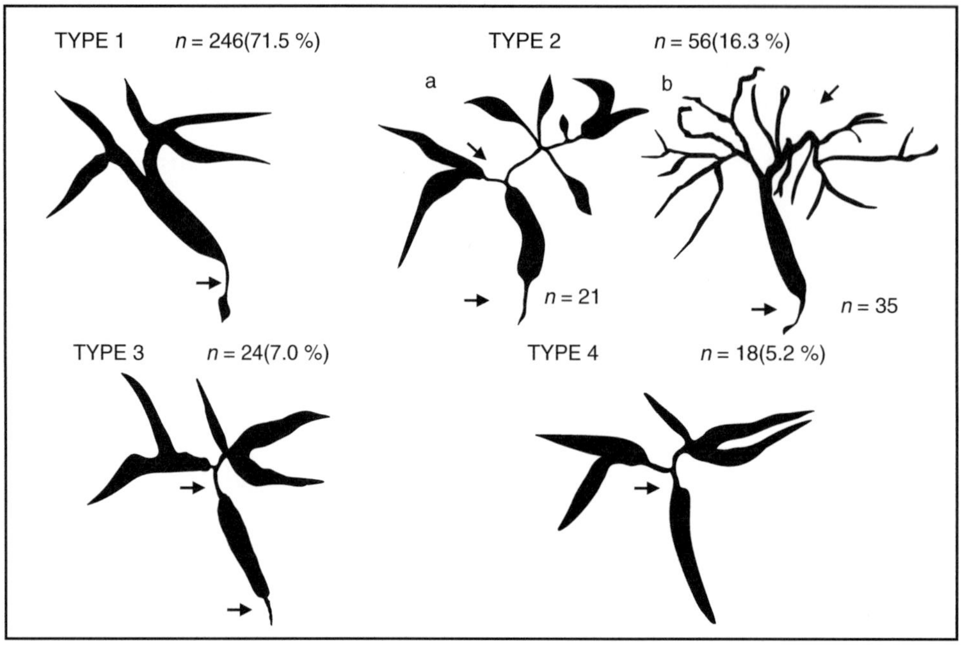

Fig. 15.1 The cholangiographic classification of IgG4-related sclerosing cholangitis. Stenosis is located only in the lower part of the common bile duct in Type 1; stenosis is diffusely distributed in the intra- and extrahepatic bile ducts in Type 2. Type 2 is further subdivided into 2 types. Extended narrowing of the intrahepatic bile ducts with prestenotic dilation is widely distributed in Type 2a. Narrowing of the intrahepatic bile ducts without prestenotic dilation and reduced bile duct branches are widely distributed in Type 2b; stenosis is detected in both the hilar hepatic lesions and the lower part of the common bile ducts in Type 3; strictures of the bile duct are detected only in the hilar hepatic lesions in Type 4

The Frequency of Associated AIP with IgG4-SC in Japanese Cohort

Recent Japanese multicenter study revealed the frequency of associated AIP with IgG4-SC [7]. A total of 344 IgG4-SC patients were enrolled in this study, and we evaluated according to our cholangiographic classification. Three hundred twenty-nine (95.6 %) out of 344 total IgG4-SC cases were associated with AIP. Two hundred forty-four out of 246 type 1 IgG4-SC cases (99.2 %) were associated with AIP. Fifty-one out of 56 type 2 IgG4-SC cases (91.1 %) were associated with AIP. Thirty-four out of 42 type 3 and 4 IgG4-SC cases (81.0 %) were associated with AIP. Type 3 and 4 IgG4-SC cases showed lower frequency of association with AIP.

Pathological Features

In IgG4-SC, fibroinflammatory involvement is observed mainly in the submucosa of the bile duct wall, whereas the epithelium of the bile duct is intact [5]. PSC should be ruled out if inflammation is observed, particularly in the epithelium of the bile duct wall. The characteristic pathological findings of IgG4-SC were first reported under the name "lymphoplasmacytic sclerosing pancreatitis with cholangitis" [8]. Abraham et al. [9] reported frequent fibroinflammatory involvement of the gallbladder and common bile duct in patients with lymphoplasmacytic sclerosing pancreatitis. Zen et al. [5] revealed that the bile duct wall in IgG4-SC had pathological features similar to those of AIP, displaying dense infiltrations of lymphocytes and IgG4-positive plasma cells, with extensive fibrosis and obliterative phlebitis. They classified IgG4-SC into 6 categories according to the extent of inflammation and association with an inflammatory pseudotumor. IgG4-positive plasma cells are sparse in the affected bile ducts in PSC, and the luminal side of the bile ducts, including the lining biliary epithelial cells, is preferentially affected compared with IgG4-SC. In PSC, the fibrosis is denser and older, whereas in IgG4-SC, the entire bile duct wall and periductal tissue are affected. However, a recent study by Zhang et al. [10] revealed that 23 (23 %) of 98 liver explants with PSC had periductal infiltration with abundant IgG4-positive plasma cells [10/high-power field (HPF)] in the hilar area.

Serum IgG4 Level

Serum IgG4 level has been reported to be a useful marker for discriminating AIP from other pancreatic diseases [11]. A cutoff IgG4 level of 135 mg/dL has been widely used as part of the diagnostic criteria for AIP. However, twice the upper limit of the normal value has also been recommended to discriminate AIP from PCa. In the International Consensus Diagnostic Criteria for AIP, once or twice the upper limit of the normal value is included in levels 1 and 2 diagnoses, respectively [12].

Only a few reports have been published concerning the cutoff IgG4 level in the diagnosis of IgG4-SC. We published for the first time, the diagnostic criteria for IgG4-SC based on a comparative study [2]. The cutoff IgG4 level of 135 mg/dL is useful in discriminating IgG4-SC from PCa and PSC. However, the level displayed lower specificity in discriminating IgG4-SC from CC. Oseini et al. [13] evaluated the utility of serum IgG4 level in distinguishing IgG4-SC from CC. They reported that among their 126 patients with CC, 17 (13.5 %) had elevated (>140 mg/dL) and 4 (3.2 %) had a >2-fold increase (>280 mg/dL) in serum IgG4 levels. PSC was present in 31/126 CC patients, of whom 7 (22.6 %) had an elevated serum IgG4 level. The authors concluded that some patients with CC, particularly PSC, had elevated serum IgG4 levels and diagnosis using a twofold higher cutoff serum IgG4 level may not reliably distinguish IgG4-SC from CC. However, a cutoff level fourfold higher than the upper limit of the normal value had 100 % specificity for IgG4-SC.

We recently established a cutoff serum IgG4 level to differentiate IgG4-SC from the 3 other diseases (type 1 IgG4-SC vs PCa, type 2 IgG4-SC vs PSC, and type 3 IgG4-SC vs CC) using serum IgG4 levels measured in 9 Japanese high-volume centers [7]. The cutoff obtained from receiver operating characteristic (ROC) curves displayed similar sensitivity and specificity to those of 135 mg/dL when all the IgG4-SC cases and controls were compared. However, a new cutoff value was established when IgG4-SC subgroups and controls were compared. A cutoff level of 182 mg/dL can increase the specificity to 96.6 % (a 4.7 % increase) for distinguishing types 3 and 4 IgG4-SC from CC. A cutoff level of 207 mg/dL might be useful for completely distinguishing types 3 and 4 IgG4-SC from CC.

Mendes et al. [14] measured the serum IgG4 level in 127 patients with PSC and found that it was elevated in 12 patients (9 %). The patients with elevated IgG4 levels had higher levels of total bilirubin and alkaline phosphatase, higher PSC Mayo risk scores, and lower incidence of inflammatory bowel disease. It is important to note that the time to liver transplantation was shorter in patients with elevated IgG4 levels (1.7 vs 6.5 years, $P=0.0009$). As only one of the patients in their series had an abnormal pancreatogram, the documented cases appeared to conform to the diagnosis of IgG4-SC. Therefore, clinical trials in which patients with PSC are evaluated for IgG4 and patients presenting elevated levels are treated with corticosteroids should be considered.

Diagnostic Criteria

Only 3 sets of diagnostic criteria for IgG4-SC have been proposed [2, 15, 16]. AIP should be clinically discriminated only from PCa. However, IgG4-SC should be discriminated from all of the 3 intractable diseases (PCa, PSC, and CC). Therefore, we should take into account these 3 intractable diseases for differential diagnosis in the diagnostic criteria for IgG4-SC.

We summarize three diagnostic criteria for the abovementioned IgG4-SC. The Research Committee of IgG4-related Diseases and the Research Committee of Intractable Diseases of Liver and Biliary Tract, in association with the Ministry of Health, Labour, and Welfare, Japan, and the Japan Biliary Association, proposed clinical diagnostic criteria for IgG4-SC in 2012 [15] (Table 15.1). The diagnosis of IgG4-SC is based on the combination of the following 4 criteria: (1) characteristic biliary imaging findings, (2) elevation of serum IgG4 concentrations, (3) the coexistence of IgG4-related diseases except those of the biliary tract, and (4) characteristic histopathological features. Furthermore, the effectiveness of steroid therapy is an optional extra diagnostic criterion to confirm accurate diagnosis of IgG4-SC.

The HISORt criteria for the diagnosis of IgG4-SC [3] are based on the characteristic features of IgG4-SC on histological, imaging, and serological examination; other organ involvement; and response to steroid therapy, which parallel the HISORt criteria established for AIP [16].

Our original diagnostic criteria provide a concrete diagnostic algorithm for IgG4-SC (Fig. 15.2) [2]. Association with AIP and other organ involvements are common useful diagnostic parameters in all three IgG4-SC types. Characteristic cholangiogram, liver biopsy, and exclusion of IBD are useful parameters in type 2 IgG4-SC. IDUS findings, exclusion of malignancy by bile duct biopsy, and a serum IgG4 cutoff level of 207 mg/dL were useful parameters in type 3 and 4 IgG4-SC. Although, generally, diagnosis should be made before starting therapy, a steroid trial is needed in some cases.

Differential Diagnosis Based on Cholangiographic Classification

IgG4-SC displays various cholangiographic features similar to those of PCa, PSC, and CC. The differential diagnosis based on cholangiographic classification is sufficient in clinical practice because the useful modalities depend on the cholangiographic types (Fig. 15.3) [18].

Type 1 IgG4-SC should be differentiated from chronic pancreatitis, PCa, and CC. The modalities useful for differential diagnosis are IDUS [6], endoscopic ultrasound-guided fine-needle aspiration for the pancreas [19], and cytological examination and/or biopsy of the bile duct [6].

Table 15.1 Clinical diagnostic criteria of IgG4-related sclerosing cholangitis 2012

Diagnostic criteria of IgG4-related sclerosing cholangitis
A. Diagnostic items
1. Biliary tract imaging reveals diffuse or segmental narrowing of the intrahepatic and/or extrahepatic bile duct associated with the thickening of bile duct wall
2. Hematological examination shows elevated serum IgG4 concentrations (≥135 mg/dl)
3. Coexistence of autoimmune pancreatitis, IgG4-related dacryoadenitis/sialadenitis, or IgG4-related retroperitoneal fibrosis
4. Histopathological examination shows:
① Marked lymphocytic and plasmacyte infiltration and fibrosis
② Infiltration of IgG4-positive plasma cells: >10 IgG4-positive plasma cells/HPF
③ Storiform fibrosis
④ Obliterative phlebitis
Option: Effectiveness of steroid therapy
A specialized facility, in which detailed examinations such as endoscopic biliary biopsy and endoscopic ultrasound-guided fine-needle aspiration (EUS-FNA) can be administrated, may include in its diagnosis the effectiveness of steroid therapy, once pancreatic or biliary cancers have been ruled out
B. Diagnosis
Definite diagnosis: 1+3, 1+2+4①②, 4①②③, 4①②④
Probable diagnosis: 1+2+Option
Possible diagnosis: 1+2
It is necessary to exclude PSC, malignant diseases such as pancreatic or biliary cancers, and secondary sclerosing cholangitis caused by the diseases with obvious pathogenesis. If IgG4-SC cannot be clinically ruled out, a patient must not be treated with facile steroid therapy but should be referred to a specialized medical facility

Cited from Ohara et al. [15]

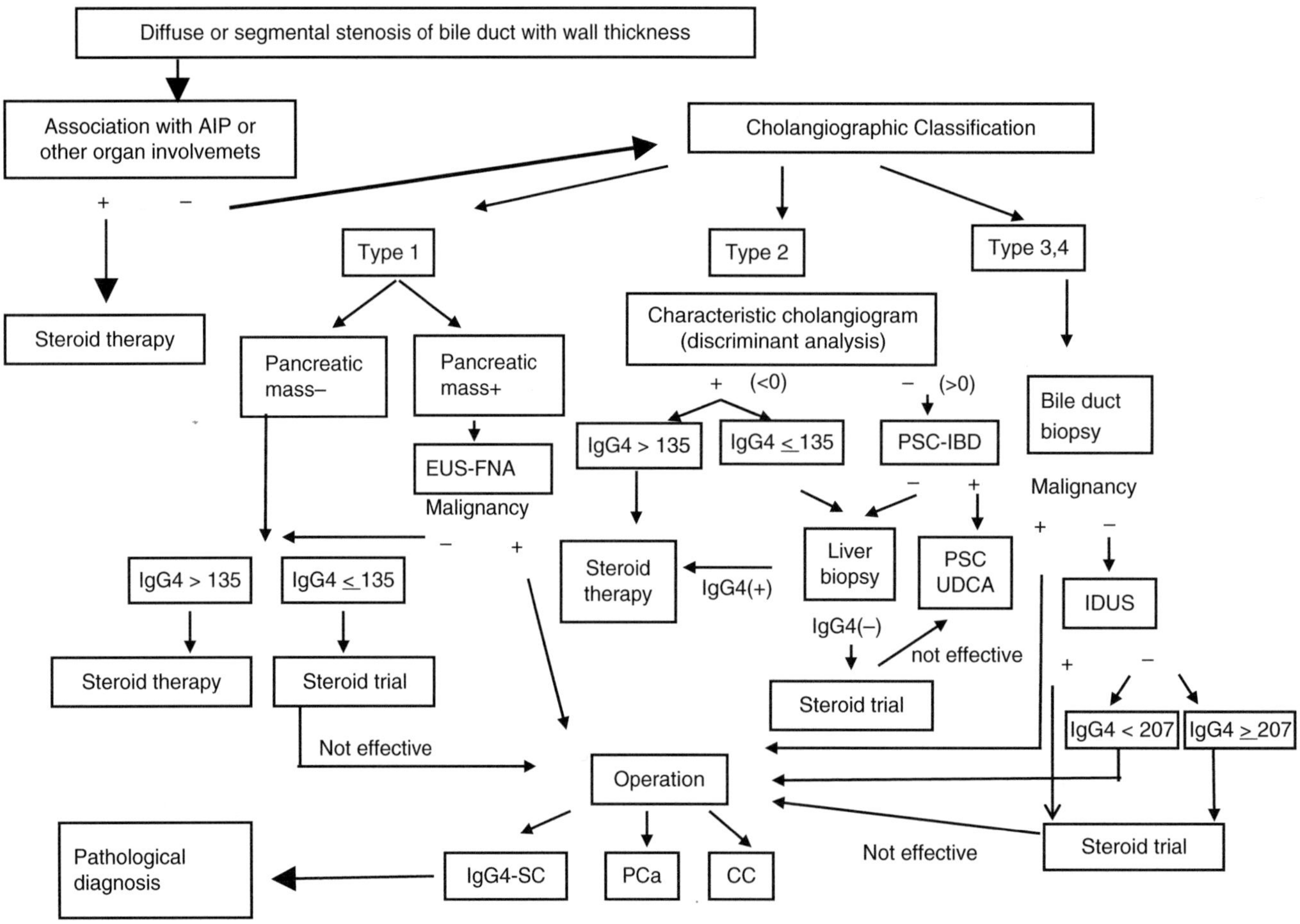

Fig. 15.2 Algorithm for management of IgG4-SC (Cited from Nakazawa et al. [17])

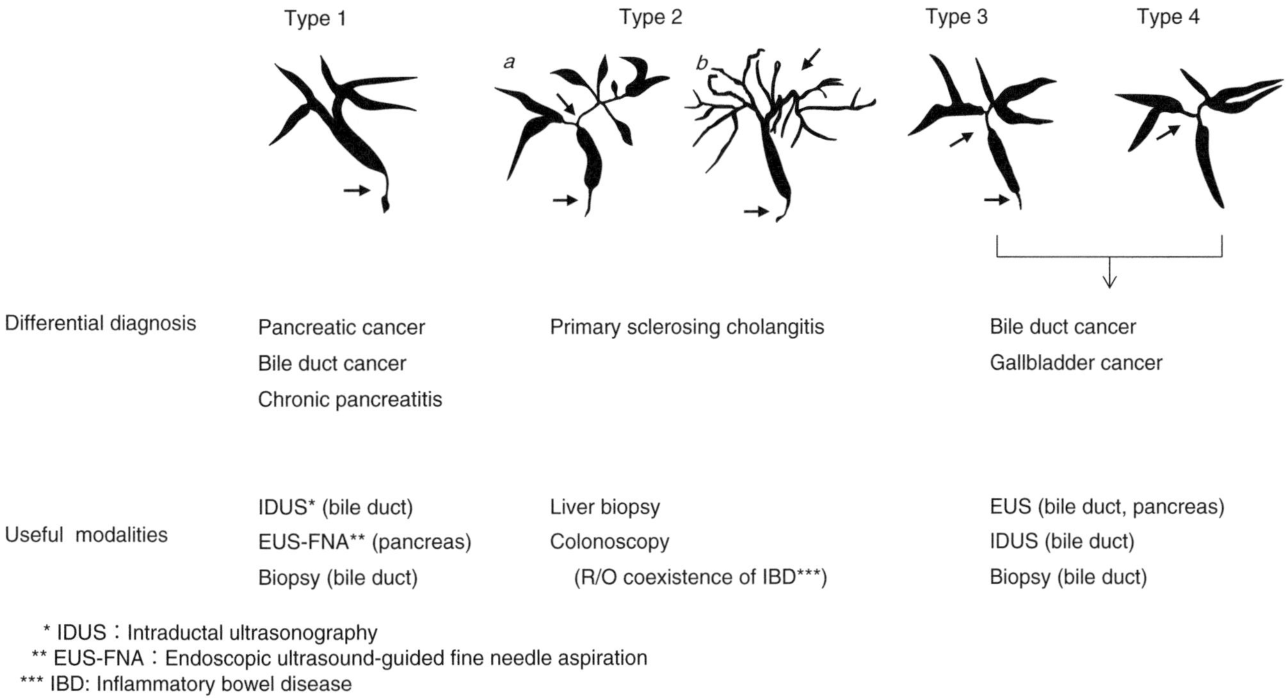

Fig. 15.3 The cholangiographic classification and differential diagnosis. *IDUS* intraductal ultrasonography, *EUS-FNA* endoscopic ultrasound-guided fine-needle aspiration, *IBD* inflammatory bowel disease

Type 2 IgG4-SC should be differentiated from PSC and secondary sclerosing cholangitis (SSC). After ruling out SSC, differential diagnosis between Type 2 IgG4-SC and PSC is necessary [20]. The modalities useful for differential diagnosis are cholangiography [17], evaluations for associated IBD [21, 22], and liver biopsy [23, 24]. Our discriminant analysis formula for cholangiographic features, including age, was able to efficiently discriminate type 2 IgG4-SC from PSC [17]. Band-like strictures, a beaded or "pruned tree" appearance, and diverticulum-like outpouching are significantly more frequent in PSC cases. In contrast, segmental strictures, long strictures with prestenotic dilation, and strictures of the lower common bile duct are significantly more common in IgG4-SC. These differences are illustrated in Fig. 15.4. The characteristic cholangiographic features reflect the underlying pathological processes involved in each condition. In PSC, obliterative fibrosis is the main cause of biliary stenosis, creating short strictures. In contrast, in IgG4-SC, severe lymphoplasmacyte infiltration into bile ducts in the long region is the main cause of biliary stenosis, resulting in long strictures.

Associated ulcerative colitis is suggestive of PSC. IBD is present in only 0–6 % of patients with IgG4-SC [3, 25, 26]. IBD is usually not a feature associated with type 1 AIP, unlike the frequent association of IBD with type 2 AIP [12]. IBD associated with PSC showed characteristic findings different from ordinary IBD [21, 22]. Backwash ileitis, rectal sparing, and low disease activity appear to be features that characterize IBD when it is associated with PSC [21, 22].

The histological features of IgG4-SC on liver biopsy are distinctive and, in conjunction with IgG4 immunohistochemical staining, help distinguish IgG4-SC from PSC [23, 24]. We have already reported that liver needle biopsy is especially useful for distinguishing IgG4-SC from PSC in patients with cholangiographically evident intrahepatic biliary strictures [24]. Four (57 %) of 7 patients with type 2 IgG4-SC presented infiltration ≥10 IgG4+plasma cells per HPF in liver biopsy samples, whereas none of the PSC patients presented this feature.

Types 3 and 4 IgG4-SC need to be discriminated from CC. The modalities useful for the differential diagnosis of types 3 and 4 IgG4-SC are endoscopic procedures [6] such as endoscopic ultrasonography, IDUS [6], cytological examination, and/or biopsy of the bile duct [6, 27]. Although we described how type 2 IgG4-SC could be discriminated from PSC on the basis of characteristic cholangiographic features, cholangiography cannot discriminate the segmental stricture of types 3 and 4 IgG4-SC from CC. Therefore, we applied our discriminant analysis formula for cholangiographic features to discriminate between only type 2 IgG4-SC and PSC.

IDUS findings such as circular symmetrical wall thickening, smooth outer margin, smooth inner margin, and homogeneous internal echo at the stenotic area were useful for the diagnosis of IgG4-SC. The most characteristic IDUS finding in the IgG4-SC cases was thickening of the bile duct wall, which appeared normal on a cholangiogram [6] (Fig. 15.5). Bile duct wall thickening spread continuously from the intrapancreatic bile duct to the upper bile duct in most cases. To differentiate IgG4-SC from CC, a 0.8 mm thickness of the bile duct wall that appears normal on a cholangiogram was the best cutoff as indicated by ROC curves. The sensitivity, specificity, and accuracy were 95, 90.9, and 93.5 %,

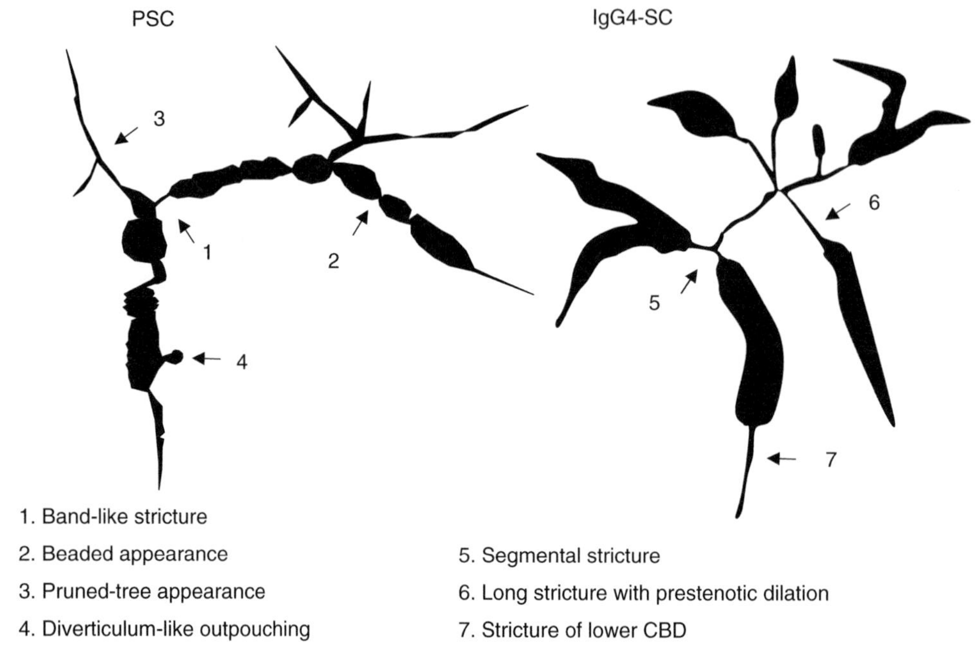

Fig. 15.4 Schematic illustration of comparison of cholangiographic (primary sclerosing cholangitis vs IgG4-related sclerosing cholangitis) findings [25]. The schematic comparison of cholangiographic findings between IgG4-related sclerosing cholangitis and primary sclerosing cholangitis. IgG4-related sclerosing cholangitis displaying segmental and long stricture and stricture of the lower common bile duct, primary sclerosing cholangitis displaying band-like stricture (short stricture 1–2 mm), beaded appearance (short and annular stricture alternating with normal or minimally dilated segments), pruned tree appearance (diminished arbolization of intrahepatic duct and pruning) and diverticulum-like outpouching (outpouchings resembling diverticula, often protruding between adjacent strictures)

respectively, when the cutoff value was 0.8 mm. No CC cases had a bile duct wall thicker than 1 mm. The sensitivity, specificity, and accuracy were 85, 100, and 87 %, respectively, when the cutoff value was set at 1 mm. We considered a 1-mm thickness as an optimal cutoff wall thickness to completely exclude CC.

Ghazale et al. [3] reported the usefulness of endoscopic biliary biopsy for diagnosis of IgG4-SC. They reported that 14 (88 %) of 16 patients had immunostaining results indicating abundant IgG4-positive cells (>10 IgG4-positive cells/HPF) in bile duct biopsy specimens. Furthermore, they considered that the absence of malignant cells in the presence of an inflamed mucosa with many IgG4-positive plasma cells provided histological evidence to support the diagnosis of IgG4-SC. However, we were unable to diagnose any case as IgG4-SC on the basis of hematoxylin-eosin and elastic-van Gieson staining alone [6]. Abundant IgG4-positive plasma cells were observed in only 3 (18 %) of 17 patients. We were able to diagnose IgG4-SC in only 3 patients (18 %) on the basis of its characteristic histopathological features. However, it was possible to rule out CC by transpapillary biopsy. In addition, 1 of 11 CC cases presented abundant IgG4-positive plasma cells. Zhang et al. [10] also reported that abundant IgG4-positive plasma cells were evident in 7 (18 %) of 38 cases of CC. Harada et al. [28] reported that CC cells could play the role of nonprofessional antigen-presenting cells and Foxp3-positive regulatory cells, inducing IgG4 reactions via the production of IL-10 indirectly and directly, respectively.

We could rule out CC by transpapillary biopsy. The superficial nature of endoscopic biopsy specimens limits their usefulness for demonstrating the characteristic histological features of IgG4-SC. However, Kawakami et al. [27] reported that the diagnostic rate from ampullary and bile duct biopsies was 52 % (15/29 cases) based on the threshold of 10 IgG4-positive plasma cells per HPF and that bile duct biopsy was significantly valuable for patients with swelling of the pancreatic head. Ampullary biopsy is sometimes useful in the diagnosis of AIP and IgG4-SC [29, 30].

Treatment

Although some patients responded to biliary drainage or surgical resection, IgG4-SC displays a good response to steroid therapy, as is the case for pancreatic lesions (Figs. 15.5 and 15.6).

Nishino et al. [31] reported that bile duct stricture improved to various degrees in all 10 patients treated by steroid therapy but persisted in the lower part of the bile duct in 4 patients (4/10, 40 %). Hirano et al. [32] reported that steroid therapy could reduce AIP-related unfavorable events

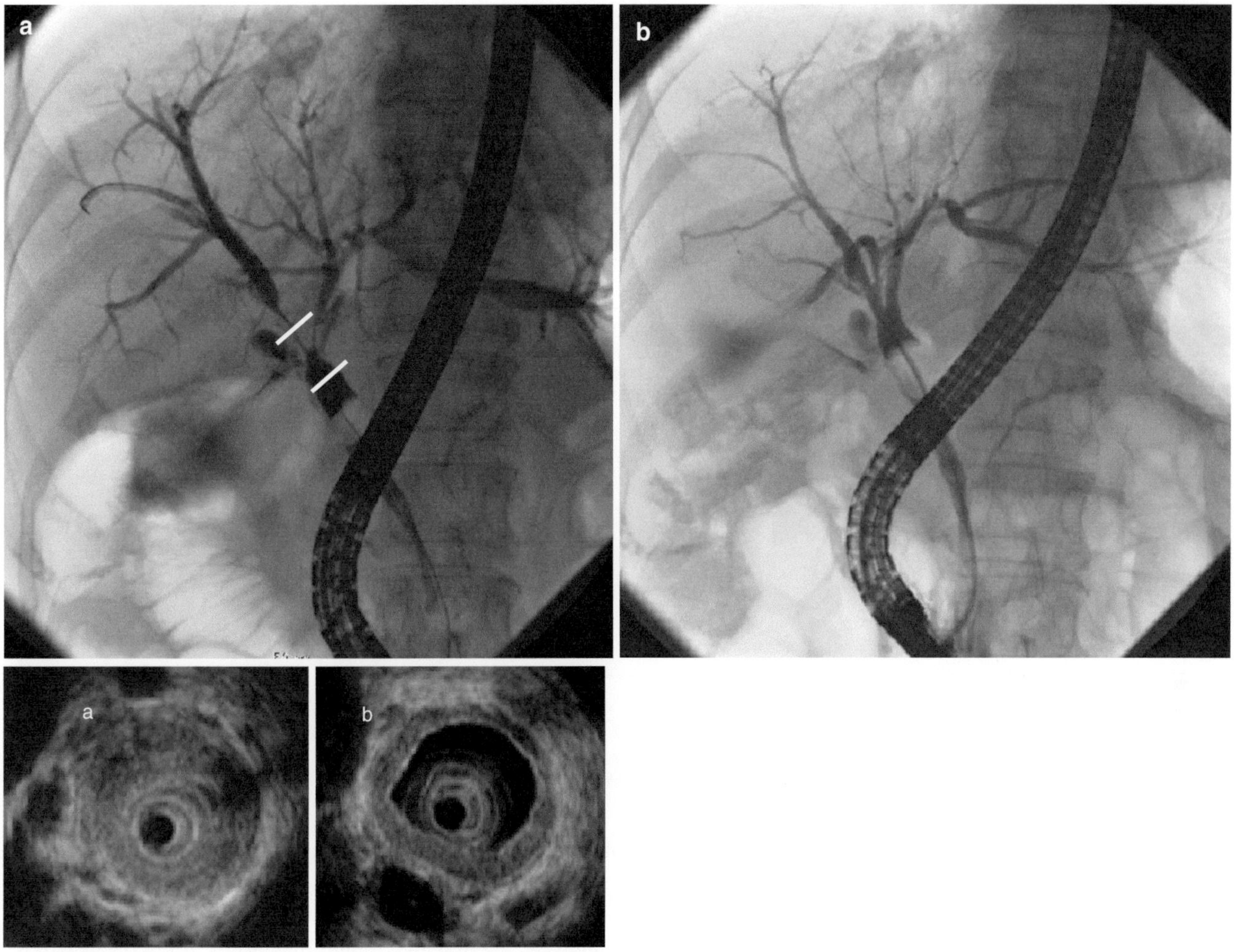

Fig. 15.5 Cholangiogram of type 4 IgG4-SC. Cholangiogram showed stenosis in hilar hepatic lesions (**a**); intraductal ultrasonography revealing bile duct wall thickening in areas with stenosis (**a**-*a*) and without (**a**-*b*). After steroid therapy, the stenosis remarkably improved (**b**)

and that multivariate analysis indicated that steroid therapy and obstructive jaundice at onset were significant factors predictive of unfavorable events. Thus, early introduction of steroid therapy is recommended, especially for patients with obstructive jaundice. Ghazale et al. [3] reported the clinical courses after steroid treatment ($n=30$), surgical resection ($n=18$), and conservative management ($n=5$). Relapses occurred in 53 % of cases after steroid withdrawal, whereas 44 % relapsed after surgery and were further treated with steroids. The presence of proximal extrahepatic/intrahepatic strictures was predictive of relapse. Steroid therapy normalized liver enzyme levels in 61 % of the patients, and it was possible to remove biliary stents in 17 of 18 patients. Fifteen patients treated with steroids for relapse after steroid withdrawal responded to the treatment, and 7 patients treated with additional immunomodulatory drugs reportedly remained in steroid-free remission. Topazian et al. [33] reported that biliary strictures in 1 patient improved after rituximab therapy and thus the biliary stents were removed. However, the role of immunomodulatory drugs for relapse warrants further study. In one of our series, 6 of 7 cases of IgG4-SC without steroid therapy and IgG levels >2,000 mg/dL were associated with significantly higher incidence of recurrence or progression [34].

Although, generally, diagnosis should be made before starting therapy, a steroid trial is needed in some cases [35]. If a diagnosis cannot be clearly established in type 2 IgG4-SC, then a steroid trial is recommended. If malignancy is not confirmed by bile duct biopsy in types 3 and 4 IgG4-SC and bile duct wall thickening that appears normal on a cholangiogram, a steroid trial is an option. No reports on any steroid trial for IgG4-SC have been published thus far. A short-term steroid trial should be performed carefully only by specialists in pancreatic and biliary diseases. The time frame for a steroid trial for IgG4-SC remains unknown. When a cholangiogram is indicative of type 1, 3, or 4 IgG4-SC, IgG4-SC should be discriminated from PCa or CC. It is important not to delay the timing of surgery by

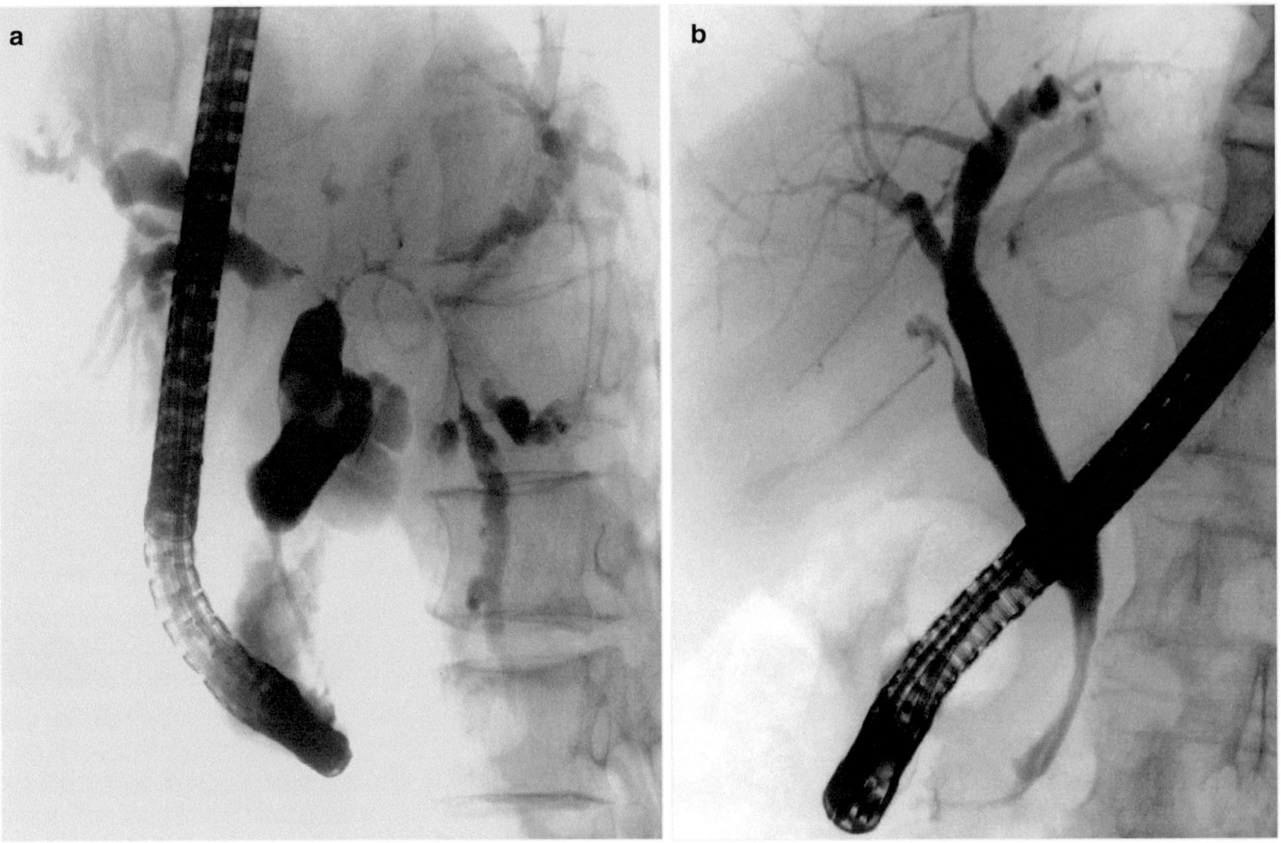

Fig. 15.6 Cholangiogram of type 2a IgG4-SC. Cholangiogram displayed diffuse stenosis in the intrahepatic ducts (**a**). After steroid therapy, the diffuse stenosis remarkably improved (**b**)

performing a long-term steroid trial. If a cholangiogram is indicative of type 2 IgG4-SC, IgG4-SC should be discriminated from PSC. Sufficient time should be devoted to a steroid trial only if an increased risk of biliary infection can be avoided.

Advanced-stage IgG4-SC may sometimes be unresponsive to steroid therapy because cases of AIP and IgG4-SC show predominant inflammatory nature at the early stage followed by relatively less inflammation but marked fibrous scarring later in the course of the disease. This should be kept in mind when attempting a steroid trial for IgG4-SC diagnosis [36].

Prognosis

Morphological and functional changes in the liver and bile ducts in IgG4-SC during long-term observation have not yet been reported. Our long-term follow-up of IgG4-SC cases without steroid therapy revealed that 2 patients developed portal obstruction and liver atrophy but no sign of liver cirrhosis or liver failure [37]. Ghazale et al. [3] reported that 4 of 53 patients displayed portal hypertension and liver cirrhosis during their clinical courses. It is possible that persistent jaundice without steroid administration would result in liver failure, thus necessitating orthotopic liver transplantation. However, further study is needed to elucidate the long-term outcome of IgG4-SC.

Simultaneous occurrences of AIP and PC have been occasionally reported [38, 39]. There are only two case reports about IgG4-SC cases with CC [40, 41] However, none of the 344 IgG4-SC cases in Japanese multicenter study were not associated with CC.

Conclusions

The concept of IgG4-SC makes it possible to avoid liver transplantation under a diagnosis of PSC and hepatectomy under a diagnosis of bile duct cancer. Therefore, we should discriminate between these diseases before selecting the most appropriate therapy. During the last decade, a large amount of new knowledge about IgG4-SC has been reported. Here we have reviewed and summarized the diagnostic procedures and treatments of IgG4-SC. However, the most important consideration for clinicians is to be aware of IgG4-SC when encountering patients with obstructive jaundice. Further understanding of the pathogenesis of IgG4-SC will pave the way for disease prevention and new treatment strategies.

References

1. Nakazawa T, Ohara H, Sano H, Ando T, Joh T. Schematic classification of sclerosing cholangitis with autoimmune pancreatitis by cholangiography. Pancreas. 2006;32:229.
2. Nakazawa T, Naitoh I, Hayashi K, Okumura F, Miyabe K, Yoshida M, Yamashita H, Ohara H, Joh T. Diagnostic criteria for IgG4-related sclerosing cholangitis based on cholangiographic classification. J Gastroenterol. 2012;47:79–87.
3. Ghazale A, Chari ST, Zhang L, Smyrk TC, Takahashi N, Levy MJ, Topazian MD, Clain JE, Pearson RK, Petersen BT, Vege SS, Lindor K, Farnell MB. Immunoglobulin G4-associated cholangitis: clinical profile and response to therapy. Gastroenterology. 2008;134:706–15.
4. Hirano K, Tada M, Isayama H, Yamamoto K, Mizuno S, Yashima Y, Sasaki T, Kogure H, Togawa O, Arizumi T, Matsubara S, Nakai Y, Sasahira N, Tsujino T, Kawabe T, Omata M. Endoscopic evaluation of factors contributing to intrapancreatic biliary stricture in autoimmune pancreatitis. Gastrointest Endosc. 2010;71:85–90.
5. Zen Y, Harada K, Sasaki M, Sato Y, Tsuneyama K, Haratake J, Kurumaya H, Katayanagi K, Masuda S, Niwa H, Morimoto H, Miwa A, Uchiyama A, Portmann BC, Nakanuma Y. IgG4-related sclerosing cholangitis with and without hepatic inflammatory pseudotumor, and sclerosing pancreatitis-associated sclerosing cholangitis: do they belong to a spectrum of sclerosing pancreatitis? Am J Surg Pathol. 2004;28:1193–203.
6. Naitoh I, Nakazawa T, Ohara H, Ando T, Hayashi K, Tanaka H, Okumura F, Takahashi S, Joh T. Endoscopic transpapillary intraductal ultrasonography and biopsy in the diagnosis of IgG4-related sclerosing cholangitis. J Gastroenterol. 2009;44:1147–55.
7. Ohara H, Nakazawa T, Kawa S, Kamisawa T, Shimosegawa T, Uchida K, Hirano K, Nishino T, Hamano H, Kanno A, Notohara K, Hasebe O, Muraki T, Ishida E, Naitoh I, Okazaki K. Establishment of a serum IgG4 cut-off value for the differential diagnosis of IgG4-related sclerosing cholangitis: a Japanese cohort. J Gastroenterol Hepatol. 2013;28:1247–51.
8. Kawaguchi K, Koike M, Tsuruta K, Okamoto A, Tabata I, Fujita N. Lymphoplasmacytic sclerosing pancreatitis with cholangitis: a variant of primary sclerosing cholangitis extensively involving pancreas. Hum Pathol. 1991;22:387–95.
9. Abraham SC, Cruz-Correa M, Argani P, Furth EE, Hruban RH, Boitnott JK. Lymphoplasmacytic chronic cholecystitis and biliary tract disease in patients with lymphoplasmacytic sclerosing pancreatitis. Am J Surg Pathol. 2003;27:441–51.
10. Zhang L, Lewis JT, Abraham SC, Smyrk TC, Leung S, Chari ST, Poterucha JJ, Rosen CB, Lohse CM, Katzmann JA, Wu TT. IgG4+ plasma cell infiltrates in liver explants with primary sclerosing cholangitis. Am J Surg Pathol. 2010;34:88–94.
11. Hamano H, Kawa S, Horiuchi A, Unno H, Furuya N, Akamatsu T, Fukushima M, Nikaido T, Nakayama K, Usuda N, Kiyosawa K. High serum IgG4 concentrations in patients with sclerosing pancreatitis. N Engl J Med. 2001;344:732–8.
12. Shimosegawa T, Chari ST, Frulloni L, Kamisawa T, Kawa S, Mino-Kenudson M, Kim MH, Klöppel G, Lerch MM, Löhr M, Notohara K, Okazaki K, Schneider A, Zhang L. International consensus diagnostic criteria for autoimmune pancreatitis: guidelines of the International Association of Pancreatology. Pancreas. 2011;40:352–8.
13. Oseini AM, Chaiteerakij R, Shire AM, Ghazale A, Kaiya J, Moser CD, Aderca I, Mettler TA, Therneau TM, Zhang L, Takahashi N, Chari ST, Roberts LR. Utility of serum immunoglobulin G4 in distinguishing immunoglobulin G4-associated cholangitis from cholangiocarcinoma. Hepatology. 2011;54:940–8.
14. Mendes FD, Jorgensen R, Keach J, Katzmann JA, Smyrk T, Donlinger J, Chari S, Lindor KD. Elevated serum IgG4 concentration in patients with primary sclerosing cholangitis. Am J Gastroenterol. 2006;101:2070–5.
15. Ohara H, Okazaki K, Tsubouchi H, Inui K, Kawa S, Kamisawa T, Tazuma S, Uchida K, Hirano K, Yoshida H, Nishino T, Ko SB, Mizuno N, Hamano H, Kanno A, Notohara K, Hasebe O, Nakazawa T, Nakanuma Y, Takikawa H. Clinical diagnostic criteria of IgG4-related sclerosing cholangitis 2012. J Hepatobiliary Pancreat Sci. 2012;19:536–42.
16. Chari ST, Smyrk TC, Levy MJ, Topazian MD, Takahashi N, Zhang L, Clain JE, Pearson RK, Petersen BT, Vege SS, Farnell MB. Diagnosis of autoimmune pancreatitis: the Mayo Clinic experience. Clin Gastroenterol Hepatol. 2006;4:1010–106; quiz 934.
17. Nakazawa T, Ohara H, Sano H, Aoki S, Kobayashi S, Okamoto T, Imai H, Nomura T, Joh T, Itoh M. Cholangiography can discriminate sclerosing cholangitis with autoimmune pancreatitis from primary sclerosing cholangitis. Gastrointest Endosc. 2004;60:937–44.
18. Nakazawa T, Ando T, Hayashi K, Naitoh I, Ohara H, Joh T. Diagnostic procedures for IgG4-related sclerosing cholangitis. J Hepatobiliary Pancreat Sci. 2011;18:127–36.
19. Mizuno N, Bhatia V, Hosoda W, Sawaki A, Hoki N, Hara K, Takagi T, Ko SB, Yatabe Y, Goto H, Yamao K. Histological diagnosis of autoimmune pancreatitis using EUS-guided trucut biopsy: a comparison study with EUS-FNA. J Gastroenterol. 2009;44:742–50.
20. Nakazawa T, Naitoh I, Hayashi K, Miyabe K, Simizu S, Joh T. Diagnosis of IgG4-related sclerosing cholangitis. World J Gastroenterol. 2013;19:7661–70.
21. Loftus EV, Harewood GC, Loftus CG, Tremaine WJ, Harmsen WS, Zinsmeister AR, Jewell DA, Sandborn WJ. PSC-IBD: a unique form of inflammatory bowel disease associated with primary sclerosing cholangitis. Gut. 2005;54:91–6.
22. Sano H, Nakazawa T, Ando T, Hayashi K, Naitoh I, Okumura F, Miyabe K, Yoshida M, Takahashi S, Ohara H, Joh T. Clinical characteristics of inflammatory bowel disease associated with primary sclerosing cholangitis. J Hepatobiliary Pancreat Sci. 2011;18:154–61.
23. Umemura T, Zen Y, Hamano H, Kawa S, Nakanuma Y, Kiyosawa K. Immunoglobulin G4-hepatopathy: association of immunoglobulin G4-bearing plasma cells in liver with autoimmune pancreatitis. Hepatology. 2007;46:463–71.
24. Naitoh I, Zen Y, Nakazawa T, Ando T, Hayashi K, Okumura F, Miyabe K, Yoshida M, Nojiri S, Kanematsu T, Ohara H, Joh T. Small bile duct involvement in IgG4-related sclerosing cholangitis: liver biopsy and cholangiography correlation. J Gastroenterol. 2011;46:269–76.
25. Nakazawa T, Ohara H, Sano H, Ando T, Aoki S, Kobayashi S, Okamoto T, Nomura T, Joh T, Itoh M. Clinical differences between primary sclerosing cholangitis and sclerosing cholangitis with autoimmune pancreatitis. Pancreas. 2005;30:20–5.
26. Nishino T, Oyama H, Hashimoto E, Toki F, Oi I, Kobayashi M, Shiratori K. Clinicopathological differentiation between sclerosing cholangitis with autoimmune pancreatitis and primary sclerosing cholangitis. J Gastroenterol. 2007;42:550–9.
27. Kawakami H, Zen Y, Kuwatani M, Eto K, Haba S, Yamato H, Shinada K, Kubota K, Asaka M. IgG4-related sclerosing cholangitis and autoimmune pancreatitis: histological assessment of biopsies from Vater's ampulla and the bile duct. J Gastroenterol Hepatol. 2010;25:1648–55.
28. Harada K, Shimoda S, Kimura Y, Sato Y, Ikeda H, Igarashi S, Ren XS, Sato H, Nakanuma Y. Significance of immunoglobulin G4 (IgG4)-positive cells in extrahepatic cholangiocarcinoma: molecular mechanism of IgG4 reaction in cancer tissue. Hepatology. 2012;56:157–64.
29. Kubota K, Kato S, Akiyama T, Yoneda M, Fujita K, Ogawa M, Inamori M, Kobayashi N, Saito S, Kakuta Y, Ohshiro H, Nakajima A. Differentiating sclerosing cholangitis caused by autoimmune pancreatitis and primary sclerosing cholangitis according

to endoscopic duodenal papillary features. Gastrointest Endosc. 2008;68:1204–8.

30. Sepehr A, Mino-Kenudson M, Ogawa F, Brugge WR, Deshpande V, Lauwers GY. IgG4+ to IgG + plasma cells ratio of ampulla can help differentiate autoimmune pancreatitis from other "mass forming" pancreatic lesions. Am J Surg Pathol. 2008;32:1770–9.
31. Nishino T, Toki F, Oyama H, Oi I, Kobayashi M, Takasaki K, Shiratori K. Biliary tract involvement in autoimmune pancreatitis. Pancreas. 2005;30:76–82.
32. Hirano K, Tada M, Isayama H, Yagioka H, Sasaki T, Kogure H, Nakai Y, Sasahira N, Tsujino T, Yoshida H, Kawabe T, Omata M. Long-term prognosis of autoimmune pancreatitis with and without corticosteroid treatment. Gut. 2007;56:1719–24.
33. Topazian M, Witzig TE, Smyrk TC, Pulido JS, Levy MJ, Kamath PS, Chari ST. Rituximab therapy for refractory biliary strictures in immunoglobulin G4-associated cholangitis. Clin Gastroenterol Hepatol. 2008;6:364–6.
34. Nakazawa T, Ohara H, Ando T, Hayashi K, Naitoh I, Okumura F, Tanaka H, Sano H, Joh T. Clinical course and indications for steroid therapy of sclerosing cholangitis associated with autoimmune pancreatitis. Hepatogastroenterology. 2009;56:584–8.
35. Tomiyama T, Uchida K, Matsushita M, Ikeura T, Fukui T, Takaoka M, Nishio A, Okazaki K. Comparison of steroid pulse therapy and conventional oral steroid therapy as initial treatment for autoimmune pancreatitis. J Gastroenterol. 2011;46:696–704.
36. Nakazawa T, Naitoh I, Ando T, Hayashi K, Okumura F, Miyabe K, Yoshida M, Ohara H, Joh T. A case of advanced-stage sclerosing cholangitis with autoimmune pancreatitis not responsive to steroid therapy. JOP. 2010;11:58–60.
37. Hirano A, Nakazawa T, Ohara H, Ando T, Hayashi K, Tanaka H, Naito I, Okumura F, Yokoyama Y, Joh T. Liver atrophy and portal stenosis in two cases of sclerosing cholangitis associated with autoimmune pancreatitis. Intern Med. 2008;47:1689–94.
38. Inoue H, Miyatani H, Sawada Y, et al. A case of pancreas cancer with autoimmune pancreatitis. Pancreas. 2006;33:208–9.
39. Pezzilli R, Vecchiarelli S, Di Marco MC, et al. Pancreatic ductal adenocarcinoma associated with autoimmune pancreatitis. Case Rep Gastroenterol. 2011;5:378–85.
40. Douhara A, Mitoro A, Otani E, Furukawa M, Kaji K, Uejima M, Sawai M, Yoshida M, Yoshiji H, Yamao J, Fukui H. Cholangiocarcinoma developed in a patient with IgG4-related disease. World J Gastrointest Oncol. 2013;5:181–5.
41. Oh H-C, Kim JG, Kim JW, Lee KS, Kim MK, Chi KC, Kim YS, Kim KH. Early bile duct cancer in a background of sclerosing cholangitis and autoimmune pancreatitis. Inter Med. 2008;47:2025–8.

Sialadenitis and Dacryoadenitiss: IgG4-Related Mikulicz's Disease Would Precede Autoimmune Pancreatitis and Be Likely to Relapse

16

Kensuke Kubota, Kunihiro Hosono, and Atsushi Nakajima

Introduction

Mikulicz's disease (MD) was confirmed as an IgG4-related disease (IgG4-RD) in 2011 and in view of its characteristic clinical features of bilateral and symmetrical swelling of the lacrimal and salivary glands, it may be appropriate to revise the disease's name as IgG4-related dacryoadenitis and sialadenitis (IgG4-DS) [1]. IgG4-DS was the same concept as IgG4-related Mikulicz's disease [1]. IgG4-DS could be diagnosed according to the Japanese consensus criteria established in 2008 [2]. Until recently, IgG4-DS was regarded as a subtype of Sjögren's syndrome (SS); however, now, we consider IgG4-DS, which is responsive to corticosteroid treatment (CST) as quite a different disease entity from SS (Fig. 16.1).

To understand the concept of IgG4-DS, it may be important to know its histological background. First, in 1888, Dr. Johann von Mikulicz published a paper about a patient with symmetrical swelling of the lacrimal, parotid, and submandibular glands, characterized pathologically by mononuclear cell infiltration, the so-called MD [3]. Then· in 1933, Dr. Henrik Sjögren published a case series of patients with rheumatoid arthritis associated with keratoconjunctivitis sicca and severe swelling of the parotid glands, the so-called SS [4]. Subsequently, in 1953, Morgan and Castleman classified IgG4-DS as a subtype of SS [5]. Since then, little attention has been paid to IgG4-DS for over 50 years. In 2004, Yamamoto unearthed the definitive differences between IgG4-DS and SS based on clinical data [6]. They revealed that IgG4-DS responded well to CST therapy and that was a reversible condition, unlike SS. In 2012, Umehara proposed the novel clinical entity IgG4-RD, encompassing autoimmune pancreatitis (AIP) and IgG4-DS. Thereafter, IgG4-DS has been regarded as one manifestation of IgG4-RD [7]. It has been suggested that lacrimal gland involvement in IgG4-RD should be referred to as IgG4-related dacryoadenitis, and submandibular gland involvement in IgG4-RD should be referred to as IgG4-related Küttner tumor (IgG4-KT) [1] (Fig. 16.2).

AIP, a major component of IgG4-RD, mainly manifesting as obstructive jaundice and/or deterioration of diabetes mellitus, was first reported by Sarles in 1961 [8] and proposed as a clinical entity by Yoshida et al. in 1995 [9]. Hamano revealed serum IgG4 elevation as a useful finding in the diagnosis for AIP [10]. Although the etiology and mechanism of AIP are still unknown, overproduction of Th2 and regulatory cytokines may play an important role [11, 12]. The characteristic findings of AIP such as elevation of the serum IgG4, infiltration of the affected organs such as the pancreas, bile duct, and gallbladder by IgG4-bearing plasma cells, and its reversibility with CST therapy are similar to those of IgG4-DS. However, AIP is associated with IgG4-DS only in a minority of patients. We describe some patients with AIP associated with IgG4-DS, preceded by dacryoadenitis and sialadenitis [13].

In this section, we summarize the features of IgG4-DS and IgG4-KT from the perspective of AIP because of the paucity of data on the clinical relationship between IgG4-DS/KT and AIP.

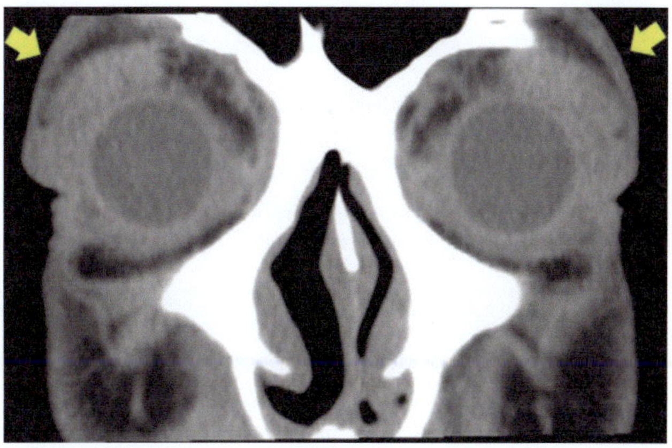

Fig. 16.1 MRI showed IgG4-related dacryoadenitis

K. Kubota, MD, PhD (✉) • K. Hosono, MD, PhD
A. Nakajima, MD, PhD
Division of Hepatogastroenterology,
Yokohama City University Graduate School of Medicine,
Fukuura 3-9, kanazawa, Yokohama 236-0004, Japan
e-mail: kubotak@yokohama-cu.ac.jp

T. Kamisawa, J.B. Chung (eds.), *Autoimmune Pancreatitis*,
DOI 10.1007/978-3-642-55086-7_16, © Springer-Verlag Berlin Heidelberg 2015

Discrimination Between IgG4-Related Mikulicz's Disease and Sjögren's Syndrome

Table 16.1 shows the consensus criteria for the diagnosis of IgG4-related Mikulicz's disease (IgG4-DS) approved by the Japanese society for Sjögren's syndrome (SS) in 2008 [2]. IgG4-DS is regarded as a component of IgG4-RD characterized by lacrimal gland and/or salivary gland involvement. IgG4-DS must be distinguished from disorders such as sarcoidosis, Castleman's disease, Wegener's granulomatosis, lymphoma, and cancer [2] (Table 16.2).

There are several marked symptomatic differences between IgG4-DS and SS, such as IgG4-DS being characterized by bilateral salivary gland/lacrimal gland swelling without tenderness, while SS tends to show unilateral involvement. Sicca is modest in IgG4-DS. In regard to the sex distribution, SS tends to occur predominantly in females, whereas no gender difference in incidence has been reported in patients with IgG4-DS [15].

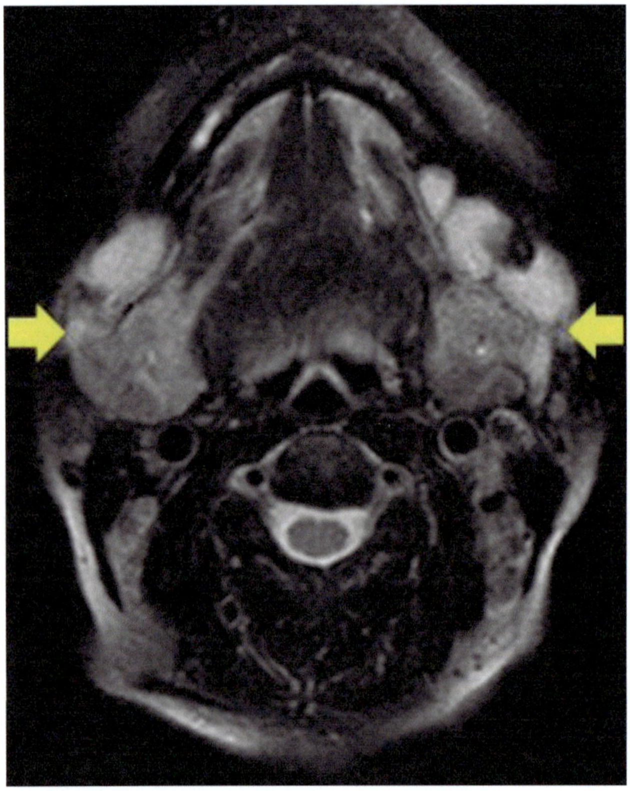

Fig. 16.2 MRI depicted IgG4-related Küttner tumor

Table 16.1 Diagnostic criteria of IgG4-related Mikulicz's disease

1. Symmetrical swelling of at least 2 pairs of lacrimal, parotid, or submandibular glands for at least 3 months
AND
2. Elevated serum IgG4 (>135 mg/dl)
OR
3. Histopathological features including lymphocyte and IgG4+plasma cell infiltration (IgG4+plasma cells/IgG+plasma cells >50 %) with typical tissue fibrosis or sclerosis

Masaki et al. [2]
Approved by the Japanese Society for Sjögren's syndrome 2008

Histopathologically, IgG4-DS had been believed to be a subgroup of SS based on histopathologic similarities between the two entities, such as degeneration and disappearance of the glandular acini due to severe mononuclear cell infiltration, proliferation of the ductal epithelial cells and duct stenosis, formation of myoepithelial islands, and cystic dilatation of the peripheral ducts [5]. However, it has been confirmed that these histopathological features can only be detected in SS, and not in IgG4-DS [15]. The most remarkable difference between IgG4-DS and SS is the marked infiltration of the affected organs by IgG4-bearing plasma cells, with the percentage of IgG4-positive cells relative to the total IgG cell population being characteristically more than 40 % in IgG4-DS [2, 15]. On the other hand, infiltration of the salivary glands by IgG4-bearing plasma cells is almost not noted in SS. In the diagnosis of IgG4-DS, the IgG4+/IgG+plasma cell ratio, whose cutoff value is organ-dependent, is reported as a more powerful tool than the total IgG4+ plasma cell count, which is useful for establishing the diagnosis of IgG4-RD [16]. In addition, apoptosis of the acinar and/or duct cells is reported to be frequent and extensive in SS, but not in IgG4-DS [17]. It might be said that the inflammatory reaction is more potent and irreversible in SS than in IgG4-DS.

In regard to the clinical features, symmetric and persistent swelling of more than two of the lacrimal and major salivary glands is seen in IgG4-DS. Most importantly, parotid gland is the major organ affected in SS, while lacrimal and submandibular glands tend to be mainly involved in IgG4-DS. The swelling is short-lived, usually resolving in about a week in IgG4-DS [14].

In regard to the gland function, salivary secretion is severely impaired in SS, while salivary gland function is either normal or only slightly disturbed in IgG4-DS, and the function can usually be improved by CST therapy [15]. Serologically, strongly positive results for anti-SSA/Ro and anti-SSB/La antibodies are obtained in patients with SS, but not in those with IgG4-DS [2]. Not only serum IgG4 but also serum total IgG, IgG2, and IgE concentrations are significantly elevated in IgG4+MOLPS (multiorgan lymphoproliferative syndrome), now accepted as being equivalent to IgG4-RD which includes IgG4-DS, as compared to SS [2].

Regarding therapy, IgG4-DS is mainly treated with CST and resolution of the gland manifestations is immediately obtained; however, CST therapy is not as effective in most patients of SS as in those with IgG4-DS. However, the relapse rate of IgG4-DS is high as also well-recognized in cases of IgG4-RD.

Table 16.2 Differential diagnosis between IgG4-related Mikulicz's disease (IgG4-DS) and Sjögren's syndrome (SS)

	IgG4-related Mikulicz's disease	Sjögren's syndrome
Age	50–70	40–50
Sex	Male = Female?	Female ≫ Male
Gland swelling	Lacrimal/submandibular/parotid	Parotid
	Lower frequency of apoptosis	Apoptosis of acinar/ductal
Keratoconjunctivitis sicca	Reversible	Mild-severely impaired
Salivary secretion	Reversible	Mild-severely impaired
Sclerosing pancreatitis	7–10 %	No
Retroperitoneal fibrosis	20 %	No
Serum IgG4 (>135 mg/dl)	>80 %	Negative
Anti-SSA/SSB antibodies	Negative	Positive 70 %
Corticosteroid response	Prompt	Almost ineffective

Modified from Yamamoto et al. [14]

Differences Between IgG4-Mikulicz's Disease and IgG4-Küttner Tumor Based on Our Case Series

IgG4-related sialadenitis is observed in IgG4-DS and IgG4-related Küttner tumor (IgG4-KT; gland swelling is noted only in the submandibular glands; IgG4-related submandibular disease) [1]. Because sialadenitis is a common manifestation in both IgG4-MD and IgG4-KT, as in IgG4-RD, it is said to be difficult to set a strict boundary between IgG4-MD and IgG4-KT [7]. Histological evidence is needed to differentiate between these two clinical entities. Küttner tumor was first described in 1896 as a rarely occurring chronic inflammatory disorder of the salivary glands, most commonly the submandibular glands, manifesting as a palpable hard tumor; this condition is also referred to as unilateral sclerosing sialadenitis [18]. As the differential diagnosis between IgG4-KT and neoplasm is difficult, the entity came to be referred to as KT. Prior to proposition of the concept of IgG4-RD, a significant proportion of cases may have been diagnosed as KT [1]. As KT has also been recognized to result from stones in the Wharton duct [18], it has been classified into classical KT and IgG4-KT. Geyer JT clarified the histopathologic differences between classical KT and IgG4-KT [19]. Tiemann et al. revealed a monoclonal cytotoxic T-cell population in the affected salivary glands [20], which suggested that in such cases, KT is IgG4-RD. Takano revealed serologic and histopathologic differences between IgG4-DS and IgG4-KT, such as the mean IgG4 concentration was significantly higher in IgG4-DS than in IgG4-KT [21]. It may be said that the disease activity in IgG4-KT is less than that in IgG4-DS. We diagnosed IgG4-KT based on findings such as persistent bilateral swelling of only the submandibular glands detectable by computed tomography and/or FDG-PET, abundant IgG4-bearing plasma cell infiltration with fibrosis in the submandibular glands on histopathologic examination, and elevated serum IgG4 concentrations (>135 mg/dl) on serological testing (Figs. 16.3 and 16.4).

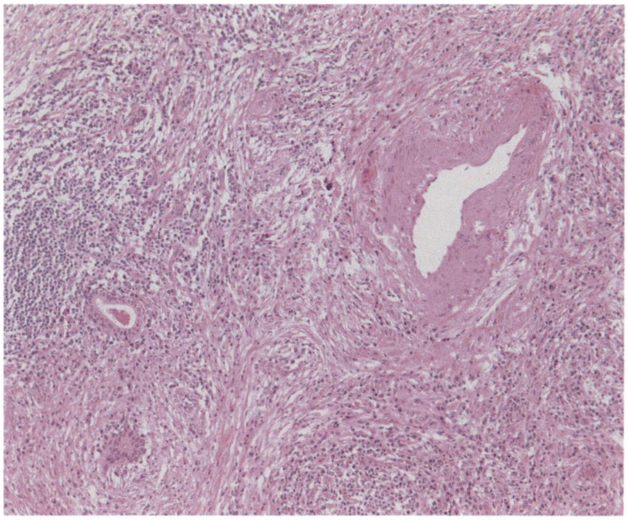

Fig. 16.3 Submandibular gland biopsy specimen showed dense lymphoplasmacytic infiltration with fibrosis

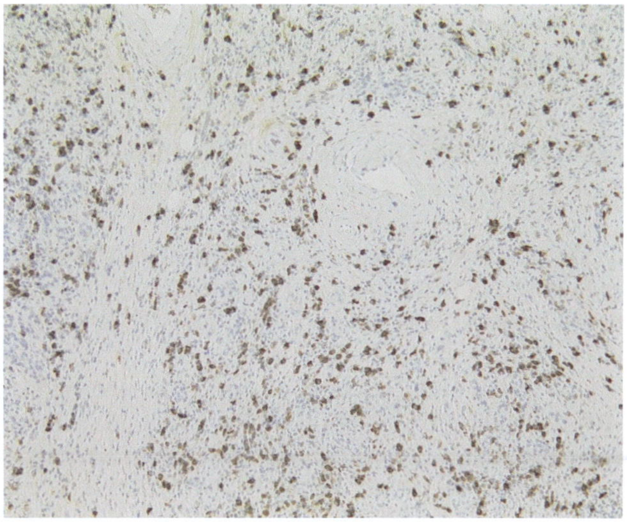

Fig. 16.4 IgG4-bearing plasma cell infiltrations were noted in biopsy specimen of the submandibular gland

Table 16.3 IgG4-related Mikulicz's disease (IgG4-DS) and IgG4-related Küttner disease (IgG4-KT)

Differences between AIP with IgG4-DS and IgG4-KT			
	IgG4-DS ($n=10$)	IgG4-KT ($n=13$)	p
Mean age at onset	63 (52–72)	68 (51–77)	N.S.
Gender ratio (M/F)	6/4 (60 %)	9/4 (69.2 %)	N.S.
Serum IgG (mg/dl)	2,839	2,923	N.S.
Serum IgG4 (mg/dl)	976	888	N.S.
DS/KT precede	*10/2 (83 %)*	*3/10 (23 %)*	*0.005*
Jaundice	5/5 (50 %)	10/3 (76.9 %)	N.S.
Diffuse pancreas swelling	1/9 (90 %)	9/4 (69.2 %)	N.S.
OOI (other than DS/KT)	5/5 (50 %)	11/2 (84.6 %)	N.S.
Relapse	5/5 (50 %)	4/9 (30.8 %)	N.S.
Cancer development	0/10 (0 %)	3/10 (23.1 %)	N.S.

N.S. not significant, *AIP* autoimmune pancreatitis, *IgG4-DS* IgG4-related dacryoadenitis and sialadenitis, *IgG4-KT* IgG4-related Küttner tumor, *M F* male female, *DS/KT precede* IgG4-related dacryoadenitis and sialadenitis/IgG4-related Küttner tumor precede, *OOI* other organ involvement (sclerosing cholangitis, retroperitoneal fibrosis, idiopathic intestinal pneumonitis)

In order to clarify the differences, we retrospectively studied 13 patients with IgG4-KT and 10 patients with IgG4-DS, the patient characteristics illustrated in Table 16.3. All of the patients had been admitted to the Department of Gastroenterology of our hospital; therefore, we could not include IgG4-KT cases without associated AIP, which was a limitation of our study. There were no differences between the two conditions in the mean age at onset, gender ratio, serum IgG level, serum IgG4 level, presence/absence of jaundice, presence/absence of diffuse pancreatic swelling, other organ involvement, relapse, and cancer development. However, IgG4-DS tended to precede the AIP, and in many cases, IgG4-KT was accidentally detected on PET-CT performed during the course of AIP. Diffuse pancreatic swelling tended to be recognized more frequently in patients with IgG4-DS than in patients with IgG4-KT. However, other organ involvement was detected more frequently in IgG4-KT than in IgG4-DS. It could also be said that the inflammation is more aggressive in IgG4-MD than in IgG4-KT. Regarding treatment, IgG4-KT is also treated with CST.

IgG4-Mikulicz's Disease and Autoimmune Pancreatitis Based on Our Case Series

IgG4-DS has been regarded as a component of other organ involvement (OOI) in cases with type 1 AIP. AIP is sometimes associated with Mikulicz's disease (MD; IgG4-DS); however, the significance of IgG4-DS appearing during the clinical course of AIP remains uncertain. We reported that AIP patients with IgG4-DS occurring during the clinical course might show a more hyperactive disease state as compared to AIP patients without IgG4-DS [13]. Although this study was small and retrospective in nature, we clarified that AIP patients presenting with IgG4-DS ($n=5$) tended to manifest different clinical features as compared to AIP patients without IgG4-DS ($n=23$), such as earlier onset, predilection for females, diffuse pancreatic swelling, and high serum titers of IgG4. In addition, in AIP patients with IgG4-DS, the latter tends to precede the gastroenterological event, suggesting that IgG4-DS may serve as a warning sign of subsequent AIP development [13].

Recently, Kuruma et al. compared patients with AIP associated with IgG4-DS, with AIP not associated with IgG4-DS, and IgG4-DS not associated with AIP. They concluded that the relapse rate in the patients with AIP plus IgG4-DS was significantly higher than that in the AIP patients without IgG4-DS; therefore, maintenance CST therapy might be indicated in the former group to reduce the likelihood of relapse [22]. Based on the results of this study, we might say that AIP associated with IgG4-DS is a potentially hyperactive disease state, showing a strong tendency toward relapse [13, 23].

What is the incidence of AIP occurring in association with IgG4-DS? A multicenter long-term outcome study of AIP was published, which showed that IgG4-DS and/or IgG4-KT occurred at a frequency of only 7 % in patients with AIP [23]. Until now, we have encountered 126 type 1 AIP patients, of which 10 (10/126; 7.9 %) had IgG4-DS and 13 (13/126; 10.3 %) had IgG4-KT (Table 16.4). On the other hand, Yamamoto reported that IgG4-DS was associated with AIP in 20 % of cases [17]. This represented a discrepancy of about 10 % in the incidence; however, the patients who initially developed AIP showed a tendency towards subsequently development of IgG4-DS. IgG4-DS preceded AIP in 80 % (8/10) of the cases. This could be a reflection of the author's subspecialty.

We investigated the differences in the features between AIP patients with/without IgG4-DS. There were no significant differences in the mean age of onset, gender ratio, presence/absence of jaundice, extent of pancreatic swelling detected on computed tomography, presence/absence of

Table 16.4 Differences between autoimmune pancreatitis (AIP) with/without IgG4-DS.

Differences between AIP with/without IgG4-DS			
	AIP + IgG4-DS (n = 10)	AIP (n = 100)	p
Mean age at onset	63 (52–72)	64 (25–93)	N.S.
Gender ratio (M/F)	6/4 (60 %)	76/24 (76 %)	N.S.
Serum IgG (mg/dl)	*2,733*	*1,936*	*0.021*
Serum IgG4 (mg/dl)	*976*	*384*	*0.0004*
Jaundice	5/5 (50 %)	50/50 (50 %)	N.S.
Duodenal papillitis	*9/9 (100 %)*	*36/60 (60 %)*	*0.0198*
Diffuse pancreas swelling	9/1 (90 %)	64/31 (67.3 %)	N.S.
OOI (SC, RPF, IIP)	5/5 (50 %)	45/55 (45 %)	N.S.
Relapse	5/5 (50 %)	34/66 (34 %)	N.S.
Cancer development	0/10 (0 %)	22/78 (22 %)	N.S.

N.S. not significant, *AIP* autoimmune pancreatitis, *IgG4-DS* IgG4-related dacryoadenitis and sialadenitis, *M/F* male/female, *OOI* other organ involvement (*SC* sclerosing cholangitis, *RPF* retroperitoneal fibrosis, *IIP* idiopathic intestinal pneumonitis)

other organ involvements, such as sclerosing cholangitis at the hilar part of the bile duct, relapse rate, or incidence of cancer between the two groups. The serum IgG and IgG4 levels were significantly higher in the AIP patients with IgG4-DS than in those without IgG4-DS. In addition, duodenal papillitis, a suggested risk factor for relapse [24], was recognized significantly more frequently in AIP patients with IgG4-DS than in those without IgG4-DS. These results suggest that AIP-associated IgG4-DS is a hyperactive disease state with a propensity to relapse. Therefore, we agree that CST therapy, including maintenance CST therapy, is required in such patients [22].

Prognosis and Prospects of IgG4-Mikulicz's Disease

IgG4-DS is a benign disease that is not fatal and can be controlled by CST; however, relapses are common [25]. Our data showed that AIP with IgG4-DS was a more hyperactive disease state than AIP without IgG4-DS. The reported relapse rate of AIP is 30–40 %, and relapse usually occurs within 3 years of initiation of CST therapy [26]. Therefore, maintenance CST treatment for a sufficient duration is of value, and low-dose CST therapy for more than 3 years is recommended to reduce the relapse rate [26]. We believe that CST is the standard treatment for IgG4-DS, while spontaneous remission (SR) can occur of AIP [24]; there are no case reports of IgG4-DS showing SR.

What should we do in cases of IgG4-DS showing relapse? Readministration of CST may be effective; however, refractory cases might be encountered among AIP patients with IgG4-DS. The mechanism underlying the onset of IgG4-RD, including IgG-DS, remains unknown, Th2-dominant disease has been suggested as one of the aspects of IgG4-RD. Zen et al. described that AIP was characterized by infiltration of helper 2 and regulatory T (Treg) cells, which secrete various cytokines, such as interleukin 10 (IL-10) and tumor growth factor-β (TGF-β). Furthermore, the expression level of FOXP-3 messenger RNA (mRNA) was significantly increased in patients with AIP, and immunohistochemical staining revealed increases in the number of CD4+ CD25+ FOXP3+ cells. Treg may be involved in in situ production of IL-10 and TGF-β, which could be followed by IgG4 class switching and fibroplasia [11].

Recently, the efficacy of immunomodulators or rituximab for the treatment of refractory AIP was studied. B-cell deletion therapy using rituximab, a monoclonal antibody directed against the CD20 antigen on the B cells, has been tried and appears promising [25]. Therefore, although standard treatment for IgG4-DS has been CST, immunomodulator or rituximab therapy should also be evaluated for refractory cases of IgG4-DS.

Is IgG4-DS a risk factor for cancer? There have been only a few papers on the risk of cancer associated with IgG4-DS. Regarding cancer development, there are two reports of an association [27, 28]. Shiokawa mentioned that AIP might develop as a paraneoplastic syndrome in some patients based on a study of the standardized incidence ratio for cancer development, the risk during the first year after AIP diagnosis [27]. Yamamoto also stressed that recognition of the possible risk of cancer development in patients with IgG4-RD is essential and that these patients need to be carefully followed up [28]. In our series of 126 patients, 22 developed cancer (22/126; 17 %; data not published). Out of these, four patients developed pancreatic cancer within 5 years of the onset of AIP, which was not associated with IgG4-DS. We believe that cancer could develop by chance in patients with IgG4-RD, because the latter is usually diagnosed in elderly patients who are already predisposed to cancer. However, due to the tendency for cancer development in these patients, irrespective of the nature of the association, close surveillance for cancer is recommended [28].

References

1. Stone JH, Khosrroshahi A, Desphande V, et al. IgG4-related disease: recommendations for the nomenclature of this condition and its individual organ system manifestations. Arthjritis Rheum. 2012;64:3061–7.
2. Masaki Z, Sugai S, Umemura H. IgG4-related diseases including Mikulicz's disease and sclerosing Pancreatitis: diagnostic insight. J Rheum. 2010;37:1380–5.
3. Mikulicz J.Über eine eigenartige symmetrishe Erkrankung der Tranen und Mundspeicheldrusen. Stuttgart: Beitr.z. Chir. Fesrschr. F. Theodor Billroth;1892. pp. 610–30.
4. Sjögren H. Zur Kenntnis der Keratocojunctivitis Sicca (Keratitis filiformis bei Hypofunktion der Tranendrusen). Acta Ophthalmol. 1933;11(suppl II):1–151.
5. Morgan WS, Castleman B. A clinicopathologic study of "Mikulicz's disease". Am J Pathol. 1953;29:471–503.
6. Yamamoto M, Ohara M, Suzuki C, et al. Elavated IgG4 concentrations in serum of patients with Mikulicz's disease. Scand J Rheumatol. 2004;33:432.
7. Umehara H, Okazaki K, Masaki Y, et al. A novel clinical entity, IgG4-related disease (IgG4RD): general concept and details. Mod Rheumatol. 2012;22:1–14.
8. Yoshida K, Toki F, Takeuti T, et al. Chronic pancreatitis caused by an autoimmune abnormality. Proposal of the concept of autoimmune pancreatitis. Dig Dis Sci. 1995;40:1561–8.
9. Sarles H, Sarles JC, Muratore R, Guien C. Chronic inflammatory sclerosis of the pancreas-an autonomous pancreatic disease? Am J Dig Dis. 1961;6:688–98.
10. Hamano H, Kawa S, Horiuchi A, et al. High serum IgG4 concentrations in patients with sclerosing pancreatitis. N Engl J Med. 2001;344:732–8.
11. Zen Y, Fujii T, Harada K, et al. Th2 and regulatory immune reactions are increased in immunoglobin G4-related sclerosing pancreatitis and cholangitis. Hepatology. 2007;45:1538–46.
12. Tanaka A, Moriyama M, Nakashima H, et al. Th2 and regulatory immune reactions contribute to IgG4 production and the initiation of Mikulicz's disease. Arthritis Rheum. 2012;64(1): 254–63.
13. Kubota K, Wada T, Kato S, et al. Highly active state of autoimmune pancreatitis with Mikulicz's disease. Pancreas. 2010;39: e6–10.
14. Yamamoto M, Takahashi H, Ohara M, et al. A new conceptualization for Mikulicz's disease as an IgG4-related plasmacytic disease. Mod Rheumatol. 2006;16:335–40.
15. Yamamoto M, Takahashi H, Sugai S, et al. Clinical and pathological differences between Mikulicz's disease and Sjogren's syndrome. (IgG4-related plasmacytic exocrinopathy). Autoimmunity Rev. 2005;4:195–200.
16. Zen Y, Nakamura Y. IgG4-related disease: cross sectional study of 114 cases. Am Surg Pathol. 2010;34:1812–9.
17. Tubota K, Fujita H, Tadano K. Abnormal expression and function Fas ligand of lacrimal glands and peripheral blood in Sjogren's syndrome patients with enlarged exocrine glands. Clin Exp Immunol. 2002;129:177–82.
18. Küttner H. Ueber entzundliche tumoren der submaxillar-speicheldruse. Beitr Klin Chir. 1896;15:815–34.
19. Geyer JT, Ferry JA, Harris NL, et al. Chronic sclerosing sialadenitis (Kuttner) is an IgG4-associated disease. Am J Surg Pathol. 2010;34:202–10.
20. Tiemann M, Teymoortash A, Schrader C, et al. Chronic sclerosing sialadenitis of the submandibular gland is mainly due to a T lymphocytic immune reaction. Mod Pathol. 2002;15:845–52.
21. Takano K, Yamamoto M, Takahashi H, et al. clinicopathologic similarities between Mikulicz disease and Kuttner tumor. Am J Otolaryngology. 2010;31:429–34.
22. Kuruma S, Kamisawa T, Tabata T, et al. Clinical characteristics of patients with autoimmune pancreatitis with or without Mikulicz's disease and Mikulicz's disease alone. Gut Liver. 2013;7:96–9.
23. Hart PA, Kamisawa T, Witzig TE, Clain JE, Gleeson FC, Klebig RR, et al. Long term outcomes of autoimmune pancreatitis :multicenter, international analysis. Gut. 2013;62:1771–6.
24. Kubota K, Iida H, Fujusawa T, et al. Clinical factors predictive of spontaneous remission or relapse of autoimmune pancreatitis. GIE. 2007;66:1142–51.
25. Hart PA, Topazian MD, Witzig TE, et al. Treatment of relapsing autoimmune pancreatitis with immunomodulators and rituximab: the Mayo Clinic experience. Gut. 2013;62:1607–15.
26. Kamisawa T, Shimosegawa T, Okazaki W, et al. Standard steroid treatment for autoimmune pancreatitis. Gut. 2009;58:1504–7.
27. Shiokawa M, Kodama Y, Yoshimura K, et al. Risk of cancer in patients with autoimmune pancreatitis. Am J Gastroenterol. 2013;108:610–7.
28. Yamamoto M, Takahashi H, Tabeya T, et al. Risk of malignancies in IgG4-related disease. Mod Rheumatol. 2012;22:414–8.

Retroperitoneal Fibrosis

17

Kazuro Chiba, Terumi Kamisawa, Taku Tabata, and Susumu Iwasaki

Introduction

A rare disease, retroperitoneal fibrosis (RF) is characterized by the presence of fibroinflammatory tissue that develops around the abdominal aorta and iliac arteries, often entrapping the ureters. RF has been divided into 2 types: idiopathic RF for which no clear cause is found and secondary RF, whose causes include drugs, radiotherapy, infections, malignant diseases, and trauma [1, 2]. Two patients with anuria caused by bilateral ureteral obstruction due to envelopment and compression of the ureters by an inflammatory retroperitoneal process were reported by Ormond in 1948 [3]. Consequently, idiopathic RF is referred to as Ormond's disease.

Based on the study of autoimmune pancreatitis (AIP), the concept of a new systemic entity of IgG4-related disease (IgG4-RD) was developed [4, 5]. RF occasionally occurs as an extrapancreatic lesion of AIP [6]. RF associated with AIP is currently considered to be IgG4-related retroperitoneal fibrosis (IgG4-RF), a retroperitoneal lesion of IgG4-RD [5, 6].

Concept

It has become clear that many previously diagnosed cases of idiopathic RF were actually IgG4-RF [7, 8].

Several cases of IgG4-RF without AIP and several cases of non-IgG4-related RF have been reported [7, 9]. It has also become apparent that some cases of inflammatory thoracic and abdominal periaortitis are a manifestation of IgG4-RD [8, 10]. IgG4-RF most commonly involves the areas around the abdominal aorta and ureters. Presumably, there is overlap between IgG4-related periaortitis and IgG4-RF, and this discrimination depends on the predominant locations of the lesions [10].

K. Chiba, MD • T. Kamisawa, MD, PhD (✉)
T. Tabata, MD • S. Iwasaki, MD
Department of Internal Medicine,
Tokyo Metropolitan Komagome Hospital,
3-18-22 Honkomagome, Bunkyo-ku, Tokyo 113-8677, Japan
e-mail: kamisawa@cick.jp

Epidemiology

Idiopathic RF is a rare disease, and the prevalence is reportedly 1.38 per 100,000 people [11]. However, the exact frequency of IgG4-RF is unknown. Among 17 patients with a histological diagnosis of RF, Zen et al. reported that 10 patients had increased serum IgG4 levels and extensive IgG4-positive plasma cell infiltration [7]. In the international multicenter survey of AIP [12], RF was seen in 10 (7 %) of 153 type 1 AIP patients. The prevalence of RF associated with AIP was 4 % in Japan, 16 % in Korea, 14 % in the United States, 2 % in Italy, and 7 % in the United Kingdom. Hamano et al. reported that concurrent retroperitoneal fibrosis was found in 8 (13 %) of 64 AIP patients [13]. In our series [9, 14–16], concurrent RF was found in 5 (5 %) of 100 type 1 AIP patients; the onset of RF coincided with the onset of AIP in 3 patients, preceded the onset of AIP in 1 patient, and occurred 1 year after bypass surgery performed for AIP in 1 patient.

Pathology

Histological features of IgG4-RF comprise marked fibrosis with lymphoplasmacytic infiltration and adipose tissue destruction. In fibrotic foci, storiform fibrosis is found. Obliterative phlebitis, lymph follicle formation, and eosinophilic infiltration are frequently seen. On immunostaining, numerous IgG4-positive plasma cells are identified. These histological findings are quite similar to those seen in the pancreas of AIP cases. The periureteral lesions in IgG4-RF are most prominent around the muscularis propria. The inflammation extends to the muscularis propria of the ureter in many cases, while inflammation in the epithelium is

T. Kamisawa, J.B. Chung (eds.), *Autoimmune Pancreatitis*,
DOI 10.1007/978-3-642-55086-7_17, © Springer-Verlag Berlin Heidelberg 2015

absent or extremely mild in most cases. Characteristic histological findings of IgG4-related periaortitis are formation of thick fibrotic inflammatory foci chiefly in the adventitia and extreme thickening of the vascular wall. Inflammation of the adventitia often extends to the media [8, 10, 17].

Clinical Features

IgG4-RF tends to occur in elderly males. In one review of 14 cases of IgG4-RF, all patients were males, and their mean age was 67 years [8]. In the series conducted by Zen et al., all 10 IgG4-RF patients were males, and their mean age was 66.5 years [7]. Our 10 IgG4-RF patients were 6 males and 4 females, and their mean age was 70.1 years. These findings are consistent with the predominance of elderly males among AIP cases.

Symptoms due to RF are not specific. Dull abdominal pain, back pain, general malaise, fever, edema of the lower extremities, and weight loss have been known to occur [18–21]. However, there are not a few IgG4-RF patients who have no symptoms due to RF. Serum IgG4 levels are frequently elevated. Elevation of serum IgE, eosinophilia, and autoantibodies are sometimes seen. Anemia, hypoalbuminemia, and increased CRP levels, which have been reported frequently in RF, are also detected in IgG4-RF patients [9].

Diagnosis

Considering the diagnostic criteria for definitive cases in the comprehensive clinical diagnostic criteria for IgG4-RD [22], we proposed diagnostic criteria of IgG4-RF as follows [9].

IgG4-related RF was diagnosed when all of the following three criteria were fulfilled.

1. Soft tissue masses surrounding the aorta and/or adjacent tissues on computed tomography (CT) and/or magnetic resonance imaging (MRI)
2. Elevation of the serum IgG4 levels (≥135 mg/dL)
3. Abundant infiltration of IgG4-positive plasma cells (≥10/high-power field (HPF)) in at least one organ or site

Since performing an adequate biopsy of a retroperitoneal mass is usually difficult, the histological criteria can be confirmed in extraretroperitoneal sites in the criteria.

The most useful diagnostic imaging techniques for IgG4-RF are CT and MRI. On CT images, IgG4-RF is seen as a soft tissue mass encasing the aorta (Fig. 17.1), which often spreads laterally to involve the inferior vena cava and urinary tract (Fig. 17.2), sometimes resulting in hydronephrosis [9, 10, 21]. On MRI, IgG4-RF shows low signal intensity on T1-weighted images and high signal intensity on T2-weighted images. Other IgG4-RD lesions such as AIP or IgG4-related sialadenitis are sometimes present. Most recently, IgG4-RF has sometimes been detected incidentally during diagnostic imaging in IgG4-RD patients. F-18 fluorodeoxyglucose positron emission tomography (FDG-PET) is also a useful tool for determination of the presence/absence of RF, as well as other lesions of IgG4-related disease (Fig. 17.3) [23].

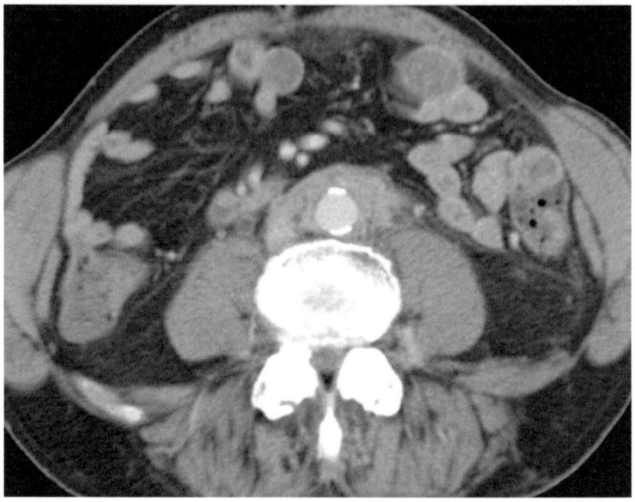

Fig. 17.1 CT imaging of IgG4-related retroperitoneal fibrosis showing a soft tissue mass encasing the aorta

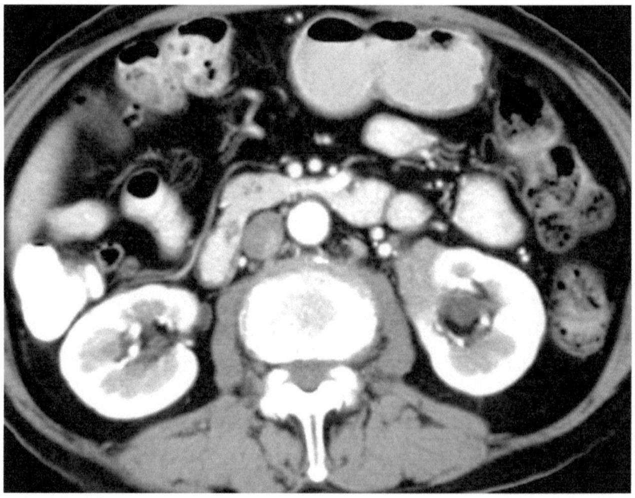

Fig. 17.2 CT imaging of IgG4-related retroperitoneal fibrosis showing a soft tissue mass in the renal hilus

The retroperitoneum is also a site where tumor lesions such as malignant lymphoma, desmoid fibromatosis, and liposarcoma often develop [24]. Histological investigation of the retroperitoneal mass is necessary to differentiate IgG4-RF from malignancy with atypical imaging or normal IgG4 levels.

Treatment

IgG4-RF responds well to steroids, and steroid therapy has become a standard therapy for IgG4-RF [25, 26]. Although a few asymptomatic patients might need only monitoring, ste-

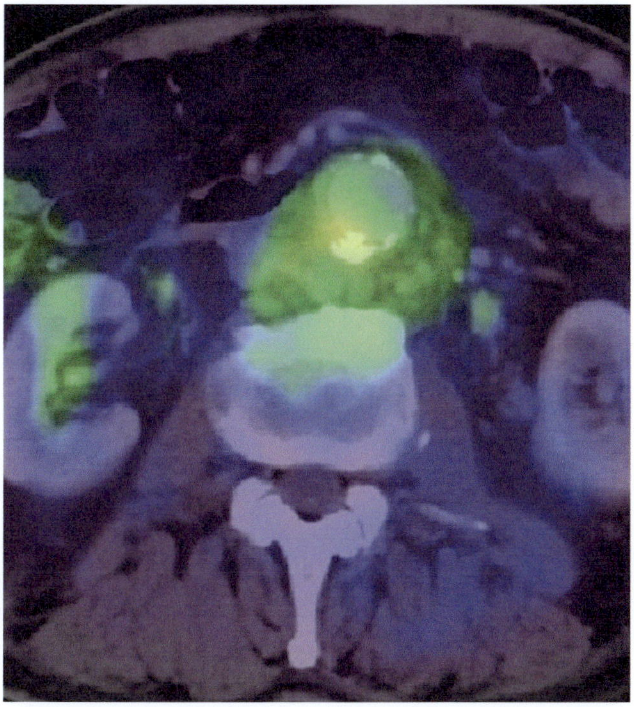

Fig. 17.3 FDG-PET/CT showing uptake of FDG around the aorta

roid therapy is necessary for patients with clinical symptoms or those with hydronephrosis. Zen et al. reported that steroid therapy was effective regardless of the presence/absence of IgG4-related disease or serum IgG4 levels [7]. The starting dose of steroid is usually 30–40 mg/day (0.6 mg/kg/day). The response to steroid therapy is generally favorable except in a few cases [24].

The long-term prognosis of IgG4-RF is unknown.

Conclusions

Recognition of the concept of IgG4-RF has resulted in great progress in the diagnosis and therapy of RF. The diagnostic criteria for IgG4-RF described herein may be helpful in diagnosing this disease correctly.

Acknowledgment This study was partially supported by the Intractable Disease, supported by the Ministry of Health, Labour, and Welfare of Japan.

References

1. Koep L, Zuidema GD. The clinical significance of retroperitoneal fibrosis. Surgery. 1997;81:250–7.
2. Vaglio A, Salvarani C, Buzio C. Retroperitoneal fibrosis. Lancet. 2006;367:241–51.
3. Ormond JK. Bilateral ureteral obstruction due to envelopment and compression by an inflammatory retroperitoneal process. J Urol. 1948;59:950–4.
4. Kamisawa T, Funata N, Hayashi Y, et al. A new clinicopathological entity of IgG4-related autoimmune disease. J Gastroenterol. 2003;38:982–4.
5. Stone JH, Khosroshahi A, Deshpande V, et al. Recommendations for the nomenclature of IgG4-related disease and its individual organ system manifestations. Arthritis Rheum. 2012;64:3061–7.
6. Kamisawa T, Takuma K, Egawa N, Tsuruta K, Sasaki T. Autoimmune pancreatitis and IgG4-related sclerosing disease. Nat Rev Gastroenterol Hepatol. 2010;7:401–9.
7. Zen Y, Onodera M, Inoue D, et al. Retroperitoneal fibrosis: a clinicopathologic study with respect to immunoglobulin G4. Am J Surg Pathol. 2009;33:1833–9.
8. Stone JR. Aortitis, periaortitis, and retroperitoneal fibrosis, as manifestations of IgG4-related systemic disease. Curr Opin Rheumatol. 2011;23:88–94.
9. Chiba K, Kamisawa T, Tabata T, et al. Clinical features of 10 patients with IgG4-related retroperitoneal fibrosis. Intern Med. 2013;52:1545–51.
10. Inoue D, Zen Y, Abo H, et al. Immunoglobulin G4-related periaortitis and periarteritis: CT findings in 17 patients. Radiology. 2011;261:625–33.
11. Uibu T, Oksa P, Auvinen A, et al. Asbestos exposure as a risk factor for retroperitoneal fibrosis. Lancet. 2004;363:1422–6.
12. Kamisawa T, Chari ST, Giday SA, et al. Clinical profile of autoimmune pancreatitis and its histological subtypes: an international multicenter survey. Pancreas. 2011;40:352–8.
13. Hamano H, Arakura N, Muraki T, Ozaki Y, Kiyosawa K, Kawa S. Prevalence and distribution of extrapancreatic lesions complicating autoimmune pancreatitis. J Gastroenterol. 2006;41:1197–205.
14. Kamisawa T, Matsukawa M, Ohkawa M. Autoimmune pancreatitis associated with retroperitoneal fibrosis. JOP. 2005;6:260–3.
15. Kamisawa T, Chen PY, Tu Y, Nakajima H, Egawa N. Autoimmune pancreatitis metachronously associated with retroperitoneal fibrosis with IgG4-positive plasma cell infiltration. World J Gastroenterol. 2006;12:2955–7.
16. Nishimura M, Kamisawa T, Kitahara Y, et al. Improvement of a compressed inferior vena cava due to IgG4-related retroperitoneal fibrosis with steroid therapy. Intern Med. 2012;51:1705–7.
17. Notohara K. Retroperitoneal fibrosis and arterial lesions. In: Umehara H et al., editors. IgG4-related disease. Tokyo: Springer; 2014. p. 181–6.
18. Scheel PJ, Feeley N. Retroperitoneal fibrosis. The clinical, laboratory, and radiographic presentation. Medicine. 2008;88:202–7.
19. Corradi D, Maestri R, Palmisano A, et al. Idiopathic retroperitoneal fibrosis: clinicopathologic features and differential diagnosis. Kidney Int. 2007;72:742–53.
20. Bommel EFH, Jansen I, Hendriksz TR, Aarnoudse ALHJ. Idiopathic retroperitoneal fibrosis. Prospective evaluation of incidence and clinicoradiologic presentation. Medicine. 2009;88:193–201.
21. Kermani TA, Crowson CS, Achenbach SJ, Luthra HS. Idiopathic retroperitoneal fibrosis: a retrospective review of clinical presentation, treatment, and outcome. Mayo Clin Proc. 2011;86:297–303.
22. Umehara H, Okazaki K, Masaki Y, et al. Comprehensive diagnostic criteria for IgG4-related disease (IgG4-RD), 2011. Mod Rheumatol. 2012;22:21–30.
23. Ozaki Y, Oguchi K, Hamano H, et al. Differentiation of autoimmune pancreatitis from suspected pancreatic cancer by fluorine-18 fluorodeoxyglucose positron emission tomography. J Gastroenterol. 2008;43:144–51.
24. Fujimori N, Ito T, Igarashi H, et al. Retroperitoneal fibrosis associated with immunoglobulin G4-related disease. World J Gastroenterol. 2013;19:35–41.
25. Kawa S, Okazaki K, Kamisawa T, et al. Amendment of the Japanese Consensus Guidelines for Autoimmune Pancreatitis, 2013 II. Extrapancreatic lesions, differential diagnosis. J Gastroenterol. 2014;49(5):765–84.
26. Kamisawa T, Okazaki K, Kawa S, et al. Amendment of the Japanese Consensus Guidelines for Autoimmune Pancreatitis, 2013 III. Treatment and prognosis of autoimmune pancreatitis. J Gastroenterol. 2014;49(6):961–70.

Renal Lesions

18

Takako Saeki

Introduction

Autoimmune pancreatitis (AIP) is currently divided into two distinct histological types – type 1 and type 2 – the former now being recognized as a condition representative of IgG4-related disease (IgG4-RD). IgG4-RD is a recently recognized emerging clinicopathological entity characterized by a dense lymphoplasmacytic infiltrate rich in IgG4-positive plasma cells with fibrosis and usually an elevated serum IgG4 concentration [1–3]. It is now clear that various inflammatory conditions affecting multiple organs fall within the category of IgG4-RD, including sclerosing cholangitis, sialadenitis, retroperitoneal fibrosis, and periaortitis, and that these have often been described as extra-pancreatic lesions associated with type 1 AIP. In the kidney, hydronephrosis due to retroperitoneal fibrosis was first reported as a renal lesion related to type 1 AIP [4], although it was considered to be a form of secondary renal injury caused by urinary tract obstruction. Renal parenchymal lesions associated with type 1 AIP were first described in case reports of tubulointerstitial nephritis (TIN) in 2004 [5, 6]. In fact, TIN is the most dominant feature associated with IgG4-RD in the kidney and is currently referred to as IgG4-related TIN [7, 8]. However, some glomerular lesions concurrent with IgG4-related TIN have also been reported, and several radiologically identified kidney lesions including pelvic lesions have been shown to be characteristic of IgG4-RD and useful for its diagnosis, in the setting of other forms of organ involvement that have been confirmed histopathologically [9, 10]. Therefore, the term "IgG4-related kidney disease" (IgG4-RKD) has recently been proposed as a comprehensive term for the renal lesions associated with IgG4-RD, including IgG4-related TIN, glomerular lesions concurrent with IgG4-related TIN, and IgG4-related pyelitis [9, 10]. In addition, glomerular lesions without IgG4-related TIN have also recently been reported in relation to type 1 AIP. This section focuses on whole renal lesions in type 1 AIP, including IgG4-RKD.

Clinical Features

IgG4-RKD shows a striking male predominance (73–87 %), and the average patient age is about 65 years [7–9]. Systemic symptoms are relatively mild, and the condition usually comes to clinical attention because of renal dysfunction and/or renal radiographic abnormalities during a systematic survey for IgG4-RD, although edema may be evident in patients with glomerular lesions. Many patients with IgG4-related TIN concurrent with type 1 AIP have IgG4-related involvement of other organs, such as lymphadenopathy, sialadenitis, dacryoadenitis, and retroperitoneal fibrosis, and the average number of affected extrarenal organs in patients with IgG4-TIN is 3.4 [9]. In IgG4-RD, involvement of several organs can occur either synchronously or metachronously [2], and IgG4-RKD tends to be found after diagnosis of other forms of organ involvement. Indeed, 40 % of cases of IgG4-related TIN are found during the follow-up of extrarenal lesions, including the remission state of AIP with or without steroid maintenance therapy [7, 9], suggesting that regular follow-up of renal function is mandatory in any cases of AIP. Although data on the epidemiology of IgG4-RKD are sparse, one study in Japan has indicated that the number of patients with IgG4-related renal lesions who visited hospitals in Japan in 2009 was approximately 57 while that of patients with AIP was approximately 2,709 [11]. However, radiologic evidence of renal involvement in patients with AIP based on CT or MR findings is not uncommon, having been reported in 14–35 % [12, 13], and the number of reported nephrology patients with IgG4-related TIN is increasing, suggesting that a considerable proportion of patients with type 1 AIP might have IgG4-RKD.

T. Saeki, MD, PhD
Department of Internal Medicine, Nagaoka Red Cross Hospital, Senshu 2-297-1, Nagaoka, Niigata 940-2085, Japan
e-mail: saekit@nagaoka.jrc.or.jp

T. Kamisawa, J.B. Chung (eds.), *Autoimmune Pancreatitis*,
DOI 10.1007/978-3-642-55086-7_18, © Springer-Verlag Berlin Heidelberg 2015

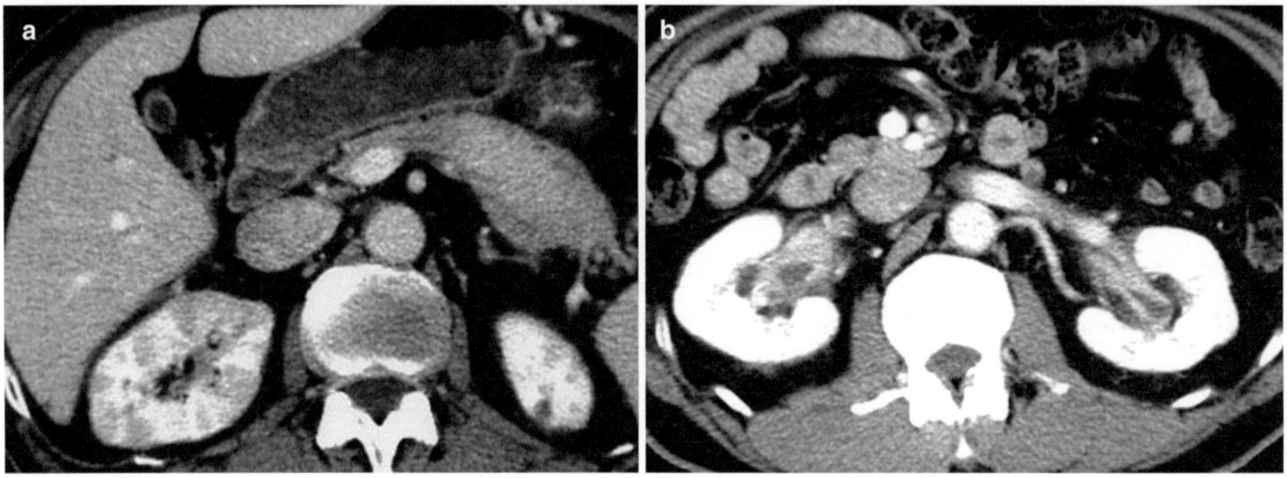

Fig. 18.1 (**a**) Contrast-enhanced renal CT finding in a patient with IgG4-related TIN. Multiple low-density lesions are evident. (**b**) Pelvic lesion in IgG4-RD. Bilateral renal pelvis wall thickening is found. The luminal surface is smooth

Laboratory Features

In type 1 AIP, the frequency of hypergammaglobulinemia and elevation of the IgG level are reported to be 34 and 56 %, respectively, and the diagnostic sensitivity of an elevated serum IgG4 level is 67–95 % [14]. Almost all patients with IgG4-related TIN have an elevated serum IgG4 level, and 90 % have an elevated serum IgG level [7, 9]. The levels of serum total IgG and IgG4 are remarkably high in many patients: in one study, the former exceeded 3,000 mg/dl in 50 % of patients, and the latter was about 1,000 mg/dl (normal <105 mg/dl) [9]. Hypocomplementemia is also remarkable in many patients with IgG4-related TIN. In type 1 AIP, low serum levels of C3, C4, and CH50 were reported to be evident in 36, 36, and 17 % of patients with active-stage type 1 AIP, respectively [15]. On the other hand, in IgG4-related TIN, the serum CH50 level was reportedly decreased in 40–70 % of patients, together with a reduction in the serum level of C3, C4, or both [7, 9]. A high serum level of IgE is also characteristic of IgG4-related TIN, being evident in 70 % of patients [7, 9]. Similar to type 1 AIP, antinuclear antibodies and rheumatoid factor are often positive, although anti-DNA, anti-SS-A, and anti-SS-B antibodies are usually negative. The level of CRP is usually low, and cryoglobulin, M-protein, and anti-neutrophil cytoplasmic antibodies are not observed [7, 9]. Although proteinuria (and sometimes hematuria) is observed in nearly half of patients with IgG4-TIN, it is mild in the majority. Nephrotic-range proteinuria is rarely detected, except when glomerular lesions such as membranous nephropathy are also present. Kidney function varies from normal to renal failure, and the development of renal dysfunction also varies from relatively acute to slowly progressive [7–9].

Imaging Features

Radiologic features are quite important for detection of renal lesions in IgG4-RD. Contrast-enhanced computed tomography (CT) is the most useful radiological tool for diagnosis, although the use of contrast medium requires careful judgment in patients with impaired renal function [9]. In the renal parenchyma, the most common feature demonstrated by enhanced CT is multiple low-density lesions, appearing as well-demarcated multiple patchy, wedge-shaped, or rounded areas that are distributed predominantly in the renal cortex (Fig. 18.1a) [9, 12, 13, 16]. In a Japanese study, 65.5 % of patients with IgG4-RKD examined by enhanced CT showed multiple low-density lesions in the kidney [9]. A hypovascular solitary mass lesion may also be observed, albeit rarely. Diffuse kidney enlargement can be recognized even by noncontrast CT examination and has been reported in 20–30 % of patients with IgG4-RKD [7–9]. Some biopsy studies have indicated that these radiological abnormalities in the renal parenchyma are due to IgG4-related TIN, even in patients with normal renal function. The radiological differential diagnosis of IgG4-related TIN includes pyelonephritis, malignancy, renal infarction, sarcoidosis, and vasculitis [9, 16]. As a pelvic lesion, diffuse thickening of the pelvic wall with a smooth intraluminal surface is reported to be characteristic of IgG4-RD (Fig. 18.1b) [9, 16]. The most important disease in the differential diagnosis is pelvic cancer, although this affects the intimal epithelium [16].

In addition to these renal lesions directly associated with IgG4-RD, hydronephrosis due to ureteral obstruction in patients with IgG4-related ureteral or periaortic/retroperitoneal lesions is sometimes evident in patients with type 1 AIP. In such cases of hydronephrosis concurrent with type 1 AIP, physicians should bear in mind that overlapping of

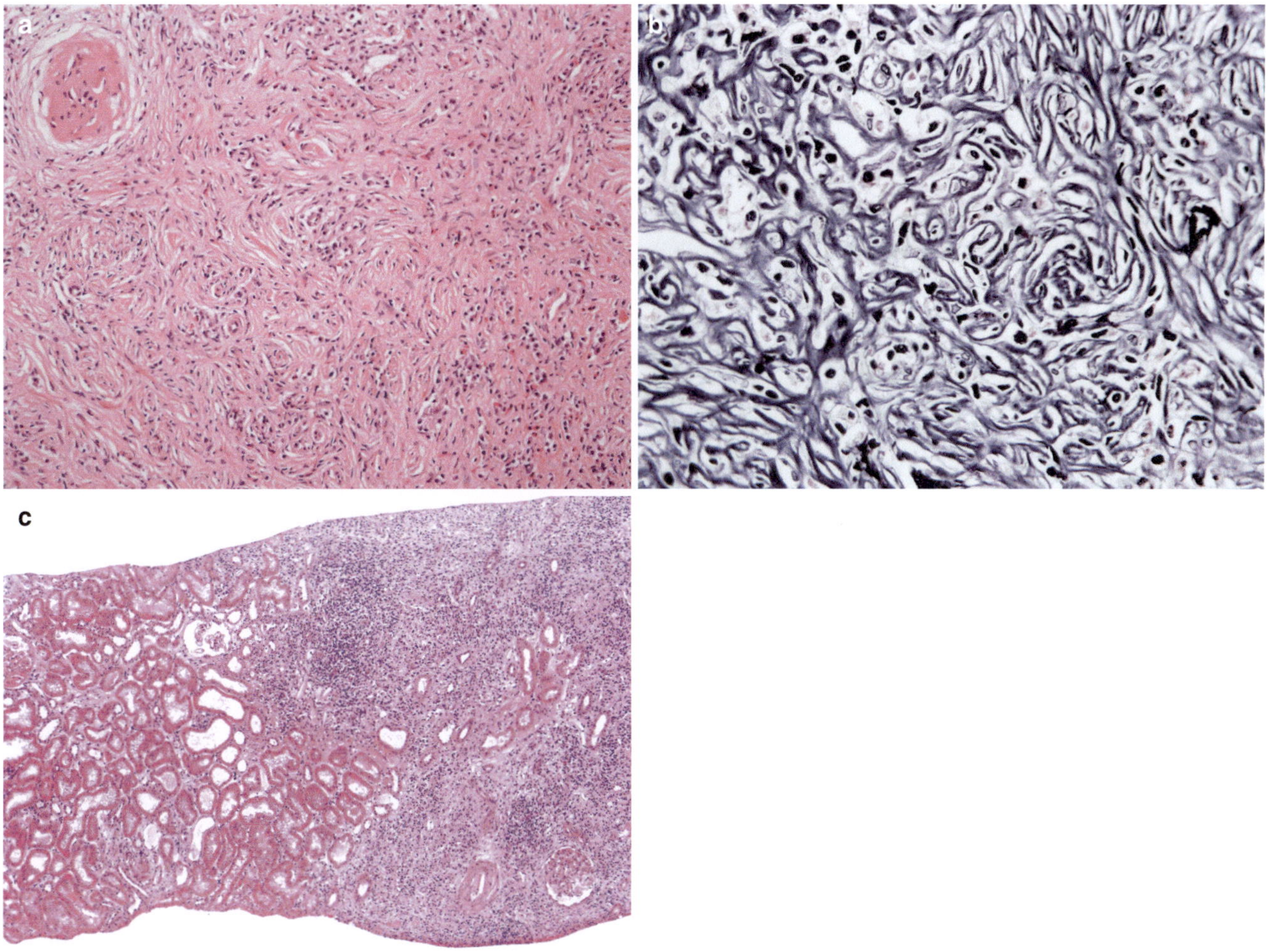

Fig. 18.2 Characteristic light microscopic findings of IgG4-related TIN. (**a**) A swirling pattern consisting inflammatory cells and collagen fibers, corresponding to storiform fibrosis in type 1 AIP, is evident (hematoxylin and eosin stain, ×100). (**b**) The "bird's eye" appearance of irregular fibers surrounding nests of inflammatory cells (periodic acid-methenamine silver stain, ×400). (**c**) A regional lesion distribution. Affected and unaffected areas are clearly demarcated (hematoxylin and eosin stain, ×60)

IgG4-TIN is possible, and renal histological examination should be considered when recovery of renal function is insufficient after resolution of the hydronephrosis following the placement of ureteral stents [17]. For cases in which contrast CT cannot be performed, MRI is also recommended to evaluate the presence, absence, or distribution of renal parenchymal lesions [16]. Gallium citrate scintigraphy and FDG-PET studies are also useful for detection of IgG4-related TIN even in patients showing no renal abnormalities by CT examination [7, 18].

Histological Features

Tubulointerstitial Lesions

IgG4-related TIN is characterized by a dense lymphoplasmacytic infiltrate associated with abundant IgG4-positive plasma cells and fibrosis, and the presence of >10 IgG4-positive plasma cells per high-power field or >40 % IgG4/IgG-positive plasma cells is required for diagnosis of renal specimens obtained by needle biopsy [8, 9]. In type 1 AIP, storiform-type fibrosis, in which bands of fibrosis radiate to various directions from the center, sometimes showing a swirling pattern, has been described as a characteristic feature [19, 20]. Also in IgG4-related TIN, such storiform fibrosis is often evident in hematoxylin and eosin (HE)-stained preparations (Fig. 18.2a) [21]. With periodic acid-methenamine silver or periodic acid-Schiff staining, which are routine in renal pathological studies, a unique so-called "bird's eye" pattern comprising nests of inflammatory cells surrounding irregular fibers is characteristic (Fig. 18.2b) [22]. The lesion distribution in IgG4-related TIN is also characteristic; affected and unaffected areas are clearly demarcated (Fig. 18.2c) [21, 22], and this correlates with the radiologic findings of well-demarcated multiple low-density lesions on enhanced CT. In addition, eosinophil infiltration or extension of lesions into the renal capsule is also positively suggestive of IgG4-related TIN [21, 22]. Conversely, necrotizing angiitis, granulomatous lesions, neutrophil infiltration, and advanced tubulitis are very rare in IgG4-related TIN [21]. Such histological characteristics are basically common to those in type 1 AIP [20], although obliterative phlebitis, which is also a critical pathologic feature of type 1 AIP [19, 20], is rarely seen in specimens of IgG4-related TIN obtained by kidney needle biopsy [22].

In addition to light microscopy, immunofluorescence and electron microscopy studies of the kidney are conducted routinely, and these often reveal deposition of immunoglobulin and/or complement or electron-dense deposits in the renal tubular basement membrane (TBM) in IgG4-related TIN [8, 22]. Raissian et al. reported immune complex deposition in the TBM in ≥80 % of patients with IgG4-related TIN [8]. Immunofluorescence microscopy demonstrates granular deposits of IgG4 (usually concurrent with other subtypes of IgG such as IgG1 and IgG3) and C3, with occasional C1q. These TBM deposits are mainly demonstrated in areas affected by fibro-inflammatory changes, and not in adjacent areas that are unaffected [8, 22].

Glomerular Lesions

Although TIN is the major lesion in IgG4-RKD, some glomerular lesions have been reported in type 1 AIP. Membranous nephropathy (MN) is the most common glomerular lesion and has been reported in 7–10 % of patients with IgG4-related TIN [8, 23]. Recently, several cases of MN without TIN in the setting of IgG4-RD, including type 1 AIP, have been reported [24], and this is attracting attention as a pathophysiological aspect other than ordinary fibro-inflammatory lesions in IgG4-RD [25]. MN is an antibody-mediated autoimmune glomerular disease and one of the most common causes of nephrotic syndrome in adults. MN occurs as an idiopathic disease or secondary to conditions such as autoimmune disease (e.g., systemic lupus erythematosus), infection (e.g., hepatitis B, hepatitis C), drug reactions, and malignancies [26]. Pathologically, MN is characterized by subepithelial deposition of immune complexes containing IgG and usually C3, and IgG4 predominance in such glomerular immune complexes has been documented in idiopathic MN [26]. Recently, the M-type phospholipase A2 receptor (PLA2R) has been identified as a target antigen common to about 70 % of patients with idiopathic MN, and the anti-PLA2R antibodies are predominantly of the IgG4 subclasses [27]. Also in MN in IgG4-RD, either with or without TIN, IgG4 is usually (but not always) predominant in glomerular immune complexes, although usually concurrent with other types of IgG subclasses [24, 28]. However, anti-PLA2R antibodies have been negative in all cases of MN in IgG4-RD [24] (and also all cases of IgG4-RD [29]) evaluated, suggesting that the condition differs from idiopathic MN and may be secondary to IgG4-RD. However, MN can be associated with malignancies, and patients with AIP are reported to be at high risk of having cancers [30]. Although IgG4 is not usually dominant in glomerular immune complexes in MN associated with malignancy, IgG4 is not always dominant in cases of MN associated with IgG4-RD. Therefore, an extensive survey for malignancy is necessary in any case of MN in type 1 AIP, especially in the absence of TIN. In addition to MN, various types of glomerular lesions have been reported to be concurrent with IgG4-related TIN, including Henoch-Schönlein purpura nephritis, IgA nephropathy, endocapillary proliferative glomerulonephritis, membranoproliferative glomerulonephritis, and mesangial proliferative glomerulonephritis [7, 9].

Pelvic Lesions

Although the number of case reports of IgG4-related pyelitis is limited, dense lymphoplasma cell infiltration with numerous IgG4-positive plasma cells and fibrosis has been described in the renal pelvis in IgG4-RD, similar to those in other affected organs [31, 32]. Lymphocytes and plasma cells markedly infiltrate beneath the urothelial epithelium of the renal pelvis, and multiple lymphoid follicles may be evident [32]. In spite of severe inflammation, the urothelial epithelium is relatively well preserved (Fig. 18.3). Storiform fibrosis, obliterative phlebitis, and eosinophil infiltration are also evident is some lesions [32].

Diagnosis

A diagnostic algorithm using a set of diagnostic criteria for IgG4-RKD has been proposed by the Japanese Society of Nephrology [9] and is useful for finding renal lesions in patients with type 1 AIP (Fig. 18.4). In this algorithm, the presence of some kidney damage, as manifested by abnormal urinalysis data or urine marker(s), abnormal radiologic findings, or decreased kidney function, with either an elevated total IgG level, hypocomplementemia, or an elevated serum IgE level, is the first step at which IgG4-RKD should be suspected. After exclusion of other renal diseases, the serum IgG4 level is confirmed, and then radiological and histological examinations are evaluated.

Treatment and Clinical Course

Similar to type 1 AIP, corticosteroid is quite effective in most cases of IgG4-RKD. Corticosteroid therapy leads to a rapid improvement in terms of renal function, radiology,

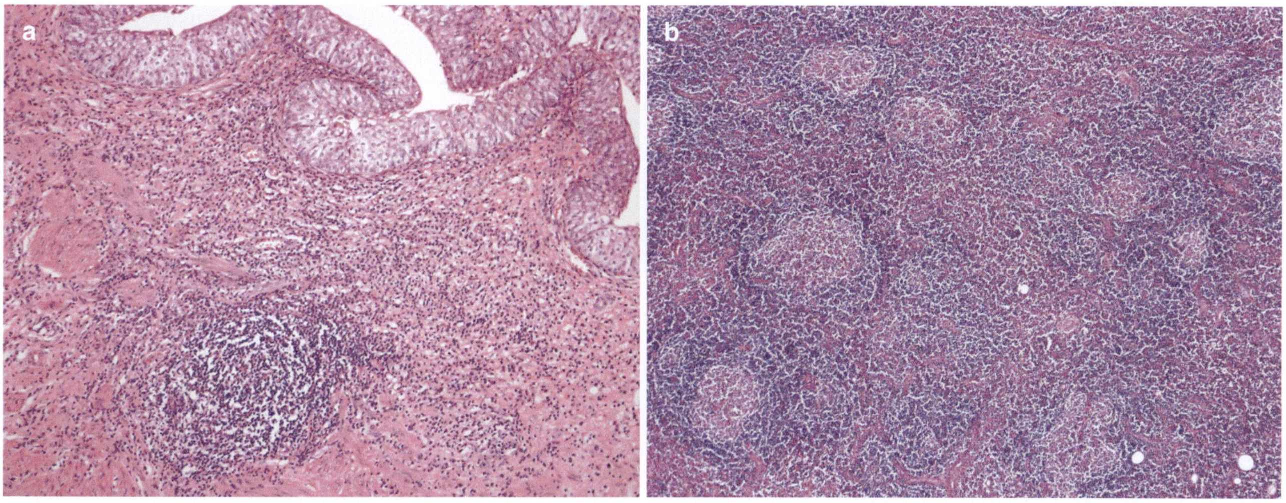

Fig. 18.3 Histological findings of IgG4-related pyelitis. (**a**) Lymphocytes and plasma cells markedly infiltrate beneath the urothelial epithelium of the renal pelvis. The urothelial epithelium is relatively well preserved (hematoxylin and eosin stain, ×100). (**b**) Lymphoid follicles are evident (hematoxylin and eosin stain, ×40)

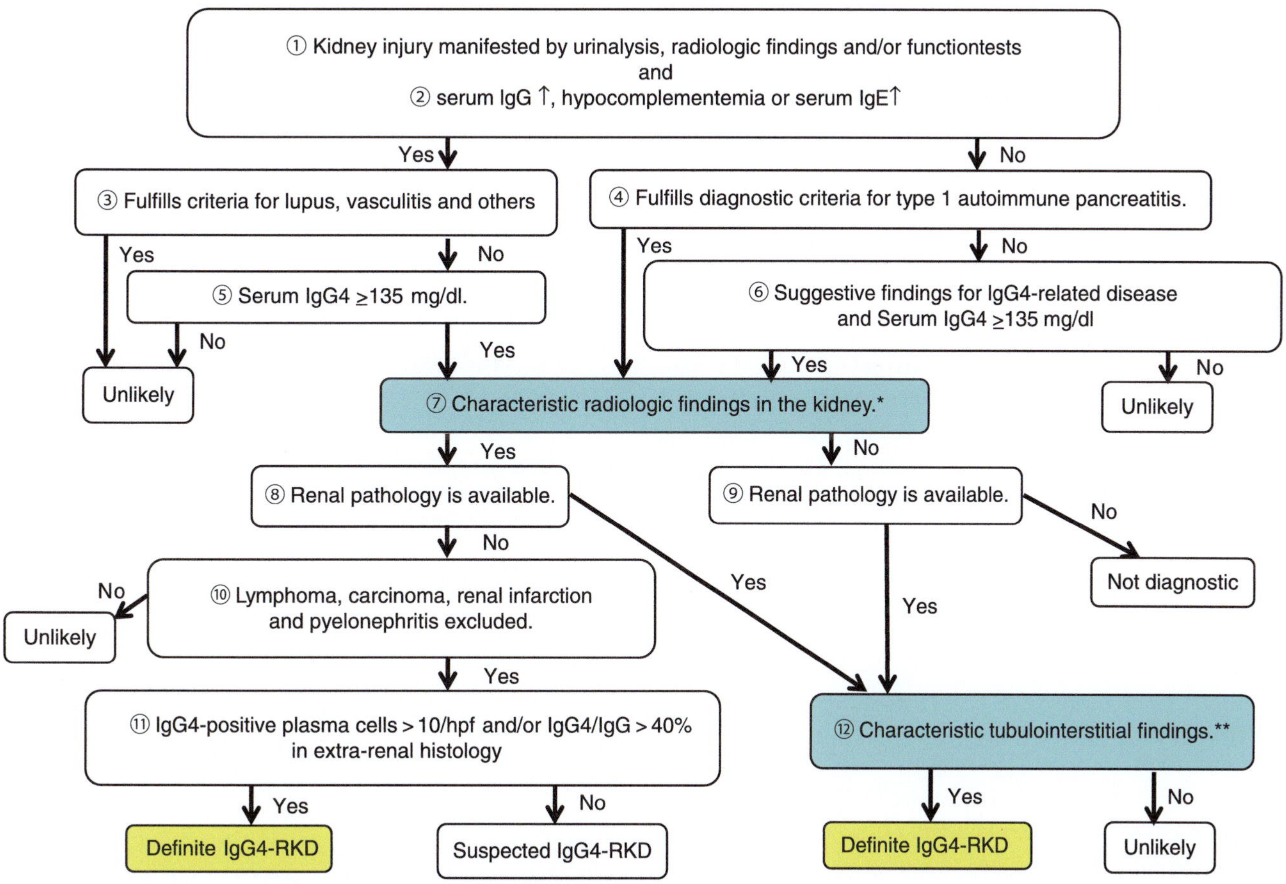

Fig. 18.4 The diagnostic algorithm for IgG4-RKD proposed by the Japanese Society of Nephrology [9] (*Characteristic radiological findings in the kidney include (a) multiple low-density lesions on enhanced computed tomography, (b) diffuse kidney enlargement, (c) hypovascular solitary mass in the kidney, (d) hypertrophic lesion of renal pelvic wall without irregularity of the renal pelvic surface. **Characteristic tubulointerstitial findings include (a) dense lymphoplasmacytic infiltration with infiltrating IgG4-positive plasma cells >10/high-power field (HPF) and/or IgG4/IgG-positive plasma cells >40 %, (b) characteristic fibrosis surrounding nests of lymphocytes and/or plasma cells)

and serology at 1 month after the start of therapy in most patients with IgG4-RKD, although the response in terms of urinalysis parameters after therapy varies [33]. However, renal function does not recover completely in patients with advanced renal damage. In patients whose estimated glomerular filtration rate (eGFR) before treatment was <60 ml/min, eGFR before treatment (34.1 ± 15.8 ml/min) was significantly improved at 1 month after the start of treatment (45.0 ± 13.8 ml/min, $p < 0.01$), but recovery of renal function reached a plateau during the initial one month of corticosteroid treatment in most cases. Thereafter, renal atrophy developed in a considerable proportion of treated patients, especially those in whom advanced renal damage had already been evident before therapy, although, fortunately, recovery of renal function persisted for a relatively long period under low-dose corticosteroid maintenance therapy [33]. These results suggest that irreversible lesions remain in patients at the advanced stage of IgG4-related TIN, despite corticosteroid therapy, and therefore early diagnosis and therapy are important. Although indications for corticosteroid therapy in IgG4-RKD have not been established, patients with renal dysfunction should receive it immediately and careful attention should be paid to patients who do not receive therapy. For induction therapy, prednisolone 0.6 mg/kg daily is recommended in Japan for type 1 AIP [34], and our data (unpublished) indicate that this therapy also seems to be appropriate for IgG4-RKD. Withdrawal of maintenance therapy for IgG4-related TIN should be considered very carefully, in view of possible progression of irreversible renal damage. The efficacy of immunosuppressant for treatment of IgG4-RKD has not been clarified, and the related data are rather sparse.

In AIP, disease relapse has been frequently reported. Also in IgG4-RKD, relapse of IgG4-related lesions occurred in 8 (20.0 %) of 40 treated patients, including 3 kidney lesions, during maintenance corticosteroid therapy [33]. Interestingly, a re-decrease of the serum complement level associated with IgG4-RD relapse occurred in all 3 patients who had shown hypocomplementemia before therapy, suggesting that such a re-decrease of the serum complement level may be useful for prediction of relapse in IgG4-RKD [33].

Summary

1. In type 1 AIP, various renal lesions including tubulointerstitial nephritis (TIN), glomerular disease, renal pyelitis, and hydronephrosis related to retroperitoneal fibrosis are observed. Among them, TIN with abundant IgG4-positive plasma cells and fibrosis is the most dominant feature and referred to as IgG4-related TIN, which may cause acute or chronic renal dysfunction. Recently, the term "IgG4-related kidney disease" (IgG4-RKD) has been proposed as a comprehensive term for the primary renal lesions associated with IgG4-related disease.
2. IgG4-RKD can develop at any time during the clinical course of type 1 AIP, including the remission period with or without maintenance therapy, and therefore, regular follow-up for renal function and urinalysis is mandatory for AIP patients. In IgG4-related TIN, mild urinary abnormalities or mild renal dysfunction is likely, and therefore, careful attention to these parameters is necessary. Massive proteinuria suggests glomerular lesions such as membranous nephropathy.
3. A diagnostic algorithm for IgG4-RKD proposed by the Japanese Society of Nephrology is useful for finding renal lesions in type 1 AIP, in which high levels of serum total IgG and IgG4 and high levels of serum IgE and hypocomplementemia are initial checkpoints for patients with some forms of kidney damage, and thereafter, renal radiological and histological findings are evaluated.
4. Characteristic histological features in IgG4-related TIN are basically the same as those in type 1 AIP: a dense lymphoplasmacytic infiltrate with abundant IgG4-positive plasma cells and fibrosis, often showing a storiform pattern. The most common glomerular lesion related to type 1 AIP is membranous nephropathy and may or may not be associated with TIN.
5. Corticosteroid therapy usually leads to a rapid improvement in terms of renal function, radiology, and serology in patients with IgG4-RKD. However, renal function does not recover completely in patients with advanced renal damage. Therefore, early diagnosis and treatment are necessary, and withdrawal of maintenance therapy for IgG4-related TIN should be considered very carefully.

Acknowledgments This work was supported in part by grants from the Health and Labour Sciences Research Grants for the Study of Intractable Disease from Ministry of Health, Labor and Welfare, Japan, and "IgG4-Related Kidney Disease" working group of the Japanese Society of Nephrology.

Disclosure
None.

References

1. Umehara H, Okazaki K, Masaki Y, et al. A novel clinical entity, IgG4-related disease (IgG4RD): general concept and details. Mod Rheumatol. 2012;22:1–14.
2. Umehara H, Okazaki K, Masaki Y, et al. Comprehensive diagnostic criteria for IgG4-related disease (IgG4-RD), 2011. Mod Rheumatol. 2012;22:21–30.
3. Stone JH, Zen Y, Deshpande V. IgG4-related disease. N Engl J Med. 2012;366:539–51.

4. Hamano H, Kawa S, Ochi Y, et al. Hydronephrosis associated with retroperitoneal fibrosis and sclerosing pancreatitis. Lancet. 2002;359:1403–4.
5. Takeda S, Haratake J, Kasai T, et al. IgG4-associated idiopathic tubulointerstitial nephritis complicating autoimmune pancreatitis. Nephrol Dial Transplant. 2004;19:474–6.
6. Uchiyama-Tanaka Y, Mori Y, Kimura T, et al. Acute tubulointerstitial nephritis associated with autoimmune-related pancreatitis. Am J Kidney Dis. 2004;43:18–25.
7. Saeki T, Nishi S, Imai N, et al. Clinicopathological characteristics of patients with IgG4-related tubulointerstitial nephritis. Kidney Int. 2010;78:1016–23.
8. Raissian Y, Nasr SH, Larsen CP, et al. Diagnosis of IgG4-related tubulointerstitial nephritis. J Am Soc Nephrol. 2011;22:1343–52.
9. Kawano M, Saeki T, Nakashima H, et al. Proposal for diagnostic criteria for IgG4-related kidney disease. Clin Exp Nephrol. 2011;25:810–9.
10. Stone JH, Khosroshahi A, Deshpande V, et al. Recommendations for the nomenclature of IgG4-related disease and its individual organ system manifestations. Arthritis Rheum. 2012;64:3061–7.
11. Uchida K, Masamune A, Shimosegawa T, Okazaki K. Prevalence of IgG4-related disease in Japan based on Nationwide Survey in 2009. Int J Rheumatol. 2012;2012:358371. p. 5.
12. Takahashi N, Kawashima A, Fletcher JG, Chari ST. Renal involvement in patients with autoimmune pancreatitis: CT and MR imaging findings. Radiollogy. 2007;242:791–801.
13. Fujinaga Y, Kadoya M, Kawa S, et al. Characteristic findings in images of extra-pancreatic lesions associated with autoimmune pancreatitis. Eur J Radiol. 2010;76:228–38.
14. Kamisawa T, Okamoto A. IgG4-related sclerosing disease. World J Gastroenterol. 2008;7:3948–55.
15. Muraki T, Hamano H, Ochi Y, et al. Autoimmune pancreatitis and complement activation system. Pancreas. 2006;32:16–21.
16. Inoue D, Kawano M, Yamada K, et al. Kidney and urinary tract lesions. In: Umehara H, Okazaki K, Stone JH, Kawa S, Kawano M, editors. IgG4-related disease. Tokyo: Springer; 2014. p. 99–105.
17. Saeki T, Ito T, Onishi T, et al. IgG4-related kidney disease with retroperitoneal fibrosis in a patient with diabetes mellitus. In: Umehara H, Okazaki K, Stone JH, Kawa S, Kawano M, editors. IgG4-related disease. Tokyo: Springer; 2014. p. 231–3.
18. Nakajima K, Inaki A, Kinuya S, et al. Scintigraphy and single-photon emission computed tomography. In: Umehara H, Okazaki K, Stone JH, Kawa S, Kawano M, editors. IgG4-related disease. Tokyo: Springer; 2014. p. 123–8.
19. Deshpande V, Zen Y, Chan JKC, et al. Consensus statement on the pathology of gG4-related disease. Mod Pathol. 2012;25:1181–92.
20. Notohara K. Pancreas. In: Umehara H, Okazaki K, Stone JH, Kawa S, Kawano M, editors. IgG4-related disease. Tokyo: Springer; 2014. p. 139–45.
21. Yoshita K, Kawano M, Mizushima I, et al. Light-microscopic characteristics of IgG4-related tubulointerstitial nephritis: distinction from non-IgG4-related tubulointerstitial nephritis. Nephrol Dial Transplant. 2012;27:2755–61.
22. Yamaguchi Y, Kanetsuna Y, Honda K, et al. Characteristic tubulointerstitial nephritis in IgG4-related disease. Hum Pathol. 2011;43:536–49.
23. Saeki T, Kawano M. IgG4-related kidney disease. Kidney Int. 2014;85:251–7.
24. Alexander MP, Larsen CP, Gibson IW, et al. Membranous glomerulonephritis is a manifestation of IgG4-related disease. Kidney Int. 2013;83:455–62.
25. Stone JH. IgG4: a tantalizing link between causes of membranous glomerulonephritis and systemic disease. Kidney Int. 2013;83:348–50.
26. Patrick H, Nachman PH, Jennette C, Falk RJ. Primary glomerular disease. In: Brenner & Rector's the kidney. 9th ed. USA: Elsevier Inc.; 2012. p. 1100–91.
27. Beck Jr LH, Bonegio RG, Lambeau G, et al. M-type phospholipase A2 receptor as target antigen in idiopathic membranous nephropathy. N Engl J Med. 2009;361:11–21.
28. Saeki T, Imai N, Ito T, et al. Membranous nephropathy associated with IgG4-related systemic disease and without autoimmune pancreatitis. Clin Nephrol. 2009;71:173–8.
29. Khosroshahi A, Ayalon R, Beck Jr LH, et al. IgG4-related disease is not associated with antibody to the phospholipase A2 receptor. Int J Rheumatol. 2012;2012:139409.
30. Shiokawa M, Kodama Y, Yoshimura K, et al. Risk of cancer in patients with autoimmune pancreatitis. Am J Gastroenterol. 2013;108:610–7.
31. Kuroda N, Nakamura S, Miyazaki K, et al. Chronic sclerosing pyelitis with an increased number of IgG4-positive plasma cells. Med Mol Morphol. 2009;42:236–8.
32. Zen Y, Nakanuma Y. IgG4-related sclerosing disease: renal lesions. Pathol Clin Med. 2009;27:50–6 (in Japanese).
33. Saeki T, Kawano M, Mizushima I, et al. The clinical course of patients with IgG4-related kidney disease. Kidney Int. 2013;84:826–33.
34. Kamisawa T, Okazaki Y, Kawa S, et al. Japanese consensus guidelines for management of autoimmune pancreatitis: III. Treatment and prognosis of AIP. J Gastroenterol. 2010; 45:471–7.

19 Pulmonary Lesions

Kenji Hirano

Introduction

Many types of extrapancreatic lesions associated with immunoglobulin G (IgG)4-related autoimmune pancreatitis (type 1 AIP) are known. IgG4-related sclerosing cholangitis, retroperitoneal fibrosis, and sclerosing sialadenitis are particularly well known. Pulmonary involvement is not rare, but the mechanism is still difficult to fully understand. Pulmonary lesions associated with AIP were described in 2 separate case reports in 2004 [1, 2] and in our case series of 4 patients in 2006 [3]. Most were reported as interstitial pneumonia. However, it gradually became evident that there were various patterns in the pulmonary lesions [4–8]. Moreover, IgG4-related lesions were found in the mediastinum and pleura [5, 7–11]. It is possible that some types of airway disease, including bronchial asthma, belong to IgG4-related disease (IgG4) [12, 13]. Because there have been no diagnostic criteria, there appears to be no consensus on the definition of "pulmonary lesions" among specialists. In this article, intrathoracic lesions, in addition to lung parenchymal lesions, are discussed.

Epidemiology

The frequency of intrathoracic lesions associated with AIP may vary depending on whether or not hilar lymphadenopathy is included. In a retrospective study in which 90 patients with AIP were studied, hilar lymphadenopathy was present in 78 % of the patients [8]; in the same study, lung lesions were found in 54 %. Thus, if hilar lymphadenopathy is included in the criteria, it follows that most patients with AIP have intrathoracic lesions. If hilar lymphadenopathy is excluded from the criteria, the lung lesion frequency of 54 % still appears very high. The authors reported that nodular lesions (3–26 mm) were observed in 39 % of patients. On the other hand, according to another study of 49 patients with IgG4-related Mikulicz's disease, hilar lymphadenopathy, pulmonary fibrosis, and pulmonary nodules were observed in 53, 4.1, and 2.0 % of patients, respectively [14]. The author speculates that these differences are simply because of differences in the size and feature criteria and methodology used to identify lesions in the various studies. As long as there are no definite criteria for intrathoracic lesions, this problem will remain.

Clinical Features

Respiratory symptoms, including cough, exertional dyspnea, and chest pain, have been described in 28–48 % of patients with IgG4-related lung disease [5, 7]. At our institute, among 11 patients in whom IgG4-related lung parenchymal lesions associated with AIP were suspected, 4 patients (36 %) were symptomatic (dyspnea in 3 and cough in 1).

Pulmonary or intrathoracic lesions may occur before or after AIP. In Zen's series, 9 patients had intrathoracic lesions and IgG4-related disease in other organs. Extrathoracic lesions preceded intrathoracic ones in 4 patients, and intrathoracic lesions preceded extrathoracic ones in 1. In the remaining 4 patients, both lesions were found at the same time [5]. According to our experience with AIP and lung lesions, AIP was identified first in 8 patients of whom lung lesions were found in 6 patients during follow-up with steroid maintenance therapy. Lung lesions preceded AIP in 1 patient. In the remaining 2 patients, both lesions were found at the same time.

Laboratory Features

There are several reports in which IgG and IgG4 were elevated in IgG4-related lung disease. The question of whether or not elevation of IgG and IgG4 is observed in patients who

K. Hirano, MD, PhD
Department of Gastroenterology, Graduate School of Medicine,
The University of Tokyo, Tokyo, Japan
e-mail: khirano-tky@umin.ac.jp

T. Kamisawa, J.B. Chung (eds.), *Autoimmune Pancreatitis*,
DOI 10.1007/978-3-642-55086-7_19, © Springer-Verlag Berlin Heidelberg 2015

developed IgG4-related lung disease during follow-up of AIP remains unanswered in previous reports. In our experience, among 6 patients who developed lung lesions during follow-up with steroid maintenance therapy, remarkable, mild, and no elevation of IgG and IgG4 were observed in 3, 1, and 2 patients, respectively.

In our previous report, we reported that elevation of Krebs von den Lungen-6 (KL-6), which is elevated in patients with various parenchymal lung diseases, such as idiopathic pulmonary fibrosis [15–17], was characteristic of IgG4-related lung disease [3]. In the first case report by Taniguchi et al., elevation of KL-6 was also documented [1]. In both reports, all of the patients were diagnosed as having interstitial pneumonia. However, another report documented that there were few patients with elevated KL-6 [7]. In that report, more than half of the patients showed nodular lesions. Thus, KL-6 may be elevated in a part of interstitial type lesions. We experienced a case in which the elevation of KL-6 was useful for diagnosis of an interstitial type lung lesion, but it was also true that KL-6 was not elevated in all cases. Although measuring KL-6 may be sometimes useful for detecting interstitial type lung lesions, it should be noted that there are many cases that do not show KL-6 elevation.

In assays of bronchoalveolar lavage (BAL) fluid, lymphocytes have been predominant, but the CD4/CD8 lymphocyte ratios were normal [7]. BAL IgG4 levels were increased relative to the levels in specimens obtained from patients with sarcoidosis and correlated with the serum IgG4 levels [6].

In pulmonary function tests, one report documented that normal, obstructive, and restrictive patterns were observed in 65 % (11/17), 24 % (4/17), and 12 % (2/17) of patients, respectively [7].

Imaging Findings

Pulmonary Lesions

There are various types of lung lesions, and according to the classification proposed by Inoue et al., there are 4 subtypes of CT findings: solid nodular type, round-shaped ground-glass opacity (GGO), alveolar interstitial type, and bronchovascular type [4]. The solid nodular type is characterized by the presence of a solitary solid lesion >1.0 cm that includes a mass (Fig. 19.1). Round-shaped GGO type is radiologically characterized by multiple round-shaped ground-glass lesions (Fig. 19.2). The alveolar interstitial type is characterized by diffuse GGO, bronchoectasia, and honeycombing (Fig. 19.3). The bronchovascular type is characterized by thickening of bronchovascular bundles and interlobular septa (Fig. 19.4). It is not rare that 2 or more types of lesions coexist [8]. Moreover, 2 or more types of lesions may often appear metachronously. It is difficult to describe the exact frequency of each type of lesion. Previous reports have emphasized the histological findings in collected cases, which may have increased the number of cases with nodular lesions because surgical biopsy was performed more often in those cases. In addition, the number of cases reported may have depended on how well small or subtle lesions are recognized. In our database, among 80 patients with AIP, 11 had pulmonary lesions. Nine patients had alveolar interstitial type lesions. However, we cannot deny the possibility that small lesions were not identified.

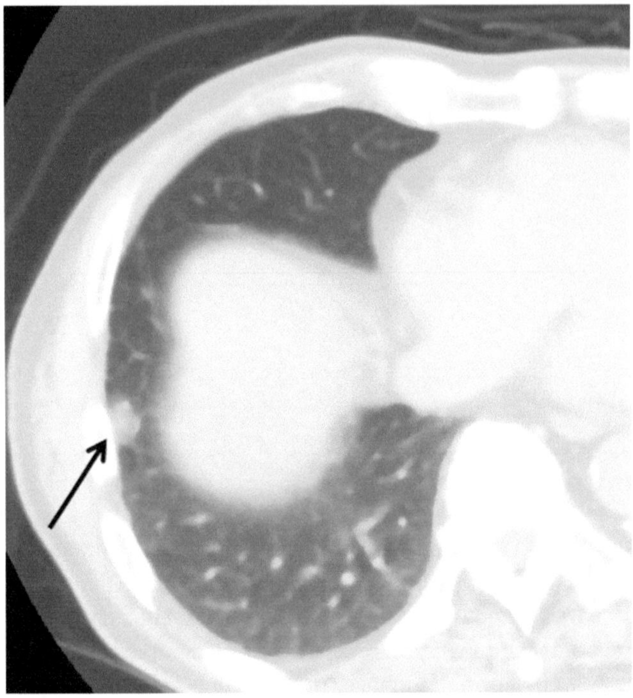

Fig. 19.1 Case 1, a 74-year-old male. A solid nodule 1.5 cm in diameter in the right lung is shown (*black arrow*). Differentiation from lung cancer is difficult. In this case, the lesion became a little smaller after steroid treatment

Extrapulmonary Lesions

Mediastinal and hilar lymphadenopathy is observed very frequently (Fig. 19.5) [6, 8]. With regard to pleural lesions, some cases have shown pleural nodular lesions in the visceral or parietal pleura [5]. Although pleural effusion is a comparatively rare feature [9, 11], pleuritis with fibrinous exudates and reactive changes are often observed in the histological findings from surgical lung biopsy specimens in patients with intrathoracic IgG4-related disease [18].

Other findings that should be noted include soft tissue mass in the paravertebral region, which may be suggestive of mediastinal fibrosis (Fig. 19.6) [7, 19, 20].

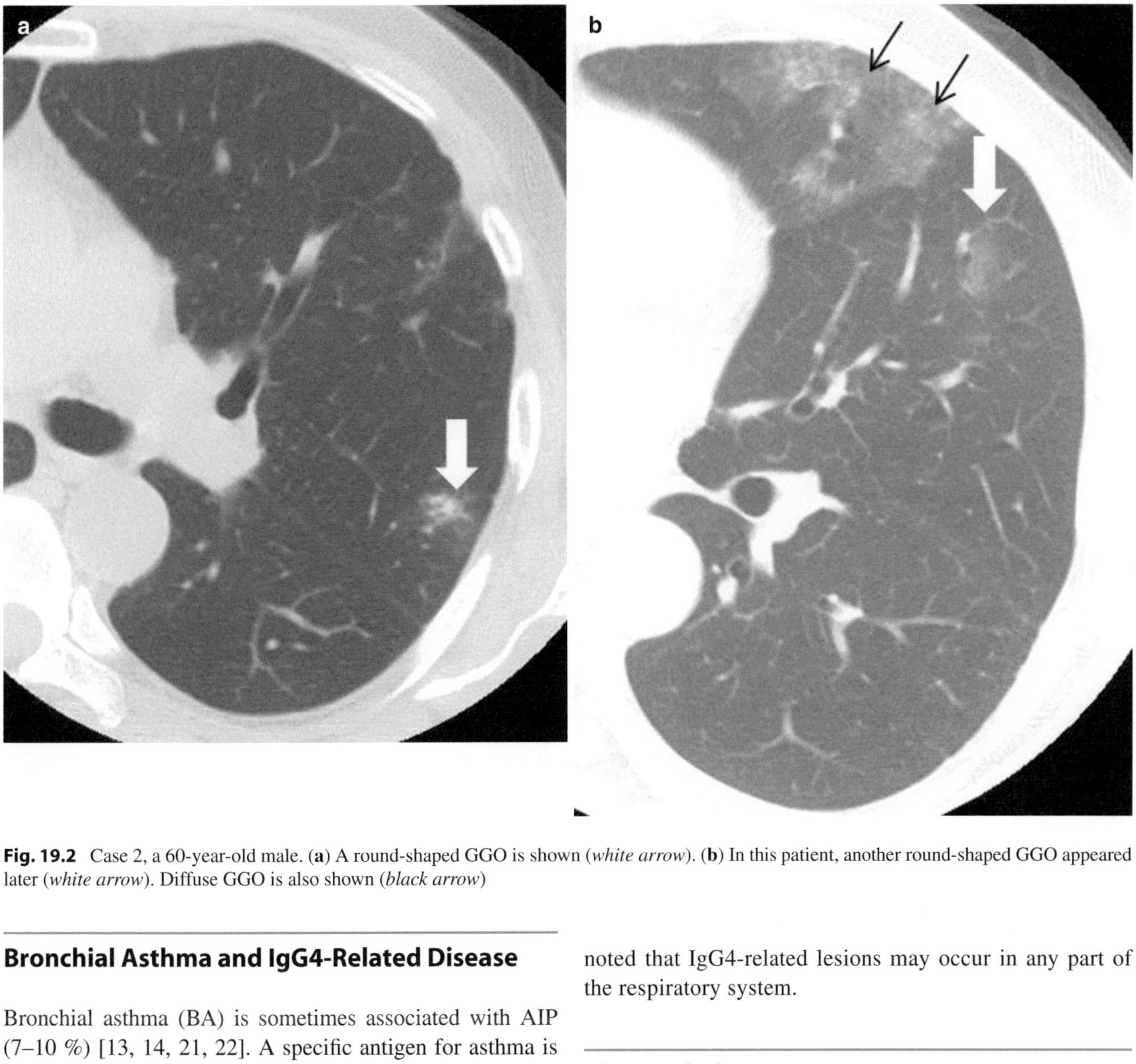

Fig. 19.2 Case 2, a 60-year-old male. (**a**) A round-shaped GGO is shown (*white arrow*). (**b**) In this patient, another round-shaped GGO appeared later (*white arrow*). Diffuse GGO is also shown (*black arrow*)

Bronchial Asthma and IgG4-Related Disease

Bronchial asthma (BA) is sometimes associated with AIP (7–10 %) [13, 14, 21, 22]. A specific antigen for asthma is not known [14]. Steroid treatment is effective for both BA and AIP. However, after tapering of the steroid, BA often becomes aggravated despite no change in the pancreas, which hinders cessation of the steroid [13]. Although BA is not included in IgG4-related pulmonary disease in general, history of BA should be noted in AIP patients.

Apart from BA, in which airway stenosis is reversible, central airway stenotic disease associated with AIP has been reported by Ito et al. [12]. In the patient in that case, bronchoscopic examination revealed an irregular tracheobronchial stenosis accompanied by an edematous mucosa and engorged vessels. Bronchial biopsy specimens demonstrated diffuse infiltrations of IgG4 positive plasma cells, lymphocytes, and eosinophils with fibrosis. CT showed marked thickness of the bronchovascular bundle. These lesions improved after steroid treatment. Thus, it should be noted that IgG4-related lesions may occur in any part of the respiratory system.

Histopathology

Histopathological findings associated with intrathoracic IgG4-related disease resemble those seen in extrapancreatic lesions, with some exceptions. That is, lymphoplasmacytic inflammation, fibrosis, phlebitis, and increased numbers of IgG4-positive plasma cells are characteristic of intrathoracic IgG4-related disease [4, 7, 11, 18, 23, 24].

Compared with the histopathological findings observed in the pancreas of AIP patients, storiform fibrosis is not as apparent in the lung, where collagenous fibrosis and active fibroblastic proliferation are more prominent [18]. Moreover, in the lung, arteries as well as veins often show intimal and mural inflammation, in contrast to the findings for an affected pancreas, which shows obliterative phlebitis with sparing of the arteries [18, 25].

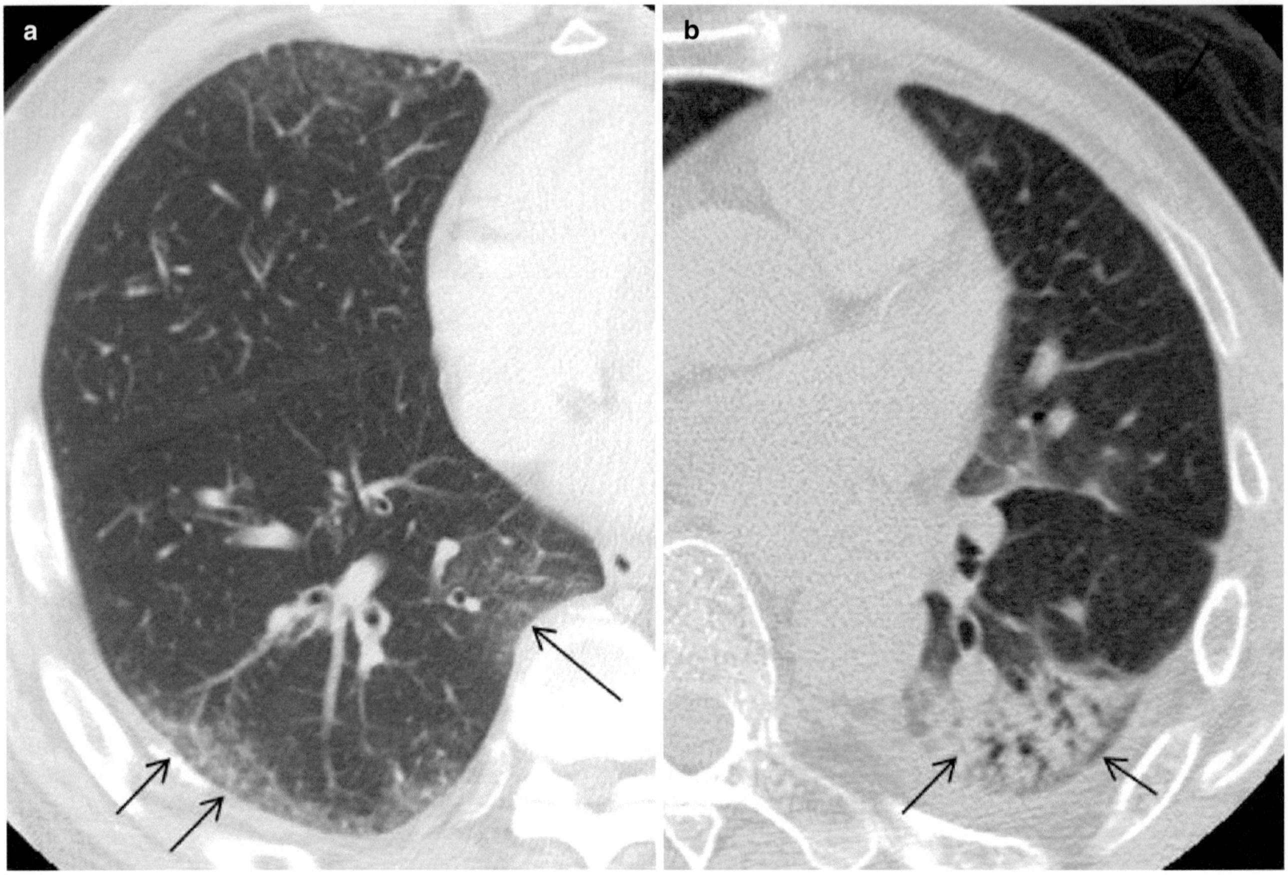

Fig. 19.3 (**a**) Case 3 (66-year-old male); (**b**) Case 3, (69-year-old male). Both cases show diffuse GGO (*arrows*)

Treatment and Prognosis

Intrathoracic lesions associated with IgG4-related disease generally respond to steroid treatment [1–7, 10–12, 18, 20, 25–27]. The exact steroid regimens have not been specified in many of the studies to date but typically consist of oral prednisolone beginning at a dose of 30–60 mg/day. Favorable response is usually observed within 2 weeks from the start of treatment. Then, the prednisolone dose is gradually tapered to a maintenance dose of 5–10 mg/day. The optimal dose and duration of steroid treatment remain undetermined. Steroid treatment for the indication of asymptomatic intrathoracic lesions is also problematic. The question arises as to whether or not it is necessary to increase the dose of prednisolone when asymptomatic lung lesions appear during maintenance steroid treatment for AIP. As far as we know, many Japanese chest physicians are not inclined to treat asymptomatic intrathoracic lesions with steroids. This is probably because for some pulmonary lesions, improvement may only be assessed by observation, at least from a short-term viewpoint [7, 28, 29]. However, the long-term prognosis of such patients is unknown. Moreover, there has been no report on the long-term prognosis of intrathoracic lesions treated with steroids. In addition, many problems remain to be solved in establishing the optimal treatment policy.

Despite good response to steroid treatment, steroid treatment for pulmonary nodular lesions without pathological diagnosis is undesirable. It is often very difficult to differentiate IgG4-related pulmonary nodular lesions from lung cancer [4]. Moreover, at our institute and affiliated hospitals, 5 cases of lung cancer have been found during follow-up of 113 patients with AIP. There were 15 malignancies, but lung cancer was observed most frequently [30]. Thus, surgical resection should be considered when differential diagnosis is difficult.

Concerning nodular lesions, the effectiveness of steroid treatment for large nodular lesions may not always be determined because many have been resected. Ito et al. reported a case in which IgG4-related pulmonary nodular lesions showed no response to steroid treatment [13]. In our experience (Fig. 19.1), nodular lesions became a little smaller but did not disappear. It should be noted that all intrathoracic lesions do not improve dramatically after steroid treatment.

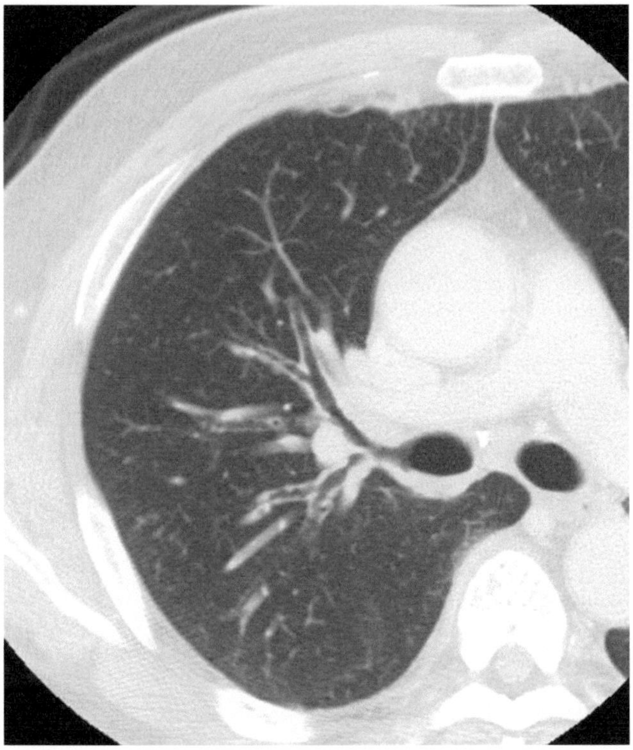

Fig. 19.4 Case 3. Thickening of the bronchovascular bundles is also observed in this case

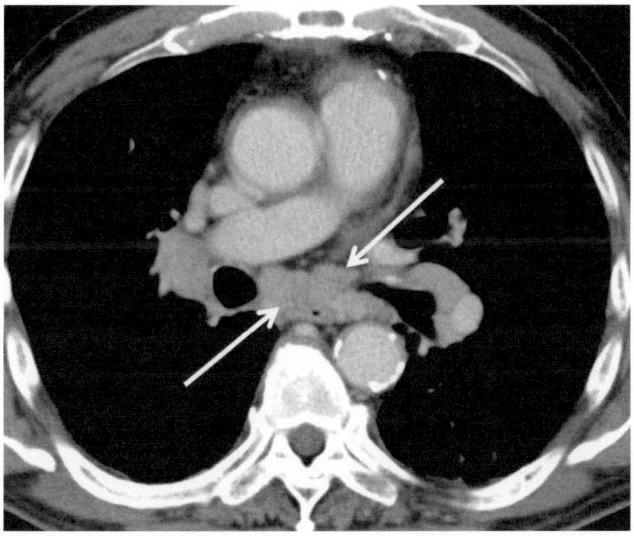

Fig. 19.5 Case 5, a 75-year-old male. Mediastinal lymphadenopathy is shown (*white arrows*)

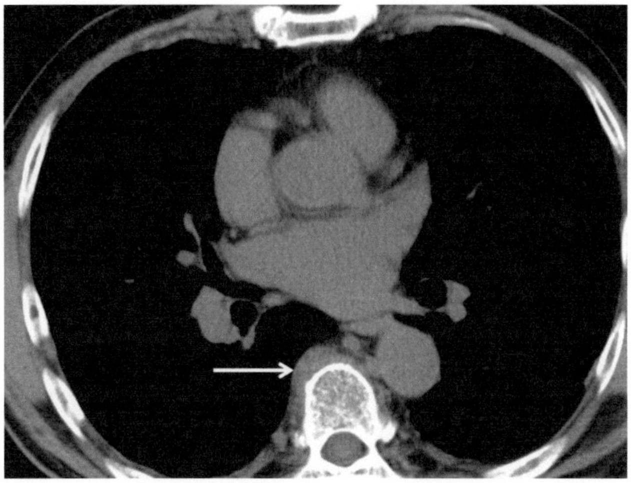

Fig. 19.6 Case 6, a 68-year-old male. A soft tissue mass is shown in the paravertebral region that is suggestive of mediastinal fibrosis (*white arrow*)

Conclusions

Intrathoracic lesions are often observed in patients with AIP even after excluding mediastinal lymphadenopathy. Gastroenterologists should perform both abdominal and chest CT for patients with AIP. The lesions may appear in the lung parenchyma, airways, and pleura as well as the mediastinum. Many diseases should be differentiated, such as lung cancer, idiopathic interstitial pneumonia, sarcoidosis, Castleman disease, and various infectious diseases. When image findings are mild, it may often be difficult to determine whether they are really IgG4 related or merely attributable to old age or heavy smoking. Thus, extrapancreatic lesions of the intrathoracic region are comparatively difficult for gastroenterologists to understand. In contrast to other extrapancreatic lesions, there appear to be fewer reports on intrathoracic lesions, which is in part because of the various patterns of these lesions. Further studies are needed to clarify the pathogenesis and establish the diagnostic criteria and optimal treatment policy.

References

1. Taniguchi T, et al. Interstitial pneumonia associated with autoimmune pancreatitis. Gut. 2004;53:770.
2. Duvic C, et al. Retroperitoneal fibrosis, sclerosing pancreatitis and bronchiolitis obliterans with organizing pneumonia. Nephrol Dial Transplant. 2004;19:2397–9.

3. Hirano K, et al. High-rate pulmonary involvement in autoimmune pancreatitis. Intern Med J. 2006;36:58–61.
4. Inoue D, et al. Immunoglobulin G4-related lung disease: CT findings with pathologic correlations. Radiology. 2009;251:260–70.
5. Zen Y, et al. IgG4-related lung and pleural disease: a clinicopathologic study of 21 cases. Am J Surg Pathol. 2009;33:1886–93.
6. Tsushima K, et al. Pulmonary involvement of autoimmune pancreatitis. Eur J Clin Invest. 2009;39:714–22.
7. Matsui S, et al. Immunoglobulin G4-related lung disease: clinicoradiological and pathological features. Respirology. 2013;18:480–7.
8. Fujinaga Y, et al. Characteristic findings in images of extrapancreatic lesions associated with autoimmune pancreatitis. Eur J Radiol. 2010;76:228–38.
9. Yamamoto H, et al. IgG4-related pleural disease diagnosed by a re-evaluation of chronic bilateral pleuritis in a patient who experienced occasional acute left bacterial pleuritis. Intern Med. 2011;50:893–7.
10. Inoue M, et al. Successful treatment of sclerosing mediastinitis with a high serum IgG4 level. Gen Thorac Cardiovasc Surg. 2007;55:431–3.
11. Yamashita K, et al. Lung involvement in IgG4-related lymphoplasmacytic vasculitis and interstitial fibrosis: report of 3 cases and review of the literature. Am J Surg Pathol. 2008;32:1620–6.
12. Ito M, et al. Central airway stenosis in a patient with autoimmune pancreatitis. Eur Respir J. 2009;33:680–3.
13. Ito S, et al. Three cases of bronchial asthma preceding IgG4-related autoimmune pancreatitis. Allergol Int. 2012;61:171–4.
14. Yamamoto M, et al. Mikulicz's disease and its extraglandular lesions. Curr Immunol Rev. 2011;7:162–71.
15. Yokoyama A, et al. Prognostic value of circulating KL-6 in idiopathic pulmonary fibrosis. Respirology. 2006;11:164–8.
16. Al-Salmi QA, et al. Serum KL-6 and surfactant proteins A and D in paediatric interstitial lung disease. Chest. 2005;127:403–7.
17. Kinoshita F, et al. Role of KL-6 in evaluating the disease severity of rheumatoid lung disease: comparison with HRCT. Respir Med. 2004;98:1131–7.
18. Shrestha B, et al. Distinctive pulmonary histopathology with increased IgG4-positive plasma cells in patients with autoimmune pancreatitis: report of 6 and 12 cases with similar histopathology. Am J Surg Pathol. 2009;33:1450–62.
19. Kitada M, et al. IgG4-related lung disease showing high standardized uptake values on FDG-PET: report of two cases. J Cardiothorac Surg. 2013;8:160.
20. Nakamura H, et al. Successful treatment of a patient with IgG4-related disease with a paravertebral mass lesion. Mod Rheumatol. 2011;21:524–7.
21. Hirano K, et al. Clinical analysis of high serum IgE in autoimmune pancreatitis. World J Gastroenterol. 2010;16:5241–6.
22. Kamisawa T, et al. Allergic manifestations in autoimmune pancreatitis. Eur J Gastroenterol Hepatol. 2009;21:1136–9.
23. Zen Y, Nakanuma YL. IgG4-related disease: a cross-sectional study of 114 cases. Am J Surg Pathol. 2010;34:1812–9.
24. Smyrk TC. Pathological features of IgG4-related sclerosing disease. Curr Opin Rheumatol. 2011;23:74–9.
25. Zen Y, et al. IgG4-positive plasma cells in inflammatory pseudotumor (plasma cell granuloma) of the lung. Hum Pathol. 2005;36:710–7.
26. Hui P, et al. Immunoglobulin G4-related lung disease: a disease with many different faces. Can Respir J. 2013;20:335–8.
27. Suzuki H, et al. Immunoglobulin G4-related lung disease accompanied by organizing pneumonia. Intern Med. 2013;52: 2105–11.
28. Seki N, et al. Spontaneous regression of lung lesions after excision of the submandibular gland in a patient with chronic sclerosing sialadenitis. Auris Nasus Larynx. 2012;39:212–5.
29. Kubota K, et al. Clinical factors predictive of spontaneous remission or relapse in cases of autoimmune pancreatitis. Gastrointest Endosc. 2007;66:1142–51.
30. Hirano K, et al. Incidence of malignancies in patients with IgG4 related disease. Inter Med. 2014;53(3):171–6.

20 Lymphadenopathy

Kazushige Uchida and Kazuichi Okazaki

Introduction

Firstly in 1961, Sarles et al. reported a case of chronic idiopathic pancreatitis with hypergammaglobulinemia in which an autoimmune mechanism was supposedly involved [1]. Kawaguchi et al. reported that the histopathological findings of AIP were characterized by the periductal infiltration of predominantly CD4-positive T cells and IgG4-positive plasma cells, storiform fibrosis with acinar cell atrophy frequently resulting in the stenosis of the main pancreatic duct, and obliterative phlebitis, as lymphoplasmacytic sclerosing pancreatitis (LPSP) in 1991 [2]. In 1995, Yoshida et al. proposed the concept of "autoimmune pancreatitis (AIP)" [3], and Hamano et al. reported that elevated serum immunoglobulin G4 (IgG4) levels were highly specific and sensitive for the diagnosis of AIP in 2001 [4]. Thereafter, many investigators including Japanese individuals have reported many literatures of AIP, and AIP has now been accepted as a new clinical entity of pancreatic disorder [5–8]. Kamisawa et al. suggested in 2003 that AIP is a systemic disease, based on their findings that the pancreas and other involved organs had abundant infiltration of IgG4-positive plasma cells and fibrosis [9].

Another unique histological pattern in the resected pancreata of patients with chronic mass-forming nonalcoholic pancreatitis with epithelial destruction by granulocytes (GEL) from western countries has been reported [10, 11]. This type histologically showed neutrophilic infiltration within the lumen and epithelium of interlobular ducts. This histological pattern is called idiopathic duct-centric pancreatitis (IDCP) [11], AIP with granulocyte epithelial lesions (AIP with GEL) [10]. In 2011, the International Consensus Diagnostic Criteria for Autoimmune Pancreatitis (ICDC) proposed the classification of AIP into type 1 AIP (LPSP) and type 2 AIP (IDCP) [12]. It is also reported that most of the Asian AIP cases are type 1 AIP; very few are type 2 AIP [13].

Various extrapancreatic lesions have been reported in patients with type 1 AIP so far, including salivary gland lesions as in IgG4-related sialadenitis (Mikulicz disease) [14]; pulmonary lesions [15]; sclerosing cholangitis [16, 17]; retroperitoneal fibrosis [18]; and kidney [19–21]; hypophysitis [22], chronic thyroiditis [23, 24]; prostatitis [25]; and aortitis [26]. These extrapancreatic lesions are usually detected by imaging study (computed tomography (CT), magnetic resonance imaging (MRI), gallium-67 scintigraphy, and 18-fluorodeoxyglucose positron emission tomography (FDG-PET)). These various extrapancreatic lesions suggest that type 1 AIP might be a part of the IgG4-related disease as Kamisawa et al. reported [9]. On the other hand, type 2 AIP involves swelling of the pancreas, but no other organ involvement, except in case of inflammatory bowel disease (approximately 30 %) [27].

Lymphadenopathy is also well known as one of the common extrapancreatic lesions in type 1 AIP. Several reports have published the incidence of lymphadenopathy accompanied with type 1 AIP to be between 7 and 80 % [28–30]. Lymphadenopathy in type 1 AIP generally takes 2 forms. First, lymphadenopathy as localized lymph nodes adjacent to pancreas is common. Second, systemic lymphadenopathy can be the major or sole component of the clinical presentation of IgG4-RD.

Clinical Features of IgG4-Related Lymphadenopathy

In IgG4-related lymphadenopathy, multiple lymph nodes are involved. In particular, mediastinal, intra-abdominal, and axillary lymph node swelling are common. Asymptomatic enlarged regional lymph nodes can be found on imaging of patients with type 1 AIP or in resected pancreas. Lymphadenopathy can develop subsequent to a diagnosis

K. Uchida, MD, PhD (✉) • K. Okazaki, MD, PhD
Division of Gastroenterology and Hepatology,
The Third Department of Internal Medicine,
Kansai Medical University, Osaka, Japan
e-mail: uchidak@hirakata.kmu.ac.jp; okazaki@hirakata.kmu.ac.jp

T. Kamisawa, J.B. Chung (eds.), *Autoimmune Pancreatitis*,
DOI 10.1007/978-3-642-55086-7_20, © Springer-Verlag Berlin Heidelberg 2015

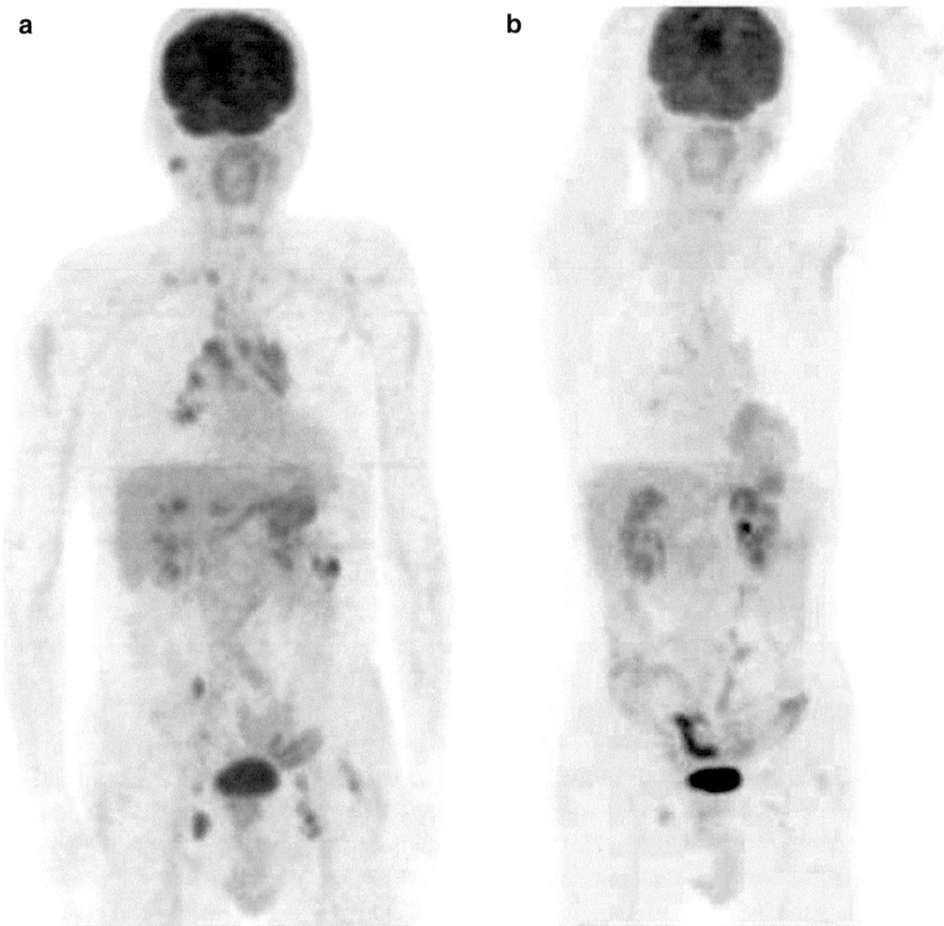

Fig. 20.1 FDG-PET scan of the patient with type 1 AIP. FDG accumulates in the pancreas body to tail, gall bladder, right parotid gland, and median and inguinal lymph nodes before steroid therapy (**a**). After steroid therapy, pancreatic enlargement and FDG accumulation are improved. Accumulation of the gall bladder, right parotid gland, and inguinal lymph nodes is disappeared. Accumulation of median lymph nodes is also decreased (**b**). FDG-PET scan is useful to detect extra pancreatic lesions and evaluate steroid therapy

of extranodal IgG4-RD. Lymphadenopathy appears synchronously or metachronously with type1 AIP, and in some patients, lymphadenopathy is the initial presentation of IgG4-related RD, and extranodal involvement can be discovered during work-up or follow-up with type 1 AIP.

Generally, IgG4-related lymphadenopathy is asymptomatic. However, patients with lymphadenopathy sometimes show a mass effect, such as hydronephrosis from compression of the ureter, but not retroperitoneal fibrosis, or lower-limb swelling due to venous compression in the pelvis [31].

IgG4-related lymphadenopathy may sometimes mimic or be misdiagnosed as lymphoma, multicentric Castleman disease, or disseminated malignancy (e.g., pancreatic cancer). In contrast with these diseases, the lymph nodes in IgG4-related lymphadenopathy are generally not very large (<2 cm); clinical symptoms (fever and body weight loss) are usually absent. Laboratory data show raised serum IgG4, IgG, and polyclonal hypergammaglobulinemia and sometimes autoantibodies [28, 31, 32]. Steroid therapy is usually effective (Fig. 20.1). These clinical manifestations are similar to type 1 AIP.

Histopathological Features of IgG4-Related Lymphadenopathy

In general, IgG4-RD (including type 1 AIP) appears to have three major histopathological features, including (1) dense lymphoplasmacytic infiltrate, (2) storiform fibrosis, and (3) obliterative phlebitis [33]. In 2011, *an international symposium on IgG4-RD was held in Boston* [34]. Consensus statement on the pathology of IgG4-related disease was proposed in 2012. This statement proposed a terminology scheme for the diagnosis of IgG4-related disease that is based primarily on the morphological appearance and importance of tissue IgG4 counts and IgG4/IgG ratios. This statement also descried that the isolated presence of IgG4-positive plasma cells or an elevated IgG4/IgG ratio constitutes relatively nonspecific findings.

Several studies of these morphological and immunohistological findings of IgG4-related lymphadenopathy have been performed [31, 32, 35–38]. Furthermore, the histopathological features of IgG4-related lymphadenopathy differ from those of extranodal sites in that there is usually no sclerosis or phlebitis. Lymph node showed no unique features of inflammation. Fibrosis is only seen in inflammatory pseudotumor-like lesions. Five histological patterns are recognized: type I, multicentric Castleman disease-like; type II, follicular hyperplasia; type III, interfollicular expansion; type IV, progressive transformation of germinal center; and type V, nodal inflammatory pseudotumor-like [31, 32, 36–38]. IgG4-positive cells are located in both the germinal centers and interfollicular zone. In case of type IV pattern, IgG4-positive cells infiltrate predominantly within the germinal centers [38].

Type I: Multicentric Castleman Disease-Like

Type I is frequently characterized by systemic lymphadenopathy. The architecture of the lymph node is preserved, and the lymph node shows varying degrees of interfollicular expansion with normal to hyperplastic germinal centers and penetration by hyalinized blood vessels. The interfollicular zone shows increased high endothelial venules, abundant plasma cells, and scattered eosinophils. These features are similar to those of multicentric Castleman disease, especially in the presence of multifocal lymphadenopathy, hypergammaglobulinemia, and elevated serum IgG4 levels [31, 32, 35–40]. Usually, multicentric Castleman disease shows small and regressive germinal centers without eosinophil infiltration. Multicentric Castleman disease sometimes fulfills the diagnostic criteria for IgG4-RD and abundant IgG4-positive plasma cell infiltration (especially an IgG4/IgG-positive plasma cell ratio >40 %) [40]. Therefore, a pathological diagnosis is difficult to make using histological findings alone. The morphological features are also similar to those of autoimmune disease-associated lymphadenopathy as seen in rheumatoid arthritis [41, 42] and the so-called idiopathic plasmacytic lymphadenopathy with polyclonal hypergammaglobulinemia [43]. Sato et al. proposed the concept of hyper IL-6 syndrome such as multicentric Castleman disease, rheumatoid arthritis, and other immune-associated conditions. In hyper-IL-6 syndromes, abnormalities of laboratory data showed elevated serum levels of IgG, IgA, and IgM; C-reactive protein (CRP); thrombocytosis; anemia; hypoalbuminemia; and hypocholesterolemia. In contrast, IgG4-RD does not show these abnormalities. They conclude that laboratory data is crucial to differentiate between IgG4-related disease and hyper IL-6 syndrome [37].

Type II: Follicular Hyperplasia

Type II is frequently showed in the regional lymph nodes of IgG4-RD. The histopathological findings of the lymph nodes usually show reactive follicular hyperplasia. The reactive follicles consist of a germinal center surrounded by a discrete mantle zone. The interfollicular zone may or may not show plasmacytosis, with eosinophils (Fig. 20.2) [31, 32, 35–38].

Type III: Interfollicular Expansion

Type III is also characterized by systemic lymphadenopathy. The lymph nodes show marked interfollicular expansion. Lymphoid follicles often are atrophic. High endothelial venules exist in expanded interfollicular zones where small lymphocytes, immunoblasts, plasmablasts, mature plasma cells, immature plasma cells, and eosinophils infiltrate. Interfollicular expansion-type lymphadenopathy is similar to angioimmunoblastic T-cell lymphoma, but definite cytologic atypia, clusters of clear cells, $CD10^+$ T cells, T-cell receptor gene rearrangement, or $CD21^+$ follicular dendritic cell proliferation is not observed (Fig. 20.3) [31, 32, 35–38].

Type IV: Progressive Transformation of Germinal Centers

Type IV is characterized as a benign reactive follicular hyperplasia of unknown origin. This type usually shows hyperplastic follicles, and lymph nodes show severalfold enlarged follicles and a distinct mantle zone but no expansion of the interfollicular zone [31, 32, 35–38].

Type V: Inflammatory Pseudotumor-Like

Type V is rare and characterized by focal replacement of the hyalinized fibrous tissue. A few residual lymphoid parenchyma shows hyperplastic germinal centers and focally dense lymphoplasmacytic infiltrations. Small lymphocytes, plasma cells, and eosinophils infiltrate the hyalinized fibrous tissue [31, 32, 35–38].

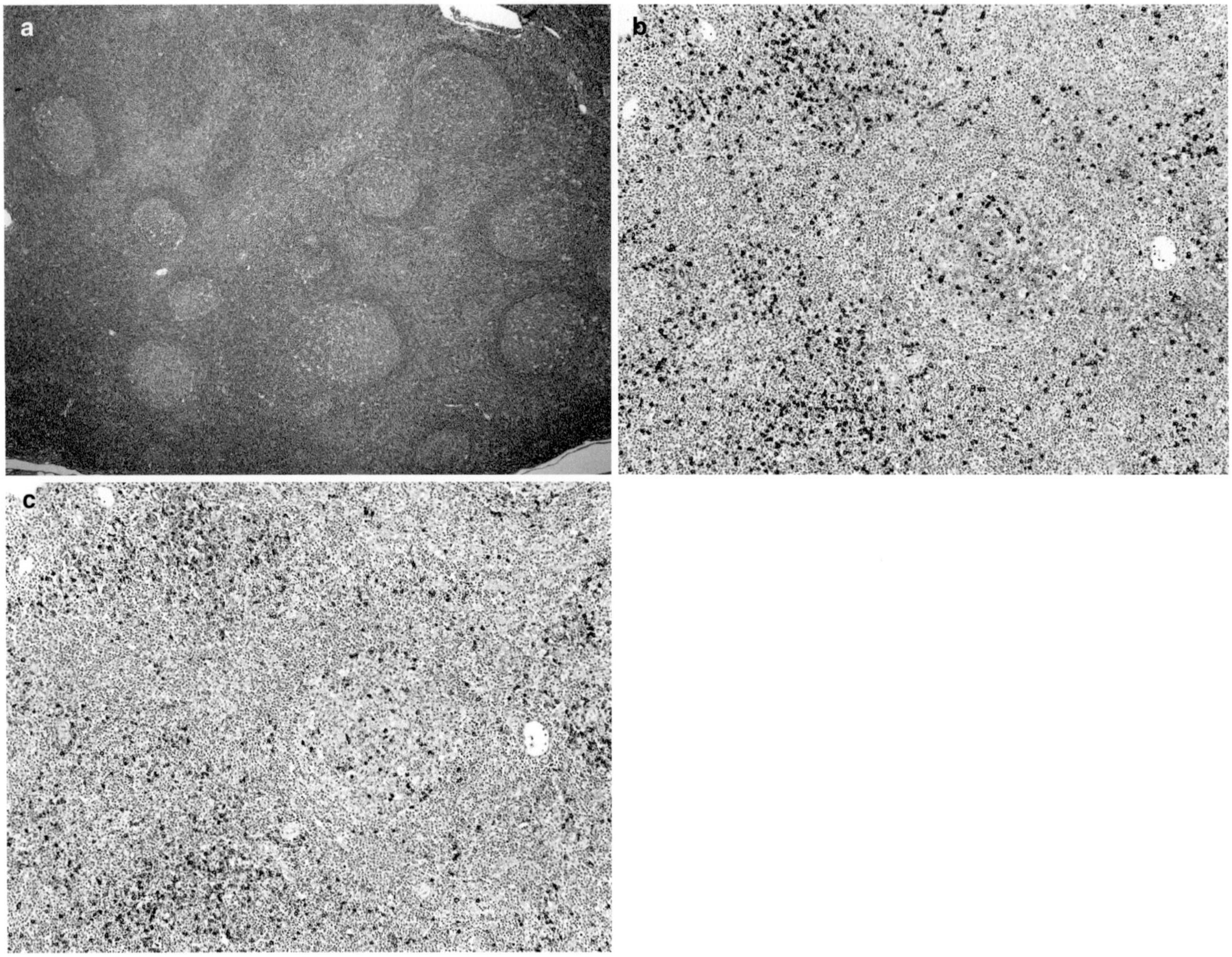

Fig. 20.2 IgG4-related lymphadenopathy (type II: follicular hyperplasia). This lymph node is surgical specimen from regional lymph nodes of IgG4-related sialadenitis. FDG-PET scan of this patient is presented in Fig. 20.1. (**a**) The lymph node shows reactive follicular hyperplasia. Immunostaining shows numerous IgG4-positive cells (**b**) and IgG-positive cells (**c**) in the interfollicular zone and germinal centers. The IgG4/IgG ratio in this case is over 40 %

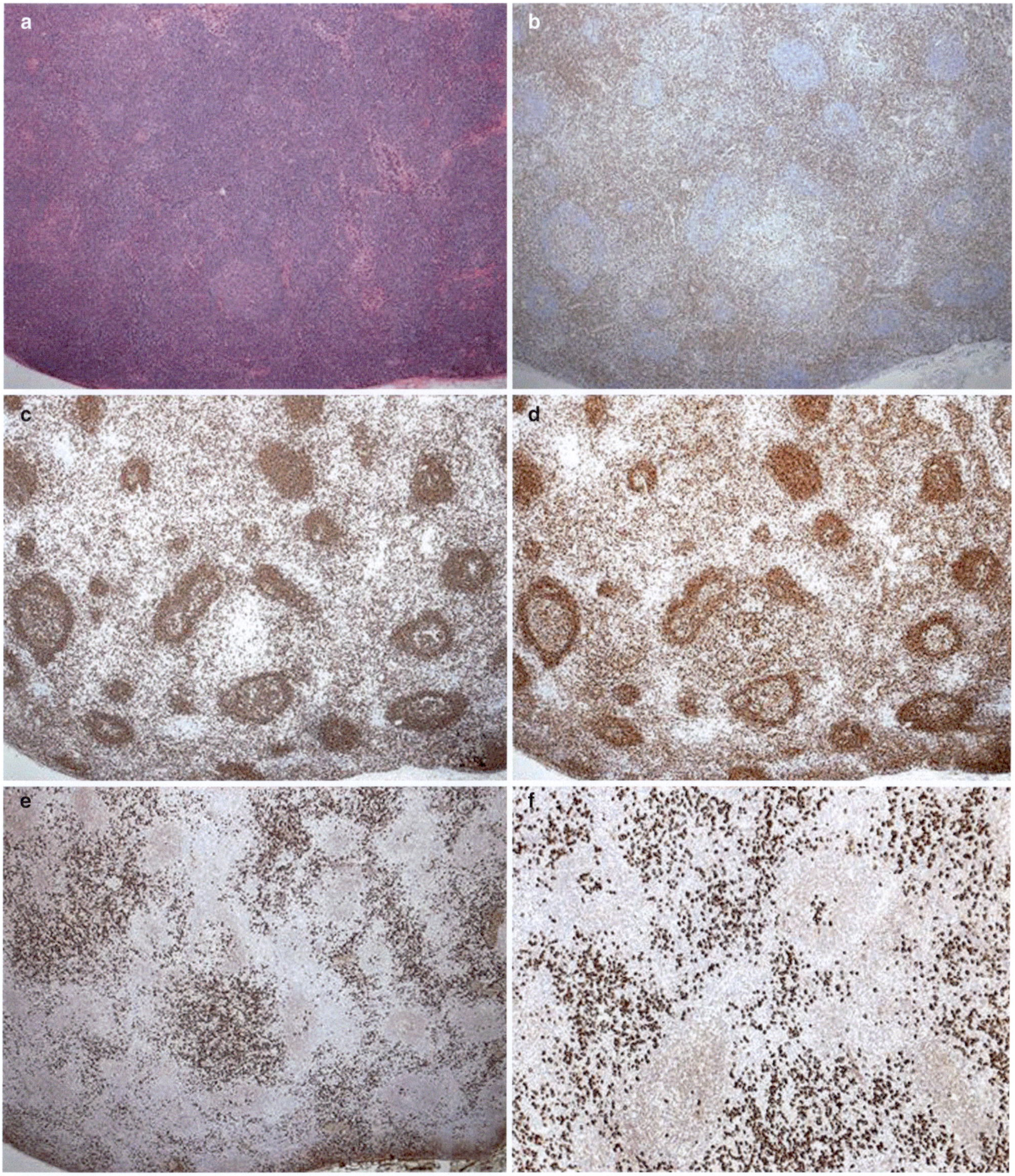

Fig. 20.3 IgG4-related lymphadenopathy (type III: interfollicular expansion). Systemic lymphadenopathy appears synchronously with type1 AIP in this patient. These figures show surgical specimen of cervical lymph nodes. The lymph node shows interfollicular expansion (**a**) Immunohistochemical staining shows that CD20 (**b**) and 79a (**c**) positive cells exist in lymphoid follicle. CD3 T cells exists in the interfollicular zone (**d**). Large numbers of IgG4-positive cells appeared mainly in the interfollicular zone (**e**, **f**)

Conclusion

AIP is a new clinical entity of pancreatic disorder. Type 1 AIP is recognized as one of pancreatic manifestations of IgG4-RD. Lymphadenopathy accompanied with type 1 AIP is well known, but that with type 2 is unclear. Further studies are needed to clarify the pathogenesis of lymphadenopathy, including the role of IgG4.

References

1. Sarles H, Sarles JC, Muratore R, et al. Chronic inflammatory sclerosis of the pancreas–an autonomous pancreatic disease? Am J Dig Dis. 1961;6:688–98.
2. Kawaguchi K, Koike M, Tsuruta K, et al. Lymphoplasmacytic sclerosing pancreatitis with cholangitis: a variant of primary sclerosing cholangitis extensively involving pancreas. Hum Pathol. 1991;22:387–95.
3. Yoshida K, Toki F, Takeuchi T, et al. Chronic pancreatitis caused by an autoimmune abnormality. Proposal of the concept of autoimmune pancreatitis. Dig Dis Sci. 1995;40:1561–8.
4. Hamano H, Kawa S, Horiuchi A, et al. High serum IgG4 concentrations in patients with sclerosing pancreatitis. N Engl J Med. 2001;344:732–8.
5. Ito T, Nakano I, Koyanagi S, et al. Autoimmune pancreatitis as a new clinical entity. Three cases of autoimmune pancreatitis with effective steroid therapy. Dig Dis Sci. 1997;42:1458–68.
6. Horiuchi A, Kawa S, Akamatsu T, et al. Characteristic pancreatic duct appearance in autoimmune chronic pancreatitis: a case report and review of the Japanese literature. Am J Gastroenterol. 1998;93:260–3.
7. Uchida K, Okazaki K, Konishi Y, et al. Clinical analysis of autoimmune-related pancreatitis. Am J Gastroenterol. 2000;95:2788–94.
8. Okazaki K, Uchida K, Chiba T. Recent concept of autoimmune-related pancreatitis. J Gastroenterol. 2001;36:293–302.
9. Kamisawa T, Funata N, Hayashi Y, et al. A new clinicopathological entity of IgG4-related autoimmune disease. J Gastroenterol. 2003;38:982–4.
10. Zamboni G, Luttges J, Capelli P, et al. Histopathological features of diagnostic and clinical relevance in autoimmune pancreatitis: a study on 53 resection specimens and 9 biopsy specimens. Virchows Arch. 2004;445:552–63.
11. Notohara K, Burgart LJ, Yadav D, et al. Idiopathic chronic pancreatitis with periductal lymphoplasmacytic infiltration: clinicopathologic features of 35 cases. Am J Surg Pathol. 2003;27:1119–27.
12. Shimosegawa T, Chari ST, Frulloni L, et al. International consensus diagnostic criteria for autoimmune pancreatitis: guidelines of the International Association of Pancreatology. Pancreas. 2011;40:352–8.
13. Hart PA, Kamisawa T, Brugge WR, et al. Long-term outcomes of autoimmune pancreatitis: a multicentre, international analysis. Gut. 2013;62:1771–6.
14. Kamisawa T, Funata N, Hayashi Y, et al. Close relationship between autoimmune pancreatitis and multifocal fibrosclerosis. Gut. 2003;52:683–7.
15. Mori S, Tokuda H, Sakai F, et al. Radiological features and therapeutic responses of pulmonary nontuberculous mycobacterial disease in rheumatoid arthritis patients receiving biological agents: a retrospective multicenter study in Japan. Mod Rheumatol. 2012;22:727–37.
16. Erkelens GW, Vleggaar FP, Lesterhuis W, et al. Sclerosing pancreato-cholangitis responsive to steroid therapy. Lancet. 1999;354:43–4.
17. Nakazawa T, Ohara H, Yamada T, et al. Atypical primary sclerosing cholangitis cases associated with unusual pancreatitis. Hepatogastroenterology. 2001;48:625–30.
18. Hamano H, Kawa S, Ochi Y, et al. Hydronephrosis associated with retroperitoneal fibrosis and sclerosing pancreatitis. Lancet. 2002;359:1403–4.
19. Saeki T, Nishi S, Imai N, et al. Clinicopathological characteristics of patients with IgG4-related tubulointerstitial nephritis. Kidney Int. 2010;78:1016–23.
20. Takeda S, Haratake J, Kasai T, et al. IgG4-associated idiopathic tubulointerstitial nephritis complicating autoimmune pancreatitis. Nephrol Dial Transplant. 2004;19:474–6.
21. Uchiyama-Tanaka Y, Mori Y, Kimura T, et al. Acute tubulointerstitial nephritis associated with autoimmune-related pancreatitis. Am J Kidney Dis. 2004;43:e18–25.
22. Shimatsu A, Oki Y, Fujisawa I, et al. Pituitary and stalk lesions (infundibulo-hypophysitis) associated with immunoglobulin G4-related systemic disease: an emerging clinical entity. Endocr J. 2009;56:1033–41.
23. Li Y, Nishihara E, Hirokawa M, et al. Distinct clinical, serological, and sonographic characteristics of Hashimoto's thyroiditis based with and without IgG4-positive plasma cells. J Clin Endocrinol Metab. 2010;95:1309–17.
24. Komatsu K, Hamano H, Ochi Y, et al. High prevalence of hypothyroidism in patients with autoimmune pancreatitis. Dig Dis Sci. 2005;50:1052–7.
25. Yoshimura Y, Takeda S, Ieki Y, et al. IgG4-associated prostatitis complicating autoimmune pancreatitis. Intern Med. 2006;45:897–901.
26. Kasashima S, Zen Y, Kawashima A, et al. A clinicopathologic study of immunoglobulin G4-related sclerosing disease of the thoracic aorta. J Vasc Surg. 2010;52:1587–95.
27. Kamisawa T, Chari ST, Giday SA, et al. Clinical profile of autoimmune pancreatitis and its histological subtypes: an international multicenter survey. Pancreas. 2011;40:809–14.
28. Okazaki K, Uchida K, Fukui T. Recent advances in autoimmune pancreatitis: concept, diagnosis, and pathogenesis. J Gastroenterol. 2008;43:409–18.
29. Vlachou PA, Khalili K, Jang HJ, et al. IgG4-related sclerosing disease: autoimmune pancreatitis and extrapancreatic manifestations. Radiographics. 2011;31:1379–402.
30. Hamano H, Arakura N, Muraki T, et al. Prevalence and distribution of extrapancreatic lesions complicating autoimmune pancreatitis. J Gastroenterol. 2006;41:1197–205.
31. Cheuk W, Yuen HK, Chu SY, et al. Lymphadenopathy of IgG4-related sclerosing disease. Am J Surg Pathol. 2008;32:671–81.
32. Sato Y, Kojima M, Takata K, et al. Systemic IgG4-related lymphadenopathy: a clinical and pathologic comparison to multicentric Castleman's disease. Mod Pathol. 2009;22:589–99.
33. Umehara H, Okazaki K, Masaki Y, et al. Comprehensive diagnostic criteria for IgG4-related disease (IgG4-RD), 2011. Mod Rheumatol. 2012;22:21–30.
34. Deshpande V, Zen Y, Chan JK, et al. Consensus statement on the pathology of IgG4-related disease. Mod Pathol. 2012;25:1181–92.
35. Grimm KE, Barry TS, Chizhevsky V, et al. Histopathological findings in 29 lymph node biopsies with increased IgG4 plasma cells. Mod Pathol. 2012;25:480–91.
36. Sato Y, Notohara K, Kojima M, et al. IgG4-related disease: historical overview and pathology of hematological disorders. Pathol Int. 2010;60:247–58.
37. Sato Y, Yoshino T. IgG4-Related Lymphadenopathy. Int J Rheumatol. 2012;2012:572539.
38. Cheuk W, Chan JK. Lymphadenopathy of IgG4-related disease: an underdiagnosed and overdiagnosed entity. Semin Diagn Pathol. 2012;29:226–34.
39. Peterson BA, Frizzera G. Multicentric Castleman's disease. Semin Oncol. 1993;20:636–47.

40. Sato Y, Kojima M, Takata K, et al. Multicentric Castleman's disease with abundant IgG4-positive cells: a clinical and pathological analysis of six cases. J Clin Pathol. 2010;63:1084–9.
41. Koo CH, Nathwani BN, Winberg CD, et al. Atypical lymphoplasmacytic and immunoblastic proliferation in lymph nodes of patients with autoimmune disease (autoimmune disease- associated lymphadenopathy). Medicine (Baltimore). 1984;63:274–90.
42. Segal GH, Clough JD, Tubbs RR. Autoimmune and iatrogenic causes of lymphadenopathy. Semin Oncol. 1993;20:611–26.
43. Kojima M, Nakamura S, Shimizu K, et al. Clinical implication of idiopathic plasmacytic lymphadenopathy with polyclonal hypergammaglobulinemia: a report of 16 cases. Int J Surg Pathol. 2004;12:25–30.

IgG4-Related Gastrointestinal Lesion

21

Satomi Koizumi, Terumi Kamisawa, and Sawako Kuruma

Introduction

IgG4-related disease has recently been recognized as a systemic condition that is characterized by increased serum IgG4 levels and responsiveness to steroid therapy. Patients with IgG4-RD show organ enlargement or nodular lesions with abundant lymphocyte and IgG4-positive plasma cell infiltration and fibrosis, and they frequently present both clinically and radiologically with findings suggestive of malignancy, which may result in unnecessary resection [1–3]. According to the comprehensive clinical diagnostic criteria for IgG4-RD [4], the diagnosis of IgG4-RD is made in the presence of a characteristic diffuse/localized swelling or mass in one or more organs with increased serum IgG4 levels or histological findings of abundant IgG4-positive plasma cell and lymphocyte infiltration associated with fibrosis.

Although there have been reports of infiltration of many IgG4-positive plasma cells in the gastric mucosa, colonic mucosa, and major duodenal papilla of some AIP patients [5–11], whether they are the lesions involved in IgG4-RD is unclear. This chapter reviews the published literature about the relationships between IgG4 and gastrointestinal diseases such as esophagitis, gastritis, colitis, and duodenal papillitis with abundant IgG4-positive plasma cell infiltration to clarify IgG4-related gastrointestinal disease.

IgG4-Related Esophageal Lesions

There have been two case reports of IgG4-related esophageal disease, which presented with dysphagia, weight loss, and recurrent esophageal strictures [12, 13]. On endoscopy, wall thickening was observed, and endoscopic ultrasound showed a submucosal lesion mass in one case. Since the possibility of malignancy and gastrointestinal stromal tumor could not be ruled out, esophageal resection was performed in both cases. Gross examination showed esophageal submucosal strictures with wall thickening. On histological examinations, transmural chronic fibrotic inflammation with abundant IgG4-positive plasma cell and lymphocyte infiltration and phlebitis were observed. The postoperative serum IgG4 level was 138 mg/dL in one case. Both cases showed no evidence of other IgG4-RD, including AIP, but they met the criteria of IgG4-RD. Thus, both cases were considered to show esophageal manifestations of IgG4-RD and could be called IgG4-related esophagitis. If unexplained esophageal stricture mimicking malignancy is seen, IgG4-related esophagitis must be considered in the differential diagnosis to avoid unnecessary surgery.

IgG4-Related Gastric Lesions

There have been nine cases in seven reports of IgG4-related gastric disease [14–20]. Seven cases were presented with abdominal symptoms like discomfort ($n=2$), abdominal pain ($n=1$), appetite loss ($n=1$), anorexia ($n=1$), weight loss ($n=1$), nausea ($n=1$), and vomiting ($n=1$). The other two cases found to have hard and fixed mass lesion in the stomach during upper endoscopy. Endoscopy findings showed submucosal tumor (SMT, $n=2$), refractory ulcer with stricture ($n=2$), and polypoid lesion ($n=4$). Endoscopic ultrasound with 2 cases showed lamina propria lesion mass. The serum IgG4 level was elevated in 2 of 4 cases. Because they could not deny the possibility of malignancy, the way of biopsy ($n=2$), endoscopic submucosal dissection ($n=1$), and resection ($n=6$) were performed. All 4 resected cases revealed dense infiltration of IgG4-positive plasma cell and marked submucosal fibrosis with storiform pattern.

Infiltration of many IgG4-positive plasma cells has been reported in the gastric mucosa of 33–47 % of AIP patients [10, 21]. After steroid therapy for AIP, most IgG4-positive plasma cells that had infiltration in the gastric mucosa disappeared

S. Koizumi, MD • T. Kamisawa, MD, PhD (✉) • S. Kuruma, MD
Department of Internal Medicine,
Tokyo Metropolitan Komagome Hospital,
3-18-22 Honkomagome, Bunkyo-ku, Tokyo 113-8677, Japan
e-mail: satokichi.048051@live.jp; kamisawa@cick.jp

T. Kamisawa, J.B. Chung (eds.), *Autoimmune Pancreatitis*,
DOI 10.1007/978-3-642-55086-7_21, © Springer-Verlag Berlin Heidelberg 2015

[22]. However, these gastric lesions cannot be called IgG4-related gastric disease, because neither dense fibrosis nor obliterative phlebitis was seen in the gastric mucosa of AIP patients.

IgG4-Related Major Duodenal Papillary Lesions

There has been only one report of an IgG4-related pseudotumor of the major duodenal papilla [23]. On duodenoscopy, a red, irregular, penile-shaped mass was seen protruding from the submucosa. Suspecting an atypical submucosal neoplastic lesion, the patient underwent pylorus-preserving pancreaticoduodenectomy. On histology, a lymphoplasmacytic granuloma with abundant IgG4-positive plasma cells localized to the major duodenal papilla was seen. In this case, no other IgG4-RD including AIP was present.

It has been reported that the duodenal major papilla is swollen in 41–65 % of AIP patients [24–26]. Abundant IgG4-positive plasma cell infiltration is detected in 55–80 % of AIP patients [8, 10, 24, 25]. Both a swollen major papilla and abundant IgG4-positive plasma cell infiltration have improved following treatment with steroids [8, 27]. In the resected pancreas of AIP patients, lymphoplasmacytic inflammation with many IgG4-positive plasma cells was found in the major duodenal papilla attached to the head of the pancreas. Therefore, the papillary lesions that are frequently detected in AIP patients are not papillary manifestations of IgG4-related RD; they represent direct spread from inflammation of the pancreatic head, although biopsy of the major papilla and histological examination with IgG4 immunostaining are useful to support a diagnosis of AIP [8, 24, 25, 28, 29].

IgG4-Related Colonic Lesions

Matsui et al. [30] reported a case of an AIP patient with a colonic polyp containing many IgG4-positive plasma cells [31] who developed colonic polyposis with many IgG4-positive plasma cells 1 year after complete remission of AIP with steroid treatment. The polyposis was markedly reduced with re-administration of steroids. They suggested that the immunopathogenesis involved enhanced T-helper type 2 responses to intestinal microflora in patients with IgG4-RD [32]. Well-circumscribed sclerosing nodular lesions of the cecum and sigmoid colon composed of hyalinized fibrocollagenous tissue with abundant IgG4-positive plasma cell infiltration were reported, and the two cases had no other IgG4-RD [20]. These polypoid or nodular lesions appear to be IgG4-related colonic lesions.

Although infiltration of many IgG4-positive plasma cells is occasionally seen in the colonic mucosa of AIP patients, dense fibrosis or obliterative phlebitis was not observed in the lesion [1, 5–7, 11, 33, 34]. While Ravi et al. [35] have suggested the possibility that inflammatory bowel disease represents an extrapancreatic manifestation of AIP, in general, ulcerative colitis (UC) is rarely seen with type 1AIP [2, 36]. Although IgG4-positive plasma cell infiltration is sometimes detected in the colonic mucosa of UC patients [11, 37–39], the mechanisms underlying IgG4-positive plasma cell infiltration in the colonic mucosa of UC patients remain unknown. Mere infiltration of many IgG4-positive plasma cells in the colonic mucosa in AIP or UC patients does not appear to be considered a colonic lesion of IgG4-RD.

IgG4-Related Ileal Lesion

There are two reports about ileal lesions involved in IgG4-related disease.

One is an IgG4-related inflammatory pseudotumor of an ileal conduit. An ill-defined, fibrotic, tumor-like mass, histologically showing fibrosis with infiltration of lymphocytes and IgG4-positive plasma cells and marked obliterative phlebitis, occurred in an ileal conduit created as part of surgery for urinary bladder cancer [40].

The other case is an isolated, stenosing chronic ulcer in the jejunum associated with necrotizing mesenteric arteries. Abundant infiltration of IgG4-positive plasma cells was identified in the jejunal wall, mesenteric artery, and mesenteric lymph nodes [41].

Discussion

IgG4-RD shows organ enlargement or nodular lesions consisting of abundant lymphocyte and IgG4-positive plasma cell infiltration and fibrosis in various organs, either simultaneously or metachronously [2, 3]. The first International Symposium on IgG4-RD held in 2011 suggested that the term “IgG4-related disease” recognizes aptly the ubiquity of IgG4 within involved organs and proposed a style that uses “IgG4-related” as a prefix to the organ system affected, along with pathological guidelines for the diagnosis of RD [3, 42]. The diagnosis of IgG4-RD rests on the combined presence of the characteristic histopathological appearance and increased numbers of IgG4-positive plasma cells. On histological examination, highly suggested IgG4-RD requires the identification of at least two of three characteristic histological features including: (1) dense lymphoplasmacytic infiltration; (2) fibrosis, usually storiform in character; and (3) obliterative phlebitis. The IgG4 counts required for the diagnosis differ among affected organs, ranging from 10 to 200 cells/hpf. The diagnosis of IgG4-RD requires corroboration between histopathological findings and clinical information such as elevated serum IgG4 levels, other organ involvement consistent with IgG4-RD, and effective response to treatment with steroids [42].

Infiltration of many IgG4-positive plasma cells is found in gastric and colonic mucosa and the major duodenal papilla of some AIP patients [1, 5–11, 21, 22, 24, 25, 33, 34]. However, since none of mass-like formation, dense fibrosis, or obliterative phlebitis was observed in these lesions, they cannot be diagnosed as gastrointestinal lesions involved in IgG4-RD. We consider both the clinical findings of mass formation and the histological findings of abundant infiltration of IgG4-positive plasma cells with fibrosis to be necessary when diagnosing IgG4-related gastrointestinal disease.

IgG4-related pseudotumors have been reported in several organs such as the liver and lung [43–45]. Based on a review of the literature, there appear to be two types in IgG4-related gastrointestinal disease. One is a gastrointestinal lesion showing marked thickening of the wall of the esophagus and stomach, consisting of dense fibrosis with abundant IgG4-positive plasma cell infiltration, which usually shows submucosal spreading. The other is an IgG4-related pseudotumor in the gastrointestinal region, such as the stomach, colon, and major duodenal papilla, that presents as a polypoid or mass-like lesion.

Most solitary IgG4-related gastrointestinal lesions that are not associated with other IgG4-RD appear to be difficult to diagnose. It is vitally important to rule out malignancy. However, these lesions may respond to steroid therapy. To avoid unnecessary resection, the differential diagnosis must include IgG4-related gastrointestinal diseases.

Conclusions

In conclusion, IgG4-related gastrointestinal disease may be part of IgG4-RD. However, this remains unclear due to its rarity, and further study is needed. Therefore, in patients with unexplained thickening or SMT, pseudotumor, nodule, polyp, ulcer, or swelling, IgG4-related gastrointestinal disease should be considered in the differential diagnosis by both clinicians and pathologists to avoid unnecessary surgery and provide appropriate treatment.

Acknowledgment This study was partially supported by the Intractable Disease, supported by the Ministry of Health, Labour, and Welfare of Japan.

References

1. Kamisawa T, Funata N, Hayashi Y, et al. A new clinicopathological entity of IgG4-related autoimmune disease. J Gastroenterol. 2003;38:982–4.
2. Kamisawa T, Takuma K, Egawa N, Tsuruta K, Sasaki T. Autoimmune pancreatitis and IgG4-related sclerosing disease. Nat Rev Gastroenterol Hepatol. 2010;7:401–9.
3. Stone JH, Khosroshani A, Deshpande V, et al. Recommendations for the nomenclature of IgG4-related disease and its individual organ system manifestations. Arthritis Rheum. 2012;64:3061–7.
4. Umehara H, Okazaki K, Masaki Y, et al. Comprehensive diagnostic criteria for IgG4-related disease (IgG4-RD), 2011. Mod Rheumatol. 2012;22:21–30.
5. Kamisawa T, Funata N, Hayashi Y, et al. Close relationship between autoimmune pancreatitis and multifocal fibrosclerosis. Gut. 2003;52:683–7.
6. Kamisawa T, Egawa N, Nakajima H, et al. Gastrointestinal findings in Patients with autoimmune pancreatitis. Endoscopy. 2005;37:1127–30.
7. Deheragoda MG, Church NI, Rodriguez-Justo M, et al. The use of immunoglobulin g4 immunostaining in diagnosing pancreatic and extrapancreatic involvement in autoimmune pancreatitis. Clin Gastroenterol Hepatol. 2007;5:1229–34.
8. Kamisawa T, Tu Y, Egawa N, Tsuruta K, Okamoto A. A new diagnostic endoscopic tool for autoimmune pancreatitis. Gastrointest Endosc. 2008;68:358–61.
9. Sepehr A, Mino-Kenudson M, Ogawa F, Brugge WR, Deshpande V, Lauwers GY. IgG4+ to IgG+plasma cells ratio of ampulla can help differentiate autoimmune pancreatitis from other "mass forming" pancreatic lesions. Am J Surg Pathol. 2008;32:1770–9.
10. Hirano K, Fukushima N, Tada M, et al. Diagnostic utility of biopsy specimens for autoimmune pancreatitis. J Gastroenterol. 2009;44:765–73.
11. Kuwata G, Kamisawa T, Koizumi K, et al. Ulcerative colitis and immunoglobulin g4. Gut Liver. 2014;8:29–34.
12. Lopes J, Hochwald SN, Lancia N, Dixon LR, Ben-David K. Autoimmune esophagitis: IgG4-related tumors of the esophagus. J Gastrointest Surg. 2010;14:1031–4.
13. Lee H, Joo M, Song TJ, et al. IgG4-related sclerosing esophagitis: a case report. Gastrointest Endosc. 2011;73:834–7.
14. Na KY, Sung JY, Jang JY, et al. Gastric nodular lesion caused by IgG4-related disease. Pathol Int. 2012;62:716–8.
15. Bateman AC, Sommerlad M, Underwood TJ. Chronic gastric ulceration: a novel manifestation of IgG4-related disease? J Clin Pathol. 2012;65:569–70.
16. Rollins KE, Mehta SP, O'Donovan M, Safranek PM. Gastric IgG4-related autoimmune fibrosclerosing pseudotumor: a novel location. ISRN Gastroenterol. 2011;2011:873087.
17. Kaji R, Okabe Y, Ishida Y, et al. Autoimmune pancreatitis presenting with IgG4-positive multiple gastric polyps. Gastrointest Endosc. 2010;71:420–2.
18. Kim do H, Kim J, Park do H, et al. Immunoglobulin G4-related inflammatory pseudotumor of the stomach. Gastrointest Endosc. 2012;76:451–2.
19. Fujita T, Ando T, Sakakibara M, Hosoda W, Goto H. Refractory gastric ulcer with abundant IgG4-positive plasma cell infiltration. World J Gastroenterol. 2010;16:2183–6.
20. Chetty R, Serra S, Gauchotte G, Markl B, Agaimy A. Sclerosing nodular lesions of the gastrointestinal tract containing large numbers of IgG4 plasma cells. Pathology. 2011;43:31–5.
21. Kamisawa T, Takuma K, Tabata T, et al. Serum IgG4-negative autoimmune pancreatitis. J Gastroenterol. 2011;46:108–16.
22. Kamisawa T, Nakajima H, Egawa N, Hayashi Y, Funata N. Autoimmune pancreatitis can be confirmed with gastroscopy. Dig Dis Sci. 2004;49:155–6.
23. Hisa T, Ohkubo H, Shiozawa S, Ishigame H, Furutake M, Takamatsu M. Lymphoplasmacytic granuloma localized to the ampulla of Vater: an ampullary lesion of IgG4-related systemic disease? Gastrointest Endosc. 2008;68:1229–32.
24. Kubota K, Iida H, Fujisawa T, et al. Clinical significance of swollen duodenal papilla in autoimmune pancreatitis. Pancreas. 2007;35:e51–60.
25. Kim MH, Moon SH, Kamisawa T. Major duodenal papilla in autoimmune pancreatitis. Dig Surg. 2010;27:110–4.

26. Unno H, Saegusa H, Fukushima M, Hamano H. Usefulness of endoscopic observation of the main duodenal papilla in the diagnosis of sclerosing pancreatitis. Gastrointest Endosc. 2002;56:880–4.
27. Kamisawa T, Anjiki H, Egawa N. Disappearance of an ampullary pseudotumor after steroid therapy for autoimmune pancreatitis. Gastrointest Endosc. 2010;71:847–8.
28. Kamisawa T, Tu Y, Nakajima H, Egawa N, Tsuruta K, Okamoto A. Usefulness of biopsying the major duodenal papilla to diagnose autoimmune pancreatitis: a prospective study using IgG4-immunostaining. World J Gastroenterol. 2006;12:2031–3.
29. Moon SH, Kim MH, Park do H, et al. IgG4 immunostaining of duodenal papillary biopsy specimens may be useful for supporting a diagnosis of autoimmune pancreatitis. Gastrointest Endosc. 2010;71:960–6.
30. Matsui H, Watanabe T, Ueno K, et al. Colonic polyposis associated with autoimmune pancreatitis. Pancreas. 2009;38:840–2.
31. Ueno K, Watanabe T, Kawata Y, et al. IgG4-related autoimmune pancreatitis involving the colonic mucosa. Eur J Gastroenterol Hepatol. 2008;20:1118–21.
32. Akitake R, Watanabe T, Zaima C, et al. Possible involvement of T helper type 2 responses to Toll-like receptor ligands in IgG4-related sclerosing disease. Gut. 2010;59:542–5.
33. Kamisawa T, Nakajima H, Egawa N, Funata N, Tsuruta K, Okamoto A. IgG4-related sclerosing disease incorporating sclerosing pancreatitis, cholangitis, sialadenitis and retroperitoneal fibrosis with lymphadenopathy. Pancreatology. 2006;6:132–7.
34. Sepehr A, Lauwers GY. Gastrointestinal evidence of autoimmune pancreatitis: a rare manifestation. Histopathology. 2008;53:358–9.
35. Ravi K, Chari ST, Vege SS, Sandborn WJ, Smyrk TC, Loftus Jr EV. Inflammatory bowel disease in the setting of autoimmune pancreatitis. Inflamm Bowel Dis. 2009;15:1326–30.
36. Hart PA, Kamisawa T, Brugge WR, et al. Long-term outcomes of autoimmune pancreatitis: a multicenter, international analysis. Gut. 2013;62:1771–6.
37. Rebours V, Le Baleur Y, Cazals-Hatem D, et al. Immunoglobulin G4 immunostaining of gastric, duodenal, or colonic biopsies is not helpful for the diagnosis of autoimmune pancreatitis. Clin Gastroenterol Hepatol. 2012;10:91–4.
38. Strehl JD, Hartmann A, Agaimy A. Numerous IgG4-positive plasma cells are ubiquitous in diverse localized non-specific chronic inflammatory conditions and need to be distinguished from IgG4-related systemic disorders. J Clin Pathol. 2011;64:237–43.
39. Kamisawa T, Tabata T, Kuwata G, Koizumi K. Extraintestinal manifestations of inflammatory bowel disease: autoimmune pancreatitis and other IgG4-related conditions. In: Baumgart DC, editor. Crohn's disease and ulcerative colitis. New York: Springer; 2012. p. 601–10.
40. Kuroda Y, Fujioka M, Kurosawa K, Ohashi K. IgG4-related inflammatory pseudotumor of the ileal conduit. Pathol Int. 2011;61:47–8.
41. Wong DD, Pillai SR, Priyanthi Kumarasinghe M, et al. IgG4-related sclerosing disease of the small bowel presenting as necrotizing mesenteric arteritis and a solitary jejunal ulcer. Am J Surg Pathol. 2012;36:929–34.
42. Deshpande V, Zen Y, Chan JK, et al. Consensus statement on the pathology of IgG4-related disease. Mod Pathol. 2012;25:1181–92.
43. Zen Y, Harada K, Sasaki M, et al. IgG4-related sclerosing cholangitis with and without hepatic inflammatory pseudotumor, and sclerosing pancreatitis-associated sclerosing cholangitis: do they belong to a spectrum of sclerosing pancreatitis? Am J Surg Pathol. 2004;28:1193–203.
44. Zen Y, Kitagawa S, Minato H, et al. IgG4-positive plasma cells in inflammatory pseudotumor (plasma cell granuloma) of the lung. Hum Pathol. 2005;36:710–7.
45. Tsuboi H, Inokuma S, Setoguchi K, et al. Inflammatory pseudotumors in multiple organs associated with elevated serum IgG4 level: recovery by only a small replacement dose of steroid. Intern Med. 2008;47:1139–42.

Part IV

Treatment and Prognosis

22 Steroid Therapy for Autoimmune Pancreatitis

Seungmin Bang and Jae Bock Chung

Introduction

Autoimmune pancreatitis (AIP) is a type of chronic pancreatitis featured by swelling of pancreas, narrowing of pancreatic duct, elevation of serum IgG4, and/or presence of several autoantibodies [1–3].

The original histologic feature of AIP revealed a distinct pattern of lymphoplasmacytic infiltrate with abundance of IgG4-positive cells in affected organs [4–6]. However, some of the pancreas specimens showed a different histologic features characterized by neutrophilic infiltration in pancreatic ductal epithelium with duct destruction. Especially, the patients showing these pathologic features do not have any IgG4 association [7]. These two different groups have now been classified type I and type II AIP, respectively [8].

Even though there are no concrete scientific evidences for medical treatment of AIP, it is definite that AIP is extremely responsive to steroid therapy irrespective of its subtypes. Consequently, oral corticosteroid therapy has been considered as a standard treatment for AIP. Furthermore, steroid responsiveness has been suggested as a diagnostic criterion in guidelines from Korea and international consensus of diagnostic criteria [9, 10]. However, the indication, dosage, and duration of steroid treatment still remain unsolved. Herein, we discuss treatment of AIP, focusing steroid treatment.

Definition of Treatment Outcomes

Remission of AIP

The ultimate treatment goal of AIP is to make the patient free from the disease. Until now, there is no generally accepted consensus on the specific single parameter for determining remission. However, remission can be defined as the resolution of symptoms along with normalizing the abnormal biochemical parameters, radiologic findings, and histology. Based on this crude concept, remission of AIP can be classified into 5 categories: (1) symptomatic remission, (2) serologic or biochemical remission, (3) radiologic remission, (4) histologic remission, and (5) functional remission [11–13]. Symptomatic remission is resolution of symptoms including abdominal pain and obstructive jaundice. Serologic or biochemical remission can be defined as normalization of serum IgG or IgG4 elevation. Radiologic remission is resolution of typical enlargement of pancreas and irregular narrowing of main pancreatic duct (Fig. 22.1). Usually, the radiologic remission can be achieved within 2–4 weeks of steroid treatment [12, 14]. Histologic remission can be defined as the restoration of normal histologic architecture of pancreas or affected organ with resolution of the histologic abnormalities including lymphoplasmacytic infiltration and fibrosis. However, histologic remission in real clinical setting is not easy to confirm. Functional remission means restoration of exocrine and/or endocrine dysfunction (Table 22.1).

In clinical setting, complete remission can be defined when symptomatic, serologic, and radiologic remissions are achieved with treatment. Incomplete remission can be defined when only 2 of the above 3 categories are satisfied.

Relapse of AIP

Even though AIP is extremely responsive to initial steroid treatment, relapse or recurrence of the disease is frequently encountered during follow-up of the patients. According to the subtypes of AIP, disease relapse is common in type 1 AIP, while type 2 AIP does not relapse [11, 15]. The exact rate of relapse for type 1 AIP has not been unveiled. In a recent international multicenter study, 31 % of patients with type 1 AIP experienced at least one disease relapse [16]. More than half of patients who experienced multiple relapses

S. Bang, MD, PhD (✉) • J.B. Chung, MD, PhD
Division of Gastroenterology, Department of Internal Medicine, Yonsei University College of Medicine, Yonsei Institute of Gastroenterology, 50-1, Yonsei-ro, Seodaemun-gu, Seoul 120-752, Republic of Korea
e-mail: bang7028@yuhs.ac; jbchung@yuhs.ac

T. Kamisawa, J.B. Chung (eds.), *Autoimmune Pancreatitis*,
DOI 10.1007/978-3-642-55086-7_22, © Springer-Verlag Berlin Heidelberg 2015

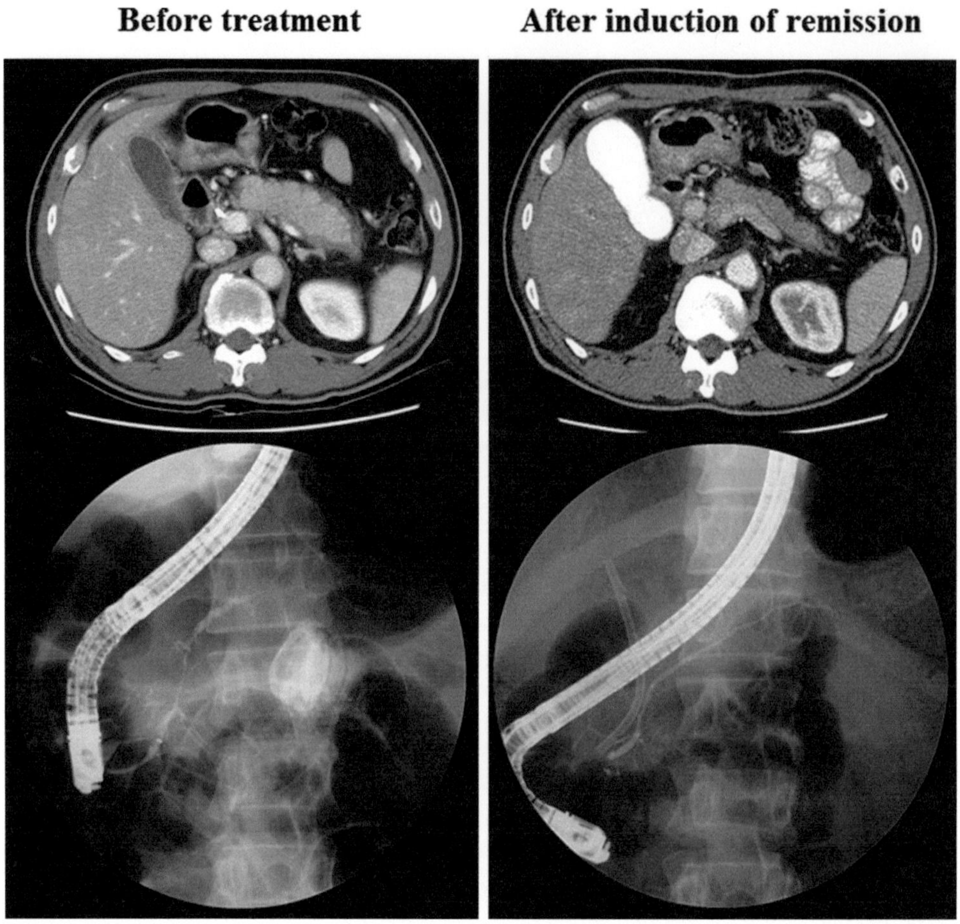

Fig. 22.1 Radiologic remission of type 1 AIP with induction of remission therapy. Before treatment, CT scan reveals diffuse swelling of pancreatic parenchyme with minimal peripancreatic haziness. The pancreatic duct visualized by ERCP shows multifocal narrowings in main pancreatic duct without remarkable poststenotic dilation. After induction of remission, pancreas on CT scan looks to have normal contour. The pancreatic duct obtained by ERCP shows normal caliber of main pancreatic duct and the multifocal stenotic segments of pancreatic duct disappeared

have permanent histologic changes (pancreatic calcifications or stones and intensive fibrosis) in pancreas and do not show steroid responsiveness [17, 18].

Theoretically, relapse of AIP can be defined as recurrence of symptomatic, serologic, radiologic, or histologic abnormalities of AIP after complete or incomplete remission has been achieved. The definition of relapse can be also categorized as (1) symptomatic, (2) serologic, (3) radiologic, and (4) histologic relapse (Table 22.1). Serologic relapse is elevation of serum IgG or IgG4 after normalization. Sometimes, serologic relapse can be observed without any evidence of symptomatic and radiologic relapse. That may mean subclinical disease activity or undetected disease activity in other organs [11, 19].

Steroid Treatment

Indication of Steroid Treatment

Patients with AIP who receive glucocorticoid treatment have significantly higher remission rates of all aspects of clinical, histopathological, and serologic findings than those who do not [20–22]. Glucocorticoid treatment has also been reported to reduce the time to remission and improve the exocrine function of the pancreas. Even though there is no consensus on the indication, steroid treatment for AIP patients can alleviate symptoms and improve radiologic and serologic abnormalities. And steroid therapy should be started when vital organs are affected for preventing severe organ dysfunction and failure. However, not all manifestations of AIP require immediate intervention, and implementation of steroid therapy should be decided based on the significance, functional status, and disease course of the organ affected. In practice, the generally accepted indications of steroid treatment include obstructive jaundice, abdominal pain, back pain, and symptomatic extrapancreatic diseases.

Induction of Remission and Withdrawal of Steroid

Steroid therapy for AIP consists of induction of remission, withdrawal of steroid, maintenance therapy, and off-steroid therapy (Fig. 22.2). For induction of remission, high dose of steroid is recommended. The exact dose of steroid and duration for remission induction have not been yet established. Most of the experts agree to use 30 mg or 40 mg of prednisolone or prednisone [3, 12, 13, 16, 20, 22–26]. Recently,

Table 22.1 Definition of remission and relapse of autoimmune pancreatitis

Classification	Subclassification	Definition
Remission	Symptom (A)	Resolution of accompanying symptoms (i.e., obstructive jaundice and abdominal pain)
	Serology (B)	Normalization of elevated serum IgG or IgG4 level
	Radiation (C)	Resolution of pancreatic enlargement and main pancreatic duct narrowing
	Histology	Restitution of abnormal histologic changes to normal architecture
	Function	Normalization of exocrine and/or endocrine function of the pancreas (diabetes mellitus)
Treatment outcome	Complete remission	A+B+C
	Incomplete remission	2 of 3 (A, B, C)
Relapse	Symptom	Occurrence of accompanying symptoms after remission
	Serology	Elevation of serum IgG or IgG4 level after remission
	Radiology	Occurrence of pancreatic enlargement and/or main pancreatic duct narrowing at the same or different locations, compared with previous disease
	Histology	Occurrence of abnormal histologic changes

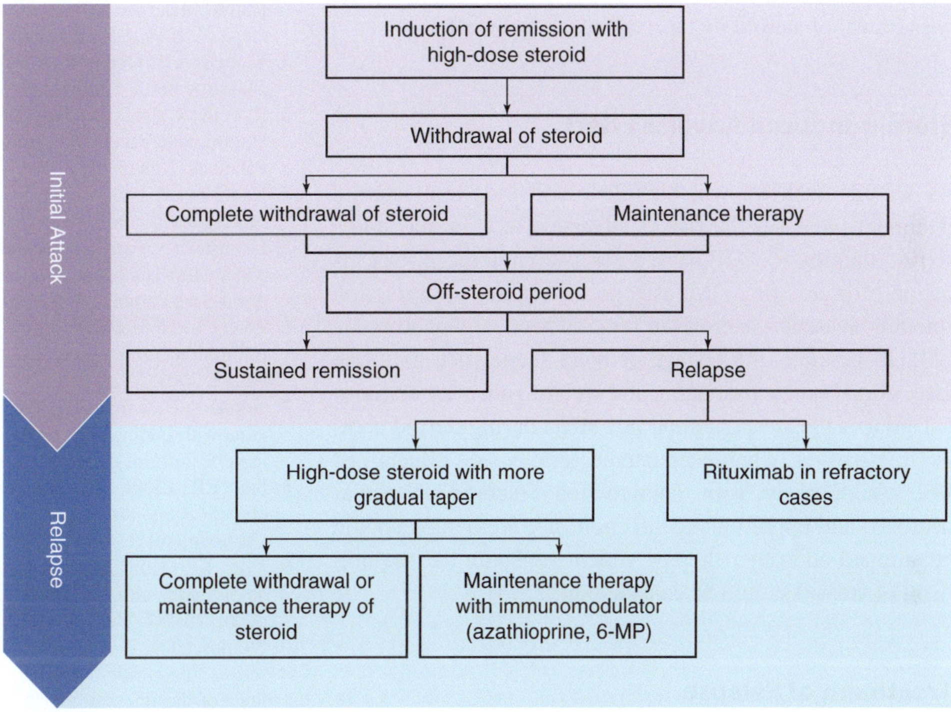

Fig. 22.2 Recommendation of steroid therapy for autoimmune pancreatitis

ICDC defines the starting dose of steroid for induction of remission as 0.6–1 mg/kg per day for type 1 AIP [10]. For the duration of induction of remission with high-dose steroid, the clinical protocols are quite different according to countries. In Korea and Japan, 30–40 mg of oral corticosteroid is usually prescribed for 1–2 months. On the contrary, 40 mg of oral steroid is used for 1 month in the USA. In general, 1 month of 30–40 mg oral corticosteroid can be used as a standard induction of remission regimen. However, the duration of high-dose steroid therapy should be tailored to each patient based on the disease activity of the involved organs.

Before starting withdrawal of steroid, it should be preceded to confirm the responsiveness of disease to the drug. Usually, symptomatic response or remission can be observed within 2–3 weeks after installation of steroid therapy. However, it usually takes several weeks to months to achieve serologic and radiologic remission. Especially, extrapancreatic lesions such as bile duct stricture and retroperitoneal fibrosis take more time to be resolved. The protocols of tapering the steroid after induction of remission are also different from medical center to center. However, most of the protocols taper the drug by 5 mg/week.

Maintenance Treatment for AIP

The goal of maintenance therapy for AIP is to prevent relapse. Theoretical reasons for need of maintenance therapy are that the relapse rate of AIP has been reported to 30–50 %

of all cases. And the serologic and radiologic remissions require more time of treatment in clinical setting. However, the issue of whether maintenance therapy should be used on all patients of AIP or confined to the patients who experienced relapse at least once remains unsolved. Furthermore, the duration of maintenance therapy is another issue to be solved.

Currently, Japanese group and several Korean groups favor the maintenance therapy after induction of remission. Japanese guidelines for AIP suggest maintenance therapy with low dose of steroid (2.5–5 mg/day) should be administered to all patients for 3 years. On the contrary, the US group recommends maintenance therapy only for the patients who experienced relapse. They recommend short course of high-dose steroid therapy for induction of remission and complete withdrawal of steroid by tapering out (5 mg/week).

Steroid-Induced Adverse Effect

As already well known, high-dose and long-term steroid treatment increases the risk of adverse effect. In one study, steroid therapy for AIP caused glucose intolerance, exacerbation of preexisting DM, osteoporosis, spinal compression fracture, avascular necrosis of femoral head, and pneumonia [22]. In practice, the change of body shape such as moon face, dorsal hump formation, and weight gain with abdominal striae is the most common side effect during steroid treatment. However, when encountered serious side effects just like osteoporosis with compression fracture, avascular necrosis, and opportunistic infection, steroid therapy should be stopped and other therapy which can spare the requirement of steroid should be considered [22, 24].

Treatment of Relapse

The patients of AIP can experience the disease relapse either during withdrawal period or after off-steroid period. Overall rate of relapse in AIP has been 30–50 %. However, these studies have several flaws such as inconsistent definition of relapse, heterogeneity of study population, and incomplete differentiation of subtype. Currently, the relapse is common in type 1 AIP and rare in type 2 disease.

The management of relapsed AIP has 3 options. The first is to reinstall high-dose steroid for induction of remission with or without maintenance therapy. Japan and Korean experts and ICDC recommend using maintenance therapy [10]. Reinstallation of steroid therapy for relapsing AIP has been effective as much as initial treatment [3, 22, 26]. The second option is to use immunomodulators (azathioprine, 6-mercaptopurine) combined with steroid. Even though recent study from Mayo group did not prove the immunomodulators (azathioprine, 6-mercaptopurine) were better than an additional course of steroid for relapsing AIP patients, the immunomodulators have been still evaluated whether to have a beneficial role for managing AIP [27–31]. The last one is to use rituximab for maintenance after reinstallation of steroid therapy. In the above study, rituximab was effective in the treatment of both immunomodulator-resistant and steroid-intolerant patients [27]. However, the real benefit of rituximab also should be evaluated with large scaled study [32–34].

References

1. Chari ST, Smyrk TC, Levy MJ, et al. Diagnosis of autoimmune pancreatitis: the Mayo Clinic experience. Clin Gastroenterol Hepatol. 2006;4:1010–6; quiz 934.
2. Kamisawa T, Okamoto A. IgG4-related sclerosing disease. World J Gastroenterol. 2008;14:3948–55.
3. Ryu JK, Chung JB, Park SW, et al. Review of 67 patients with autoimmune pancreatitis in Korea: a multicenter nationwide study. Pancreas. 2008;37:377–85.
4. Kamisawa T. IgG4-positive plasma cells specifically infiltrate various organs in autoimmune pancreatitis. Pancreas. 2004;29:167–8.
5. Kamisawa T, Funata N, Hayashi Y. Lymphoplasmacytic sclerosing pancreatitis is a pancreatic lesion of IgG4-related systemic disease. Am J Surg Pathol. 2004;28:1114.
6. Zhang L, Notohara K, Levy MJ, et al. IgG4-positive plasma cell infiltration in the diagnosis of autoimmune pancreatitis. Mod Pathol. 2007;20:23–8.
7. Notohara K, Burgart LJ, Yadav D, et al. Idiopathic chronic pancreatitis with periductal lymphoplasmacytic infiltration: clinicopathologic features of 35 cases. Am J Surg Pathol. 2003;27:1119–27.
8. Sah RP, Chari ST. Autoimmune pancreatitis: an update on classification, diagnosis, natural history and management. Curr Gastroenterol Rep. 2012;14:95–105.
9. Kim KP, Kim MH, Kim JC, et al. Diagnostic criteria for autoimmune chronic pancreatitis revisited. World J Gastroenterol. 2006;12:2487–96.
10. Shimosegawa T, Chari ST, Frulloni L, et al. International consensus diagnostic criteria for autoimmune pancreatitis: guidelines of the International Association of Pancreatology. Pancreas. 2011;40:352–8.
11. Chari ST, Murray JA. Autoimmune pancreatitis, Part II: the relapse. Gastroenterology. 2008;134:625–8.
12. Ghazale A, Chari ST. Optimising corticosteroid treatment for autoimmune pancreatitis. Gut. 2007;56:1650–2.
13. Kim HM, Chung MJ, Chung JB. Remission and relapse of autoimmune pancreatitis: focusing on corticosteroid treatment. Pancreas. 2010;39:555–60.
14. Nishino T, Toki F, Oyama H, et al. Biliary tract involvement in autoimmune pancreatitis. Pancreas. 2005;30:76–82.
15. Sah RP, Chari ST, Pannala R, et al. Differences in clinical profile and relapse rate of type 1 versus type 2 autoimmune pancreatitis. Gastroenterology. 2010;139:140–8; quiz e12–3.
16. Hart PA, Kamisawa T, Brugge WR, et al. Long-term outcomes of autoimmune pancreatitis: a multicentre, international analysis. Gut. 2013;62:1771–6.
17. Stone JH, Zen Y, Deshpande V. IgG4-related disease. N Engl J Med. 2012;366:539–51.
18. Takayama M, Hamano H, Ochi Y, et al. Recurrent attacks of autoimmune pancreatitis result in pancreatic stone formation. Am J Gastroenterol. 2004;99:932–7.

19. Horiuchi A, Kawa S, Hamano H, et al. ERCP features in 27 patients with autoimmune pancreatitis. Gastrointest Endosc. 2002;55:494–9.
20. Ito T, Nishimori I, Inoue N, et al. Treatment for autoimmune pancreatitis: consensus on the treatment for patients with autoimmune pancreatitis in Japan. J Gastroenterol. 2007;42 Suppl 18:50–8.
21. Kamisawa T, Chung JB, Irie H, et al. Japan-Korea symposium on autoimmune pancreatitis (KOKURA 2007). Pancreas. 2007;35:281–4.
22. Kamisawa T, Shimosegawa T, Okazaki K, et al. Standard steroid treatment for autoimmune pancreatitis. Gut. 2009;58:1504–7.
23. Church NI, Pereira SP, Deheragoda MG, et al. Autoimmune pancreatitis: clinical and radiological features and objective response to steroid therapy in a UK series. Am J Gastroenterol. 2007;102:2417–25.
24. Hirano K, Tada M, Isayama H, et al. Long-term prognosis of autoimmune pancreatitis with and without corticosteroid treatment. Gut. 2007;56:1719–24.
25. Nishino T, Toki F, Oyama H, et al. Long-term outcome of autoimmune pancreatitis after oral prednisolone therapy. Intern Med. 2006;45:497–501.
26. Raina A, Yadav D, Krasinskas AM, et al. Evaluation and management of autoimmune pancreatitis: experience at a large US center. Am J Gastroenterol. 2009;104:2295–306.
27. Hart PA, Topazian MD, Witzig TE, et al. Treatment of relapsing autoimmune pancreatitis with immunomodulators and rituximab: the Mayo Clinic experience. Gut. 2013;62:1607–15.
28. Matsushita M, Ikeura T, Fukui T, et al. Refractory autoimmune pancreatitis: azathioprine or steroid pulse therapy? Am J Gastroenterol. 2008;103:1834; author reply 1834–5.
29. Naitoh I, Nakazawa T, Ohara H, et al. Autoimmune pancreatitis associated with various extrapancreatic lesions during a long-term clinical course successfully treated with azathioprine and corticosteroid maintenance therapy. Intern Med. 2009;48:2003–7.
30. Sandanayake NS, Church NI, Chapman MH, et al. Presentation and management of post-treatment relapse in autoimmune pancreatitis/immunoglobulin G4-associated cholangitis. Clin Gastroenterol Hepatol. 2009;7:1089–96.
31. Sodikoff JB, Keilin SA, Cai Q, et al. Mycophenolate mofetil for maintenance of remission in steroid-dependent autoimmune pancreatitis. World J Gastroenterol. 2012;18:2287–90.
32. Khosroshahi A, Bloch DB, Deshpande V, et al. Rituximab therapy leads to rapid decline of serum IgG4 levels and prompt clinical improvement in IgG4-related systemic disease. Arthritis Rheum. 2010;62:1755–62.
33. Maithel SK, Pratt W, Kelleher T, et al. Autoimmune pancreatitis in the setting of Castleman disease. Pancreas. 2007;35:384–7.
34. Topazian M, Witzig TE, Smyrk TC, et al. Rituximab therapy for refractory biliary strictures in immunoglobulin G4-associated cholangitis. Clin Gastroenterol Hepatol. 2008;6:364–6.

Treatment: Immunomodulatory Drugs and Rituximab

23

Phil A. Hart and Suresh T. Chari

Introduction

Autoimmune pancreatitis (AIP) is the pancreatic manifestation of the multiorgan syndrome currently referred to as IgG4-related disease (IgG4-RD). Although AIP and the other organ manifestations of IgG4-RD characteristically respond to steroid treatment, a subset of individuals has disease that is difficult to control, including those who are unable to tolerate high-dose steroids, develop steroid dependence, or have frequent relapses despite maintenance treatment. Existing data suggest that immunomodulatory agents and rituximab (RTX) may be helpful for some to achieve and maintain remission; however, additional studies demonstrating efficacy are needed.

Immunomodulatory Agents

The management of AIP has evolved over the last decade; however, oral steroids remain the mainstay of treatment. Although spontaneous remissions can occur, data from observational studies suggest that patients treated with steroids achieve remission more rapidly and have fewer disease-related complications [1]. There are differing approaches to maintenance treatment. Many physicians in Asian centers provide a slow steroid taper with continuation of low-dose steroids for up to 3 years [2]. Alternatively, many in Western countries taper steroids off without a maintenance regimen. For those who relapse, a steroid-sparing approach is advocated to avoid steroid-related complications in a disease population that largely consists of older patients. In this approach, induction of disease is accomplished with a brief course of high-dose steroids overlapping with an immunomodulatory agent for maintenance of remission, which is continued for over a year. This strategy was borrowed from autoimmune hepatitis, in which patients received high-dose steroids overlapping with a low fixed dose of an immunomodulatory agent, but early experience suggested that higher doses of the immunomodulatory agent were needed for AIP.

Clinical Data

Initial studies describing the use of immunomodulatory agents for maintenance of remission in AIP published through 2010 were very promising [3–6]. Four centers collectively reported on a total of 33 patients. The most frequently used agent was azathioprine, with others including methotrexate, mycophenolate mofetil, and cyclophosphamide. The ability to achieve steroid-free remission was almost universal (30/31 patients), and only a few developed a relapse ($n=3$) after achieving remission. There were several limitations with these studies, including small sample sizes ($n \leq 10$ for each center) and limited follow-up, so the true benefit remained unclear.

More recently, we described the Mayo Clinic experience treating 41 patients with immunomodulators [7]. Again, the most commonly used agent was azathioprine (generally at a dose of 2–3 mg/kg/day), followed by 6-mercaptopurine and mycophenolate mofetil. Indications for starting one of these agents included relapsing disease or the presence of IgG4-related sclerosing cholangitis at the time of disease presentation. Of those with follow-up of more than 2 months, 21/38 (55 %) were able to successfully remain in remission. On

Conflicts of interest/disclosures: No conflicts of interest exist.

P.A. Hart, MD (✉) • S.T. Chari, MD
Division of Gastroenterology and Hepatology, Mayo Clinic,
200 First Street SW, Rochester, MN, USA
e-mail: philip.hart@osumc.edu; chari.suresh@mayo.edu

T. Kamisawa, J.B. Chung (eds.), *Autoimmune Pancreatitis*,
DOI 10.1007/978-3-642-55086-7_23, © Springer-Verlag Berlin Heidelberg 2015

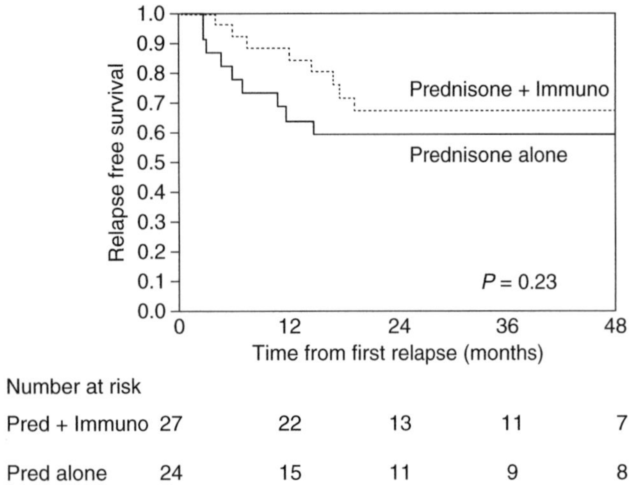

Fig. 23.1 Comparison of relapse-free survival following an initial relapse for those treated with steroids alone vs. steroids and an immunomodulatory agent (Adapted from Hart et al. [7] with permission from the BMJ Publishing Group)

the other hand, 17/38 (45 %) patients either developed a disease relapse during treatment with the immunomodulatory agent or were not able to have steroids weaned without recurrence of disease. Lastly, although there was a trend toward prolonged relapse-free survival for patients treated with an immunomodulatory agent at the time of first disease relapse, this was not statistically different from those who only received high-dose steroids (with a rapid taper) (Fig. 23.1). However, considering the small statistical sample size, a modest benefit would have been obscured (i.e., a type 2 error).

In this series, almost one-quarter ($n=9/41$) of all patients needed to discontinue the immunomodulatory agent due to side effects (including bacteremia, myelosuppression, and nausea/vomiting). This rate of discontinuation is comparable to rates in other disease populations, such as inflammatory bowel disease [8]. Depending on the indication for drug discontinuation, substitution with a different thiopurine (i.e., 6-mercaptopurine) or mycophenolate mofetil can be considered (this was successful in 6/9 patients in the previous series).

Future Studies

The decision to use azathioprine as the primary steroid-sparing agent was based on previous experience in management of autoimmune hepatitis, which does not clearly share a common pathogenic mechanism with AIP. Recently, Schwaiger et al. published a study using a murine model showing that an alternative immunomodulatory agent may be more efficacious than azathioprine [9]. They developed a model in MRL/Mp female mice that when exposed to polyinosinic:polycytidylic acid induces an inflammatory condition that mimics the histologic and phenotypic features of human type 1 AIP. Treatment with cyclosporine or rapamycin reduced histologic damage to the pancreas to a greater degree than azathioprine achieved. Thus, these data suggest that a different immunomodulatory agent may be more clinically efficacious than azathioprine, which has been the most studied in AIP. However, whether or not the findings from their animal model are relevant in humans remains to be demonstrated.

Summary Immunomodulatory agents, such as azathioprine, may have a modest benefit in maintenance of remission in patients with AIP. However, almost half of the treated patients develop disease relapse during treatment, are unable to be weaned from steroids, or require discontinuation due to side effects. Therefore, additional treatment options are needed. It is possible that alternative immunomodulatory agents (other than thiopurines) may be more effective than azathioprine; however, this remains to be demonstrated in humans.

Rituximab

Rituximab (RTX) is a monoclonal antibody to the CD20 antigen on premature and mature B cells. It is used to treat a variety of conditions including B-cell lymphoma, rheumatoid arthritis, and ANCA-associated vasculitis; however, its use in pemphigus vulgaris and orbital pseudolymphoma are most pertinent to the treatment of AIP. Pemphigus vulgaris is a bullous skin disease in which pathogenic IgG4 antibodies (antikeratinocyte cell-surface antibodies) mirror disease activity that responds to RTX [10]. Orbital pseudolymphoma is a condition that was traditionally treated with radiation treatment. However, it has also been demonstrated that treatment with RTX successfully induces remission in most patients [11]. Subsequent studies demonstrated that many patients with orbital pseudolymphoma frequently have elevated serum IgG4 levels, and now, orbital pseudolymphoma is recognized as a manifestation of IgG4-RD [12].

Treatment of AIP with RTX was first reported in a patient with relapsing IgG4-related sclerosing cholangitis [13]. He had refractory disease requiring multiple courses of high-dose steroids and developed a flare during maintenance treatment with 6-mercaptopurine. Core pancreatic biopsies revealed a modest population of CD20-positive B cells in the inflamed tissue, suggesting RTX would address at least a significant component of the inflammatory infiltrate. Thus, RTX was initiated, and subsequent cholangiography was markedly improved with almost complete resolution of liver test abnormalities. Other disease activity including pancreatic and orbital enlargement also resolved with RTX treatment. Since this initial patient, we have continued to use RTX in difficult-to-treat patients who either are resistant to an immunomodulatory agent or are unable to tolerate induction treatment with high-dose steroids.

Clinical Data

Currently, the two largest series describing the use of RTX in AIP/IgG4-RD are from the United States, including one from Massachusetts General Hospital (MGH) (Boston, MA) and the other from Mayo Clinic (Rochester, MN). The series published from MGH details the treatment of 10 patients with IgG4-RD, with predominantly extra-pancreaticobiliary involvement (one patient had pancreas involvement and two had biliary involvement) [14]. The dosing protocol consisted of two infusions of 1,000 mg intravenously on days 0 and 15. Nine of the 10 patients demonstrated significant clinical improvement within one month of therapy. All 6 patients on steroid treatment at the time of RTX initiation could be successfully tapered off of steroids. However, within 6 months of follow-up, four (40 %) patients required additional RTX treatment for disease recurrence.

In the Mayo Clinic series, a total of 12 patients were treated with a series of RTX infusions spanning a period of 2 years [7]. One patient had isolated biliary involvement, while the other 11 patients had pancreatic involvement with or without biliary disease. The treatment protocol was similar to that used to treat B-cell lymphoma, in which patients received 4 weekly infusions (375 mg/m^2), followed by a maintenance infusion every 3 months for 2 years (12 total doses). Using this regimen, 10/12 patients had a complete, clinical remission (symptomatic, biochemical, and radiographic) within 3 months of initiating treatment. Four of these patients were unable to tolerate high-dose steroids and were treated with RTX alone, demonstrating that it is an alternative induction agent to steroids. One patient had a partial response but had persistent liver test abnormalities due to another diagnosis. No patients developed a disease relapse during treatment.

Although RTX has only been used in small numbers of individuals with AIP, it has been extensively used in large numbers of patients with rheumatoid arthritis and B-cell lymphoma, so the side effect profile is well characterized. The most common side effect is a cytokine-mediated infusion reaction. This occurs in up to 10 % of patients during the first infusion and are typically mild. Otherwise, an immunologically mediated hypersensitivity reaction can produce cutaneous-, respiratory-, or joint-related symptoms. Myelosuppression (particularly lymphopenia) is an important consideration, and the median onset of abnormalities is 14 days following an infusion. However, delayed-onset cytopenias can also develop, so routine monitoring of complete blood counts is advisable during and after treatment. Finally, infectious complications are an important consideration, with infections occurring in up to 30 % of patients. Most infections are not serious, but one notable exception is progressive multifocal leukoencephalopathy (PML). PML has been described after RTX treatment, and although it is exceedingly rare, it is almost universally fatal and therefore should be discussed with patients prior to starting treatment [15].

Summary Studies to date have provided meaningful, albeit uncontrolled, data demonstrating that RTX is effective for treating AIP/IgG4-RD, including difficult-to-treat patients. For those unable to tolerate high-dose steroids, RTX was successfully used for induction of remission without steroids. Additionally, it was useful for patient who had disease relapse despite the use of maintenance treatment with either low-dose steroids or immunomodulatory agents. It is unclear how many doses are necessary for maintenance of remission, particularly since there can be persistent B-cell depletion for more than 6 months following an infusion [10]. To further understand this and study RTX in IgG4-RD (with or without pancreatic involvement), MGH and Mayo Clinic are participating in an open-label prospective treatment study to evaluate the efficacy of two doses of RTX to induce and maintain remission (NCT01584388) (Fig. 23.2). Overall, RTX is safe and well tolerated, but considering the cost and potential serious side effects is most appropriate to reserve for difficult-to-treat patients.

Treatment Approach to Management of Relapsing AIP Using Immunomodulators and Rituximab

Steroids remain the mainstay of treatment for AIP and work very well for induction of remission as well as reinduction of remission at the time of disease relapse. However, there is an important subset of patients who either are not able to tolerate high-dose steroids or require unacceptably high doses of steroids to maintain disease remission. In these difficult-to-treat patients, steroid-sparing treatment options include traditional immunomodulators and RTX. Studies supporting their use for this indication are based on uncontrolled, observational data. Many factors should be considered when an alternative to steroids is considered including patients' age, other comorbidities, severity and distribution of disease, cost and availability of the medication, and the physician's comfort with medication titration and monitoring for side effects. Considering the high cost of treatment with RTX, we feel that currently, it is reasonable to at least consider the use of an immunomodulator (such as azathioprine) prior to initiating RTX. Our current strategy for managing disease relapses is outlined in Fig. 23.3.

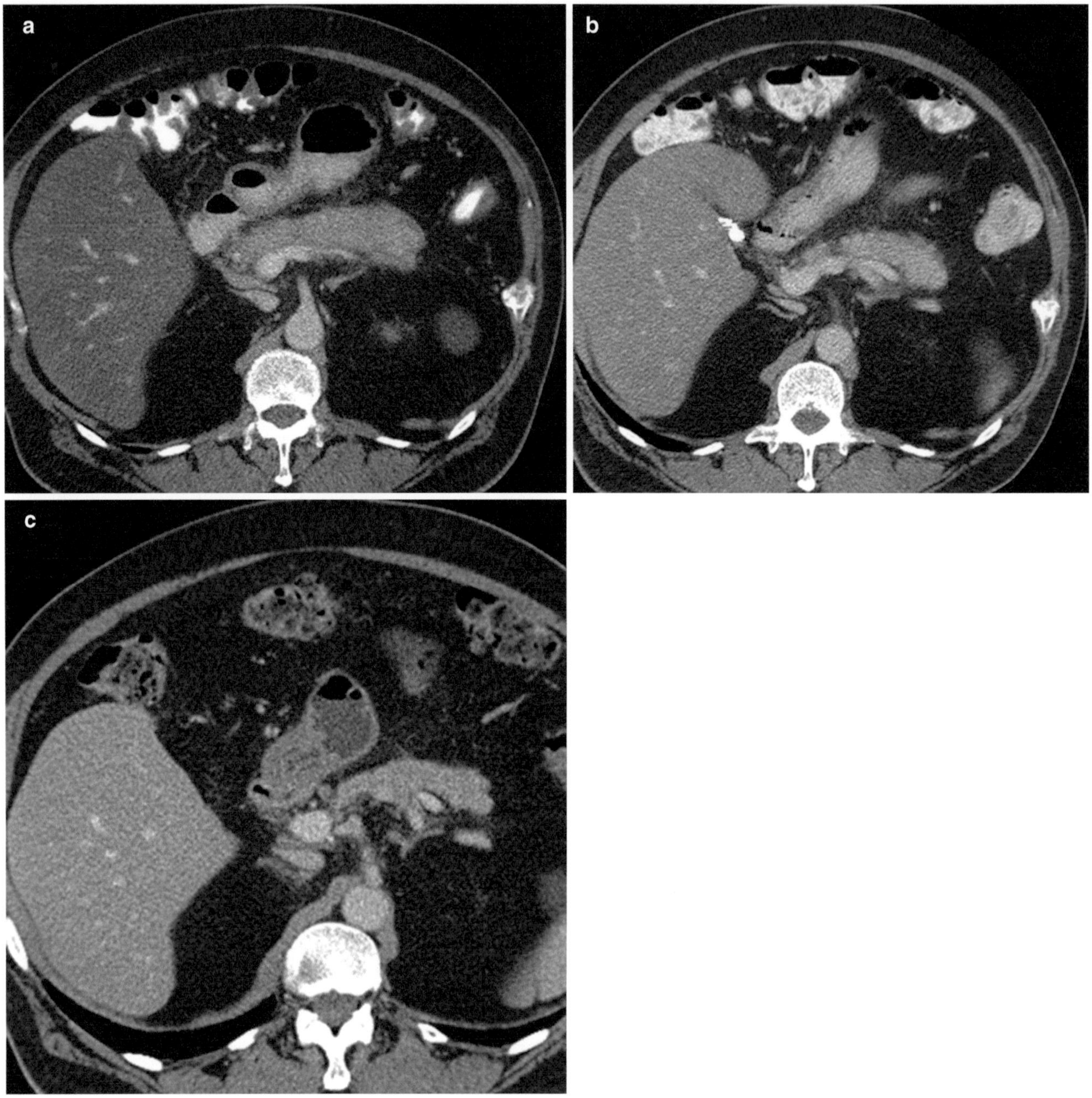

Fig. 23.2 CT scan of the abdomen of a patient with type 1 AIP at baseline (panel **a**) and one (panel **b**) and six (panel **c**) months following rituximab treatment (two doses of 1,000 mg intravenously). At baseline, the pancreas is diffusely enlarged with the presence of rim-like enhancement ("capsule sign"), which is most prominent in the tail. Follow-up images demonstrate a decrease in the size of the pancreas, resolution of the capsule sign, and increased enhancement of the pancreatic parenchyma

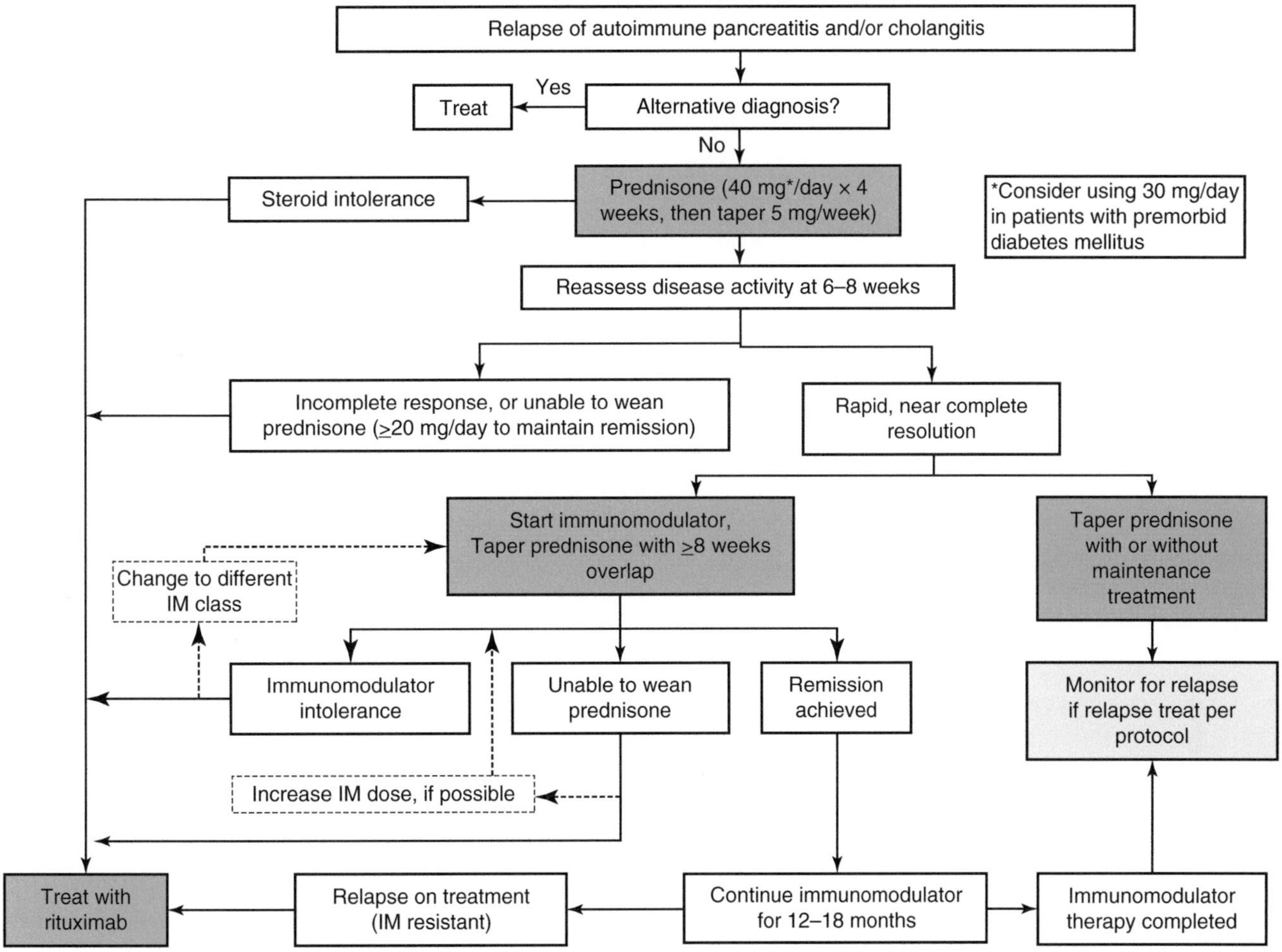

Fig. 23.3 A proposed treatment algorithm for managing disease relapses of confirmed AIP (after malignancy has been excluded) (Adapted from Hart et al. [7] with permission from the BMJ Publishing Group)

References

1. Hirano K, Tada M, Isayama H, Yagioka H, Sasaki T, Kogure H, Nakai Y, Sasahira N, Tsujino T, Yoshida H, Kawabe T, Omata M. Long-term prognosis of autoimmune pancreatitis with and without corticosteroid treatment. Gut. 2007;56:1719–24.
2. Hart PA, Kamisawa T, Brugge WR, Chung JB, Culver EL, Czako L, Frulloni L, Go VL, Gress TM, Kim MH, Kawa S, Lee KT, Lerch MM, Liao WC, Lohr M, Okazaki K, Ryu JK, Schleinitz N, Shimizu K, Shimosegawa T, Soetikno R, Webster G, Yadav D, Zen Y, Chari ST. Long-term outcomes of autoimmune pancreatitis: a multicentre, international analysis. Gut. 2012;62(12):1771–6.
3. Sandanayake NS, Church NI, Chapman MH, Johnson GJ, Dhar DK, Amin Z, Deheragoda MG, Novelli M, Winstanley A, Rodriguez-Justo M, Hatfield AR, Pereira SP, Webster GJ. Presentation and management of post-treatment relapse in autoimmune pancreatitis/immunoglobulin G4-associated cholangitis. Clin Gastroenterol Hepatol. 2009;7:1089–96.
4. Raina A, Yadav D, Krasinskas AM, McGrath KM, Khalid A, Sanders M, Whitcomb DC, Slivka A. Evaluation and management of autoimmune pancreatitis: experience at a large US center. Am J Gastroenterol. 2009;104:2295–306.
5. Ghazale A, Chari ST. Optimising corticosteroid treatment for autoimmune pancreatitis. Gut. 2007;56:1650–2.
6. Frulloni L, Scattolini C, Falconi M, Zamboni G, Capelli P, Manfredi R, Graziani R, D'Onofrio M, Katsotourchi AM, Amodio A, Benini L, Vantini I. Autoimmune pancreatitis: differences between the focal and diffuse forms in 87 patients. Am J Gastroenterol. 2009;104:2288–94.
7. Hart PA, Topazian MD, Witzig TE, Clain JE, Gleeson FC, Klebig RR, Levy MJ, Pearson RK, Petersen BT, Smyrk TC, Sugumar A, Takahashi N, Vege SS, Chari ST. Treatment of relapsing autoimmune pancreatitis with immunomodulators and rituximab: the Mayo Clinic experience. Gut. 2013;62:1607–15.
8. Su C, Lichtenstein GR. Treatment of inflammatory bowel disease with azathioprine and 6-mercaptopurine. Gastroenterol Clin North Am. 2004;33:209–34, viii.
9. Schwaiger T, van den Brandt C, Fitzner B, Zaatreh S, Kraatz F, Dummer A, Nizze H, Evert M, Broker BM, Brunner-Weinzierl MC, Wartmann T, Salem T, Lerch MM, Jaster R, Mayerle J. Autoimmune pancreatitis in MRL/Mp mice is a T cell-mediated disease responsive to cyclosporine A and rapamycin treatment. Gut. 2013;63(3):494–505.
10. Ahmed AR, Spigelman Z, Cavacini LA, Posner MR. Treatment of pemphigus vulgaris with rituximab and intravenous immune globulin. N Engl J Med. 2006;355:1772–9.
11. Witzig TE, Inwards DJ, Habermann TM, Dogan A, Kurtin PJ, Gross Jr JB, Ananthamurthy A, Ristow KM, Garity JA. Treatment of benign orbital pseudolymphomas with the monoclonal anti-CD20 antibody rituximab. Mayo Clin Proc. 2007;82:692–9.
12. Umehara H, Okazaki K, Masaki Y, Kawano M, Yamamoto M, Saeki T, Matsui S, Sumida T, Mimori T, Tanaka Y, Tsubota K, Yoshino T, Kawa S, Suzuki R, Takegami T, Tomosugi N, Kurose N, Ishigaki Y, Azumi A, Kojima M, Nakamura S, Inoue D. A novel clinical entity,

IgG4-related disease (IgG4RD): general concept and details. Mod Rheumatol. 2012;22:1–14.
13. Topazian M, Witzig TE, Smyrk TC, Pulido JS, Levy MJ, Kamath PS, Chari ST. Rituximab therapy for refractory biliary strictures in immunoglobulin G4-associated cholangitis. Clin Gastroenterol Hepatol. 2008;6:364–6.
14. Khosroshahi A, Carruthers MN, Deshpande V, Unizony S, Bloch DB, Stone JH. Rituximab for the treatment of IgG4-related disease: lessons from 10 consecutive patients. Medicine. 2012;91:57–66.
15. Carson KR, Evens AM, Richey EA, Habermann TM, Focosi D, Seymour JF, Laubach J, Bawn SD, Gordon LI, Winter JN, Furman RR, Vose JM, Zelenetz AD, Mamtani R, Raisch DW, Dorshimer GW, Rosen ST, Muro K, Gottardi-Littell NR, Talley RL, Sartor O, Green D, Major EO, Bennett CL. Progressive multifocal leukoencephalopathy after rituximab therapy in HIV-negative patients: a report of 57 cases from the Research on Adverse Drug Events and Reports project. Blood. 2009;113: 4834–40.

Treatment of Relapsed Autoimmune Pancreatitis

24

Seung Woo Park

Introduction

With the exception of earlier reports of cases, autoimmune pancreatitis (AIP) was appreciated in the early 1990s [1–4]. AIP has been well characterized in clinical, pathological, and radiologic aspects. Subsequently distinct subgroups were identified, and now AIP is categorized into types I and II [5, 6]; both are considered as an uncommon form of chronic pancreatitis. The type I AIP is caused by autoimmunity in which IgG4-positive B lymphocytes play an important role and histologically characterized by lymphoplasmacytic sclerosing lesions, obliterative phlebitis, infiltration of IgG4-positive plasmacytes, and fibrotic fascicles of fibroblasts and myofibroblasts [5]. With the appreciation of various other organ involvements and elevation of IgG4, type I AIP is now regarded as a pancreatic manifestation of IgG4-related disease [7, 8]. Type II AIP, however, is associated with inflammatory bowel disease and is not related to elevation of IgG4 and characterized by granulocytic epithelial lesions [5, 9].

Although it is not entirely clear whether the disorder is an autoimmune disease, most patients with AIP show favorable response to corticosteroid treatment. It is not uncommon to observe spontaneous remission of AIP without corticosteroid treatment. Nonetheless, remission rate is higher in patients treated with corticosteroid therapy [10], which justifies the use of corticosteroid.

Indications of corticosteroid therapy are obstructive jaundice caused by IgG4-related cholangitis and symptomatic involvement of extrapancreatic organs such as retroperitoneal fibrosis, hydronephrosis, and diabetes mellitus [7, 11, 12]. Although response rates to corticosteroid treatment approaches to 100 %, relapse of AIP is a cumbersome problem.

S.W. Park, MD, PhD
Department of Internal Medicine, Institute of Gastroenterology, Yonsei University College of Medicine, Seoul, Korea
e-mail: swoopark@yuhs.ac

Relapse of Autoimmune Pancreatitis

In sizable patients with type I AIP, the disease relapses during the course of corticosteroid treatment and maintenance or during the follow-up after cessation of corticosteroid. According to the previous studies, relapse rates widely vary from 24 to 60 % [9, 10, 13, 14]. The wide range of relapse rates is caused by inconsistent definition of relapse, variations in study design such as follow-up period, number of included patients, prospective versus retrospective studies, wrong categorization of subtypes, and ethnic difference [6]. Relapse in type II AIP, however, is not common. In a multicenter study [10], relapse rates were 31 % (302/978) and 9 % (8/85) in types I and II AIP, respectively. In a European study which enrolled 114 surgically treated AIP [9], relapse rates after surgery were 41 % (21/51) and 15.4 % (6/39) in types I and II AIP, respectively. Thus, it is reasonable to expect approximately 30–40 % of the remitted patients with type I AIP experience relapse during the course of follow-up.

Relapse of autoimmune pancreatitis accompanies reappearance of symptoms depending on the sites of relapse and serologic or radiologic findings similar to the initial manifestations. These findings are not always apparent at the time of relapse. While symptomatic relapse usually accompanies serological and radiologic abnormalities, serological abnormality can be a sole manifestation of relapse. Although some physicians prefer to include reappearance of serologic abnormality in the definition of relapse, most physicians exclude asymptomatic serologic abnormality from relapse [10, 15]. Asymptomatic serologic or biochemical abnormalities may represent incomplete remission, subclinical disease activity, or presence of undetected lesions in other organs [11, 16]. Although the pancreas is the most common site of relapse in type I AIP, extrapancreatic relapses are not uncommon. Sometimes, the relapse in the biliary system (50.6 %) outnumbers pancreatic (42.9 %) relapse, followed by salivary gland (7.3 %), lung (4.5 %), lymphadenopathy (1.6 %), and renal (1.2 %) in order of frequency [10]. In type II AIP, relapse occurs exclusively in the pancreas.

T. Kamisawa, J.B. Chung (eds.), *Autoimmune Pancreatitis*,
DOI 10.1007/978-3-642-55086-7_24, © Springer-Verlag Berlin Heidelberg 2015

In type I AIP, most relapses occur within the first 3 years [10, 13, 15, 17]. According to the Mayo Clinic data [18], cumulative relapse rates were 35 % at 1 year, 42 % at 2 years, and 46 % at 3 years in type I AIP. In a Chinese study [19], relapse episodes occurred within 1 year in 50 %, 2 years in 75 %, and 3 years in 100 %. In corticosteroid-treated patients, the majority of the relapse episodes occur following the cessation of corticosteroid (67 %), as compared with during tapering (15 %) or while on corticosteroid maintenance (18 %) [10].

Prediction of Relapse

So far, several factors have been speculated as useful findings of predicting relapse in type I AIP. According to a series of reports, presence of sclerosing cholangitis [10, 20], nonsurgical treatment [10], incomplete remission of radiologic or serological abnormalities [12], diffuse pancreatic swelling [21], and HLA DQß1 57 genotype [22] seem to be associated with relapse. Other factors than the sclerosing cholangitis, however, did not appear as consistent factors of predicting relapse. Persistent high level of IgG4, however, does not harbor higher risk of relapse (21.7 % vs. 31.4 % in abnormal and normal IgG4, respectively) [10]. Incomplete normalization of serological test may actually mean incomplete remission of autoimmunity in type I AIP. Likewise, there is no difference in relapse rate between diffuse (32.3 %) and focal (32.3 %) pancreatic parenchymal enlargement [10]. The most consistent factor of relapse is the presence of bile duct involvement [10, 13, 14, 17, 20, 23, 24]. In the largest multicenter study [10], patients with IgG4-related sclerosing cholangitis experienced at least one relapse in 56.1 % (96/171) compared to 25.7 % (142/551) in patients without sclerosing cholangitis. The relapse rates were similar in patients with or without distal biliary involvement (33.9 % vs. 31.1 %, respectively). In a Korean study [22], substitution of aspartic acid to non-aspartic acid at residue 57 of HLA class II allele DQß1 was associated with higher relapse rate of AIP (29.6 % [8/27] and 100 % [13/13] in non-relapse and relapse group, respectively), which, however, needs further verification in a larger number of patients by further investigation. There are no known factors predicting relapse in type II AIP in which relapse rate is far lower than type I AIP.

Treatment of Relapse

The role of maintenance therapy using low-dose corticosteroid after initial induction of remission has not been standardized yet. Whereas Japanese groups tend to advocate the maintenance therapy, Western groups do not. Corticosteroid maintenance after induction of remission of type I AIP up to 1 year seems to actually lower the relapse rates (28.6 % vs. 42.5 %) [19]. However, concern regarding adverse effects of long-term corticosteroid treatment and the fact that relapses do not occur in almost half of the patients without maintenance therapy render some physicians to be reluctant of administering maintenance therapy.

When type I AIP relapses during the withdrawal or maintenance of corticosteroid treatment, or off periods, there are three possible approaches of dealing with it [6, 18]. First is the readministration of induction dose of corticosteroid, second is the use of immunomodulators, and third is the use of targeted agents. Repeated course of corticosteroid is again highly effective for reinduction of remission. In this case, more gradual tapering and long-term maintenance of low-dose corticosteroid are usually recommended to prevent second relapse. The available immunomodulators are azathioprine, methotrexate, 6-mercaptopurine, mycophenolate mofetil, cyclosporine, and cyclophosphamide. These agents can be combined with corticosteroid for induction of remission and maintained up to 18 months to prevent another relapse. In the Mayo Clinic study [18], however, immunomodulators, when they were combined with corticosteroid, did not lower relapse rates of type I AIP compared to additional course of corticosteroid alone. Besides, failure or intolerance to immunomodulators occurred in 45 % (17/38). The role of immunomodulators has yet to be further evaluated by larger multicenter prospective studies.

Rituximab is an anti-CD20 antibody and depletes CD20-positive B lymphocytes. It has shown to be effective in the treatment of patients with various autoimmune diseases such as rheumatoid arthritis, Wegener's granulomatosis, pemphigus vulgaris, orbital pseudolymphoma, and microscopic polyangiitis, in which IgG4-positive B lymphocytes play an important role [8, 18, 25, 26]. When rituximab was used in 12 patients with failure or intolerance to immunomodulators, complete remission was induced in 10 (83 %) patients without any relapses while on maintenance therapy for 24 months [18]. Likely to immunomodulators, the role of rituximab needs to be further validated through larger and randomized trials.

Surveillance of Relapse

The surveillance strategy has not been standardized yet. Depending on the policies of the institutions, a 3-, 6-, or 12-month interval of symptomatic, serologic, and radiologic examinations is recommended.

Conclusion

Relapse of AIP occurs in up to 50 % of patients with type I and 10 % with type II AIP. Presence of sclerosing cholangitis at initial manifestation is associated with high risk of relapse of type I AIP. When relapse occurs, readministration of corticosteroid is effective for reinduction of remission. Addition of immunomodulators to corticosteroid did not show better outcome than corticosteroid alone. Rituximab may be a promising drug for the treatment of relapsed type I AIP. The role of these agents, however, needs to be further evaluated through larger randomized trials.

References

1. Ball WP, Baggenstoss AH, Bargen JA. Pancreatic lesions associated with chronic ulcerative colitis. Arch Pathol (Chic). 1950;50:347–58.
2. Sarles H, Sarles JC, Muratore R, Guien C. Chronic inflammatory sclerosis of the pancreas – an autonomous pancreatic disease? Am J Dig Dis. 1961;6:688–98.
3. Kawaguchi K, Koike M, Tsuruta K, Okamoto A, Tabata I, Fujita N. Lymphoplasmacytic sclerosing pancreatitis with cholangitis: a variant of primary sclerosing cholangitis extensively involving pancreas. Hum Pathol. 1991;22:387–95.
4. Yoshida K, Toki F, Takeuchi T, Watanabe S, Shiratori K, Hayashi N. Chronic pancreatitis caused by an autoimmune abnormality. Proposal of the concept of autoimmune pancreatitis. Dig Dis Sci. 1995;40:1561–8.
5. Deshpande V, Gupta R, Sainani N, et al. Subclassification of autoimmune pancreatitis: a histologic classification with clinical significance. Am J Surg Pathol. 2011;35:26–35.
6. Kamisawa T, Chari ST, Merch MM, et al. Recent advances in autoimmune pancreatitis: type 1 and type 2. Gut. 2013;62:1373–80.
7. Yamamoto M, Takahashi H, Shinomura Y. Mechanisms and assessment of IgG4-related disease: lessons for the rheumatologist. Nat Rev Rheumatol. 2014;10:148–59.
8. Detlefsen S. IgG4-related disease: a systemic condition with characteristic microscopic features. Histol Histopathol. 2013;28:565–84.
9. Detlefsen S, Zamboni G, Frulloni L, et al. Clinical features and relapse rate after surgery in type I autoimmune pancreatitis differ from type 2: a study of 114 surgically treated European patients. Pancreatology. 2012;12:276–83.
10. Hart PA, Kamisawa T, Brugge WR, et al. Long-term outcomes of autoimmune pancreatitis: a multicenter, international analysis. Gut. 2013;62:1771–6.
11. Kim HM, Chung MJ, Chung JB. Remission and relapse of autoimmune pancreatitis. Pancreas. 2010;39:555–60.
12. Kamisawa T, Okamoto A, Wakabayashi T, et al. Appropriate steroid therapy for autoimmune pancreatitis based on long-term outcome. Scand J Gastroenterol. 2008;43:609–13.
13. Kamisawa T, Shimosegawa T, Okazaki K, et al. Standard steroid treatment for autoimmune pancreatitis. Gut. 2009;58:1504–7.
14. Raina A, Yadav D, Krasinskas AM, et al. Evaluation and management of autoimmune pancreatitis: experience at a large US center. Am J Gastroenterol. 2009;104:2295–306.
15. Sah RP, Chari ST. Autoimmune pancreatitis: an update on classification, diagnosis, natural history and management. Curr Gastroenterol Rep. 2012;14:95–105.
16. Chari ST, Murray JA. Autoimmune pancreatitis, part II: the relapse. Gastroenterology. 2008;134:625–8.
17. Sah RP, Chari ST, Pannala R, et al. Differences in clinical profile and relapse rate of type 1 versus type 2 autoimmune pancreatitis. Gastroenterology. 2010;139:140–8.
18. Hart PA, Topazian MD, Witzig TE, et al. Treatment of relapsing autoimmune pancreatitis with immunomodulators and rituximab: the Mayo Clinic experience. Gut. 2013;62:1607–15.
19. Liu B, Li J, Yan LN, et al. Retrospective study of steroid therapy for patients with autoimmune pancreatitis in Chinese population. World J Gastroenterol. 2013;19:569–74.
20. Hirano K, Tada M, Isayama H, et al. Long-term prognosis of autoimmune pancreatitis with and without corticosteroid treatment. Gut. 2007;56:1719–24.
21. Kubota K, Iida H, Fujisawa T, et al. Clinical factors predictive of spontaneous remission or relapse in cases of autoimmune pancreatitis. Gastrointest Endosc. 2007;66:1142–51.
22. Park DH, Kim MH, Oh HB, et al. Substitution of aspartic acid at position 57 of the DQß1 affects relapse of autoimmune pancreatitis. Gastroenterology. 2008;134:440–6.
23. Church NI, Pereira SP, Deheragoda MG, et al. Autoimmune pancreatitis: clinical and radiological features and objective response to steroid therapy in a UK series. Am J Gastroenterol. 2007;102:2417–25.
24. Frulloni L, Scattolini C, Falconi M, et al. Autoimmune pancreatitis: differences between the focal and diffuse forms in 87 patients. Am J Gastroenterol. 2009;104:2288–94.
25. Okazaki K, Uchida K, Ikeura T, et al. Current concept and diagnosis of IgG4-related disease in the hepato-bilio-pancreatic system. J Gastroenterol. 2013;48:303–14.
26. Masaki Y, Sugai S, Umehara H. IgG4-related diseases including Mikulicz's disease and sclerosing pancreatitis: diagnostic insights. J Rheumatol. 2010;37:1380–5.

25 Development to Chronic Pancreatitis

Masahiro Maruyama, Norikazu Arakura, and Shigeyuki Kawa

Introduction

The long-term prognosis and outcomes of autoimmune pancreatitis (AIP) remain unclear. Because patients with AIP respond favorably to prednisolone (PSL) therapy in clinical, serological, imaging, and pathological settings [1–5], the disease was previously believed to be an acute condition that did not progress to an advanced stage of chronic pancreatitis. However, over the last decade, it has been revealed that some patients with AIP could progress to pancreatic stone formation, pancreatic atrophy, and/or irregular dilatation of the main pancreatic duct (MPD), which may raise new questions about whether AIP can progress to confirmed chronic pancreatitis or not.

We have proposed the working hypothesis that AIP could progress to ordinary chronic pancreatitis similar to an alcoholic type over a long-term course based on the following findings or considerations, including (1) the chronic state of this disease possibly manifesting different clinical features from those of the acute state, such as severe lymphoplasmacytic infiltration; (2) observation of pancreatic stone formation during the long-term disease course [6–14]; (3) the presence of unidentified or idiopathic chronic pancreatitis, which corresponds to approximately 30–40 % of ordinary chronic pancreatitis and might represent a chronic state of AIP; and (4) our observation of 7.4 % high serum IgG4 concentration in patients with previously diagnosed ordinary chronic pancreatitis [7]. In this chapter, we describe a series of study results to confirm our working hypothesis that AIP has the potential to develop into advanced chronic pancreatitis.

M. Maruyama, MD, PhD (✉)
Department of Gastroenterology, Shinshu University School of Medicine, 3-1-1 Asahi, Matsumoto 390-8621, Japan
e-mail: masa10_hiro15@yahoo.co.jp

N. Arakura, MD, PhD
Endoscopic Examination Center, Shinshu University School of Medicine, 3-1-1 Asahi, Matsumoto 390-8621, Japan

S. Kawa, MD, PhD
Center for Health, Safety, and Environmental Management, Shinshu University, 3-1-1 Asahi, Matsumoto 390-8621, Japan

Autoimmune Pancreatitis and Pancreatic Stone Formation

We evaluated the long-term outcomes of patients with AIP, showing that some patients with AIP had presented with pancreatic stone formation.

Development of Pancreatic Stone Formation

In 1995, Yoshida et al. first proposed the concept of AIP and reported that a characteristic feature of this condition was the lack of calcification [15]. Because of the favorable response to corticosteroid therapy, AIP was previously believed to be an acute condition that did not progress to an advanced stage of chronic pancreatitis with pancreatic stone formation. However, it has later become evident that some patients share similar clinical findings with patients who have ordinary chronic pancreatitis over a long-term course. These commonalities include pancreatic stone formation, pancreatic atrophy, and irregular dilatation of the MPD, suggesting that some patients with AIP may progress to chronic pancreatitis.

We examined 42 patients with AIP (median follow-up period, 54.5 months; range, 13–111 months) and found pancreatic calcification in eight patients (19 %) during the follow-up periods. Because about half of the patients with relapse (6/11, 54.5 %) showed calcification, pancreatic calcification was significantly associated with relapse in AIP ($P=0.0019$) [6]. Later, similar results were shown in a study with a greater number of cases, 51 patients with AIP, among whom nine had pancreatic calcification (18 %), indicating that pancreatic calcification was significantly more frequent in the recurrence group (7/21, 33 %) compared with the nonrecurrence group (2/30, 7 %) ($P=0.014$) [7]. These results suggested that pancreatic stone formation is closely related to

T. Kamisawa, J.B. Chung (eds.), *Autoimmune Pancreatitis*,
DOI 10.1007/978-3-642-55086-7_25, © Springer-Verlag Berlin Heidelberg 2015

recurrence and that AIP has the potential to transform into ordinary chronic pancreatitis after several recurrences.

Predictive Factors of the Relapse

Our observation of a close association between pancreatic stone formation in AIP and recurrence raised the notion that we should carefully predict disease recurrence and determine the necessary support at the early stage. We investigated the association between the clinical course of one female patient with AIP involving several recurrences and serum levels of IgG4 and immune complex, as determined by the monoclonal rheumatoid factor method (IC-mRF). We found that these markers tended to rise several months before each recurrence became clinically apparent [16]. For prediction of the recurrence, sequential measurement of serum IgG4 and IC-mRF concentration was helpful. With a cutoff value of 10 μg/dL, IC-mRF predicted recurrence is well, with good sensitivity (61.9 %), specificity (70.0 %), and efficacy (66.7 %). The probability of recurrence was 60 % when IC-mRF >10 mg/dL and 30 % when IC-mRF <10 mg/dL [7]. In addition, complement factors C3 and C4 have also been reported to be useful markers for monitoring disease activity or tissue damage [17].

Risk Factors for Pancreatic Stone Formation

Two mechanisms for pancreatic stone formation in AIP could be postulated: (1) severe inflammatory tissue injury specific to the disease process of AIP and (2) pancreatic juice stasis because of pancreatic duct narrowing. We sought to clarify the risk factors underlying pancreatic stone formation in AIP to confirm which mechanism is in operation. We enrolled 69 AIP patients who had been followed for at least 3 years (median follow-up period, 91 months; range, 36–230 months) [18]. During the course of this study, increased or de novo stone formation was seen in 28 patients (28/69, 40.6 %), who were defined as the stone-forming group. No stones were observed in 32 patients (32/69, 46.4 %), who were defined as the non–stone-forming group. Nine patients who had stones at diagnosis but showed no change during the course of the study were excluded. As a result, we found pancreatic stone formation in approximately 40 % of patients with AIP over a long-term course. We compared the two groups for various relevant parameters, such as clinical, laboratory, and image findings. Univariate analysis revealed no significant differences in clinical or laboratory factors associated with AIP-specific inflammation between the two groups. Relapse was more frequently seen in the stone-forming group, but not significantly so. However, pancreatic head swelling ($P = 0.006$) (Fig. 25.1a) and narrowing of both the Wirsung and Santorini ducts in the pancreatic head region ($P = 0.010$) (Fig. 25.1c) at the time of diagnosis were significantly more frequent in the stone-forming group, respectively (Table 25.1). Multivariate analysis identified the latter imaging findings as a significant independent risk factor for pancreatic stone formation (odds ratio [OR] 4.4, $P = 0.019$). Furthermore, even after corticosteroid therapy, residual pancreatic head swelling and residual narrowing of both the Wirsung and Santorini ducts were also more frequently seen in the stone-forming compared to the non–stone-forming group in our cohort [18]. These findings suggested that Wirsung and Santorini duct narrowing in the pancreatic head region provokes pancreatic juice stasis in the pancreas and results in eventual stone formation. Because there was no significant relationship between stone formation and well-known activity markers for AIP and no cases of severe pancreatitis, we suggested that the other hypothesized mechanism of severe tissue injury attributed to the specific inflammatory process of AIP had a poor association with pancreatic stone formation. Although the present study indicated that alcohol consumption including some ethanol uptake was not a risk factor for pancreatic stone formation, Hirano et al. reported that high alcohol consumption of ethanol >50 g/day increased the risk of pancreatic stone development and atrophy [19]. Further study is needed to determine the contribution of alcohol consumption.

Pancreatic Stone Formation and Pancreatic Function

It is essential to confirm whether pancreatic stone formation in AIP is associated with pancreatic exocrine or endocrine dysfunction, as is the case in ordinary chronic pancreatitis. To clarify this, we compared serum values of amylase and HbA1c (JDS) at diagnosis, 5 years, and 8 years among non–stone-forming patients, stone-forming patients, and intraductal stone-forming patients, who seemed to be at a more advanced stage of stone formation. Although we found no significant differences among the groups, both serum amylase and HbA1c values tended to be at abnormal levels in intraductal stone-forming patients compared with non–stone-forming patients (Table 25.2) [18]. We consider that further study may reveal a significant deterioration of pancreatic exocrine or endocrine function in stone-forming patients, although stone-forming AIP might have a different pathophysiology from that of ordinary chronic pancreatitis.

Epidemiology of Pancreatic Calcification

Other reports presenting the frequency of pancreatic calcification in AIP have cited ranges from 4 to 40 % [3, 6–10, 12,

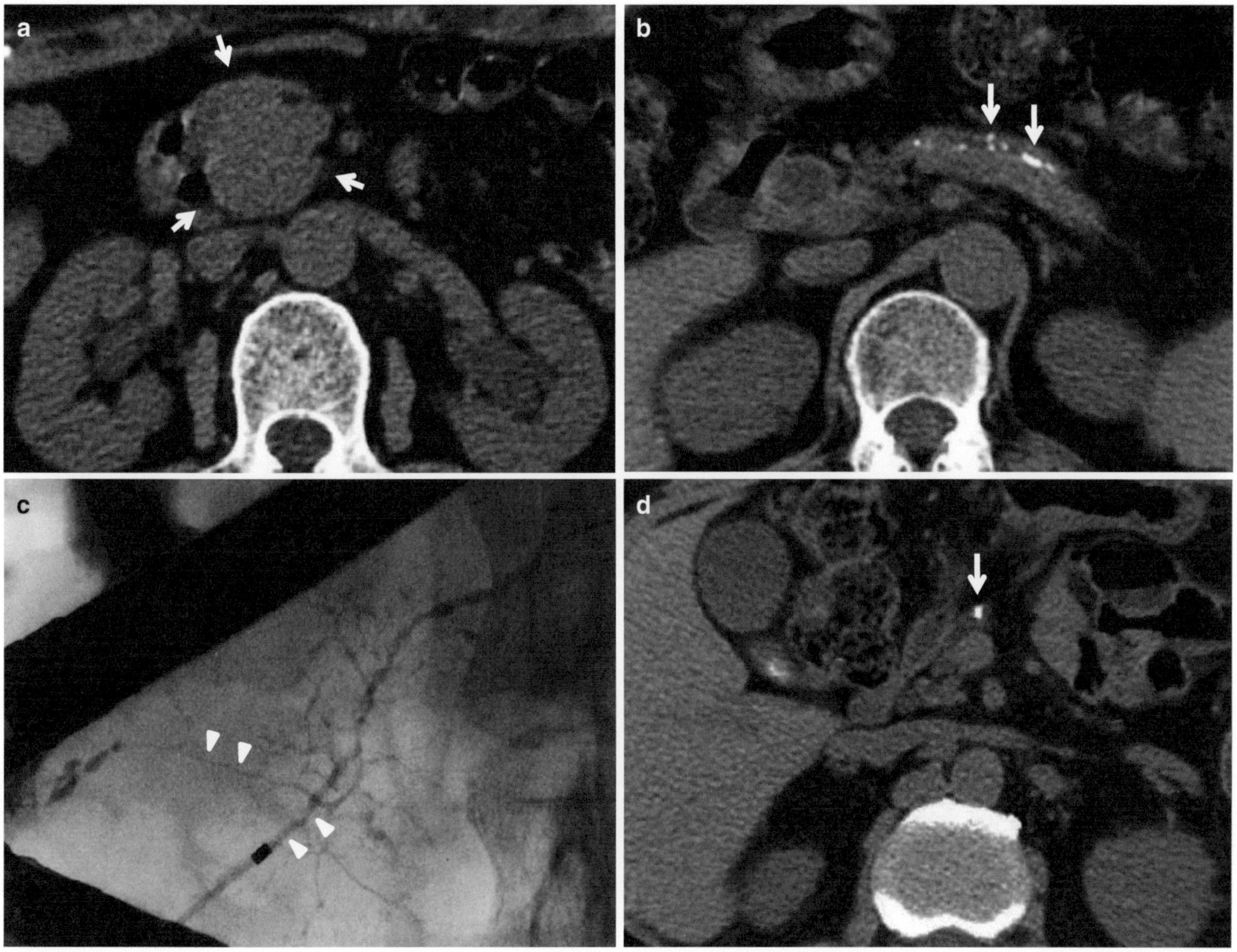

Fig. 25.1 (**a**, **b**) CT findings in a 67-year-old female with pancreatic head swelling. (**a**) CT at diagnosis in May 2005 showing pancreatic head swelling (*arrows*). (**b**) CT 27 months later in August 2007 showing pancreatic stone formation (*arrows*) and pancreatic atrophy. (**c**, **d**) ERP and CT findings in a 69-year-old male with narrowing of both the Wirsung and Santorini ducts. (**c**) ERP at diagnosis in April 2001 showing Wirsung and Santorini duct narrowing (*arrowheads*). (**d**) CT 105 months later in December 2009 showing pancreatic stone formation (*arrows*) and pancreatic atrophy (Data are reprinted from Ref. [18] with permission from the *Journal of Gastroenterology*)

18–20]. Hart et al. conducted an international investigation of 659 patients with AIP and reported that 46 patients (7 %) showed pancreatic calcification, which had a significant correlation with relapse [3]. The frequency of the pancreatic calcification in these results was generally lower than that of our findings, which might be because of differences in disease activity, observation period, therapeutic method, and especially maintenance therapy.

Autoimmune Pancreatitis Can Progress to Chronic Pancreatitis

Some patients with AIP show severe pancreatic calcifications over a long-term course, and those pancreatic stones are a characteristic feature of ordinary chronic pancreatitis, suggesting that AIP could progress to a chronic pancreatitis that fulfills the diagnostic criteria for ordinary chronic pancreatitis.

Serum Levels of IgG4 in Patients with Confirmed Chronic Pancreatitis

It is an interesting matter how many patients with advanced-stage AIP who demonstrated definite chronic pancreatitis symptoms were included with patients having ordinary chronic pancreatitis before the proposal of AIP. We previously reported that more than 60 % of AIP patients maintain high serum IgG4 concentrations even after the clinical symptoms have resolved [21]. Accordingly, if those with advanced-stage AIP are present among cases of confirmed ordinary chronic pancreatitis, these AIP patients might maintain serum IgG4 elevation even at chronic or advanced

Table 25.1 Clinical features, laboratory tests, and pancreatic morphology at diagnosis

	Stone-forming group ($n=28$)	Non–stone-forming group ($n=32$)	P value
Clinical features	Median (range)		
Observation period[a]	100 (36–165)	90 (36–230)	0.524
Age	67 (47–84)	64.5 (38–81)	0.543
Sex (M/F)	24/4	22/10	0.140
Alcohol (+/–)	20/8	19/12	0.582
Prednisolone (+/–)	25/3	28/4	1.000
Relapse (+/–)	11/17	6/26	0.093
Laboratory tests			
Amylase	94 (17–431)	86 (22–478)	0.678
IgG	2187 (892–7236)	2183 (1194–5545)	0.686
IgG4	640 (154–2855)	424 (4–2970)	0.916
C3	91 (33–157)	87 (29–199)	0.538
C4	20.1 (7.7–39.7)	21.3 (1.1–38.7)	0.627
sIL2-R	738 (132–2260)	940 (257–4695)	0.130
CIC	5.1 (1.9–40)	5.5 (1.9–27.5)	0.392
Pancreatic morphology at diagnosis			
Pancreatic swelling (by CT)			
Head (+/–)	26/2	20/12	0.006*
Body (+/–)	20/8	19/13	0.419
Tail (+/–)	17/11	19/13	1.000
Focal/segmental–diffuse	7/21	12/20	0.406
Ductal narrowing in MPD (by ERP)			
Head (+/–)	24/4	22/10	0.140
Wirsung + Santorini (+/–)	21/7	13/19	0.010*
Body (+/–)	15/13	19/13	0.795
Tail (+/–)	22/6	24/8	0.770
Focal/segmental–diffuse	6/22	11/21	0.390

From Ref. [18]
sIL2-R soluble interleukin 2 receptor, *CIC* circulating immune complex
*$P<0.05$
[a]Period from diagnosis of AIP to the most recent observation (months)

Table 25.2 Serum values of amylase and HbA1c during the study course

	Non–stone-forming patients	Stone-forming patients	P value[a]	Intraductal stone-forming patients ($n=9$)	P value[b]
Amylase	Median (range)			Median (range)	
At diagnosis	86 (22–478)	94 (17–431)	0.678	102 (62–323)	0.490
5 years later	85 (45–160)	80 (42–136)	0.497	92 (46–134)	0.569
8 years later	83 (59–130)	75 (37–128)	0.230	75 (48–98)	0.313
HbA1c (JDS)	Median (range)			Median (range)	
At diagnosis	5.7 (4.1–11.2)	5.7 (4.5–9.5)	0.536	6.0 (4.5–9.5)	0.549
5 years later	5.8 (5.1–10.4)	6.0 (4.6–10.2)	0.366	6.0 (5.4–10.2)	0.289
8 years later	5.8 (5.1–9.8)	6.0 (5.1–10.3)	0.504	6.8 (5.1–10.3)	0.293

From Ref. [18]
[a]Non–stone-forming patients vs. stone-forming patients
[b]Non–stone-forming patients vs. intraductal stone-forming patients

stages. Thus, we measured serum values of IgG4 in 175 patients with confirmed chronic pancreatitis who had been diagnosed before 1995, the year when the concept of AIP was first proposed. We found high serum IgG4 concentrations in 13 patients with confirmed chronic pancreatitis (7.4 %) (12 men and 1 woman; diagnosis of 9 alcoholic and 4 idiopathic). Among the 13 patients, three had been diagnosed with pancreatic cancer at first, and one had been

Table 25.3 Breakdown of the diagnostic imaging findings for chronic pancreatitis as determined by the revised Japanese clinical diagnostic criteria

Findings of definite chronic pancreatitis ($n=15$)	Number
(a) Stones in pancreatic ducts	9
(b) Multiple or numerous calcifications distributed in the entire pancreas	13
(c) Irregular dilatation of the MPD and irregular dilatation of pancreatic duct branches of variable intensity with scattered distribution throughout the entire pancreas on ERCP	2
(d) Irregular dilatation of the MPD and branches proximal to complete or incomplete obstruction of the MPD (with pancreatic stones or protein plugs) on ERCP	2
Findings of probable chronic pancreatitis ($n=1$)	
(a) Irregular dilatation of pancreatic duct branches of variable intensity with scattered distribution throughout the entire pancreas, irregular dilatation of the MPD alone, or protein plugs on ERCP	1
(b) Irregular dilatation of the MPD throughout the entire pancreas plus pancreatic deformity with irregular contour on CT	0

From Ref. [23]
This study did not evaluate MRCP or US (EUS) findings, so the probable chronic pancreatitis findings of (a) and (d), which are judged by these modalities, were excluded

recently diagnosed with AIP after long-term clinical follow-up. The remaining nine patients showed typical image findings consistent with ordinary chronic pancreatitis, such as pancreatic stones and irregular dilatation of the MPD [7]. This result suggested that an advanced stage of AIP might have been previously included among cases of ordinary chronic pancreatitis and might be regarded as another condition, such as chronic alcoholic pancreatitis.

Autoimmune Pancreatitis Can Progress to Chronic Pancreatitis that Meets the Revised Japanese Clinical Diagnostic Criteria for Ordinary Chronic Pancreatitis

Our observation that ordinary chronic pancreatitis cases might include a few advanced-stage AIP cases and that some patients with AIP show severe pancreatic calcifications over a long-term course suggested that AIP could progress to chronic pancreatitis that meets the definitive diagnostic criteria for ordinary chronic pancreatitis. We examined whether AIP could transform into chronic pancreatitis that met the revised Japanese clinical diagnostic criteria [22] and aimed to clarify the susceptibility factors and underlying mechanisms for AIP progressing to confirmed chronic pancreatitis [23]. We enrolled 73 patients with AIP who had been followed for at least 3 years (median follow-up period, 88 months; range, 36–230 months) and found that 16 patients (22 %) were confirmed to have chronic pancreatitis in terms of the revised Japanese clinical diagnostic criteria [22], including 15 patients with definite chronic pancreatitis and one patient with probable chronic pancreatitis during this study period (Table 25.3). Among the 15 definite cases, major imaging findings were stones in pancreatic ducts in nine (Fig. 25.2a) and multiple or numerous calcifications distributed throughout the entire pancreas in 13 patients (Fig. 25.2b) [23].

Clinical Features of Autoimmune Pancreatitis Meeting the Revised Japanese Clinical Diagnostic Criteria for Ordinary Chronic Pancreatitis: Risk Factors for Progression to Chronic Pancreatitis

We compared the clinical and laboratory factors as well as CT and ERP findings between the group of patients who progressed to chronic pancreatitis and those who did not, in which progression into chronic pancreatitis in terms of the diagnostic criteria was seen in 16 patients and no progression was seen in 52 patients [23]. Univariate analysis of data for clinical features revealed that relapse was significantly more frequent in the progression group ($P=0.030$). We found no significant differences in laboratory factors associated with the AIP activity markers between the two groups. In pancreatic imaging findings, pancreatic head swelling was more frequently seen in the progression group, although not significantly. Interestingly, MPD narrowing in the pancreatic body was significantly less frequent ($P=0.001$) in the progression group, and MPD dilatation at one pancreatic area or more was significantly more frequent ($P=0.001$) in that group (Table 25.4). Of the 13 patients with AIP who had MPD non-narrowing in the pancreatic body, eight patients with a dilated duct diameter and five with a normal diameter showed pancreatic head swelling almost simultaneously. Furthermore, multivariate analysis showed that pancreatic head swelling (OR 12.7, $P=0.023$) (Fig. 25.2c) and MPD non-narrowing in the pancreatic body (OR 12.6, $P=0.001$) (Fig. 25.2d) were significant independent risk factors for progression to chronic pancreatitis [23]. We found a difference in the risk factors between pancreatic stone formation and progression to chronic pancreatitis. The reason for this discrepancy might be that the former included small pancreatic calculi that could not fulfill the diagnostic criteria of chronic pancreatitis.

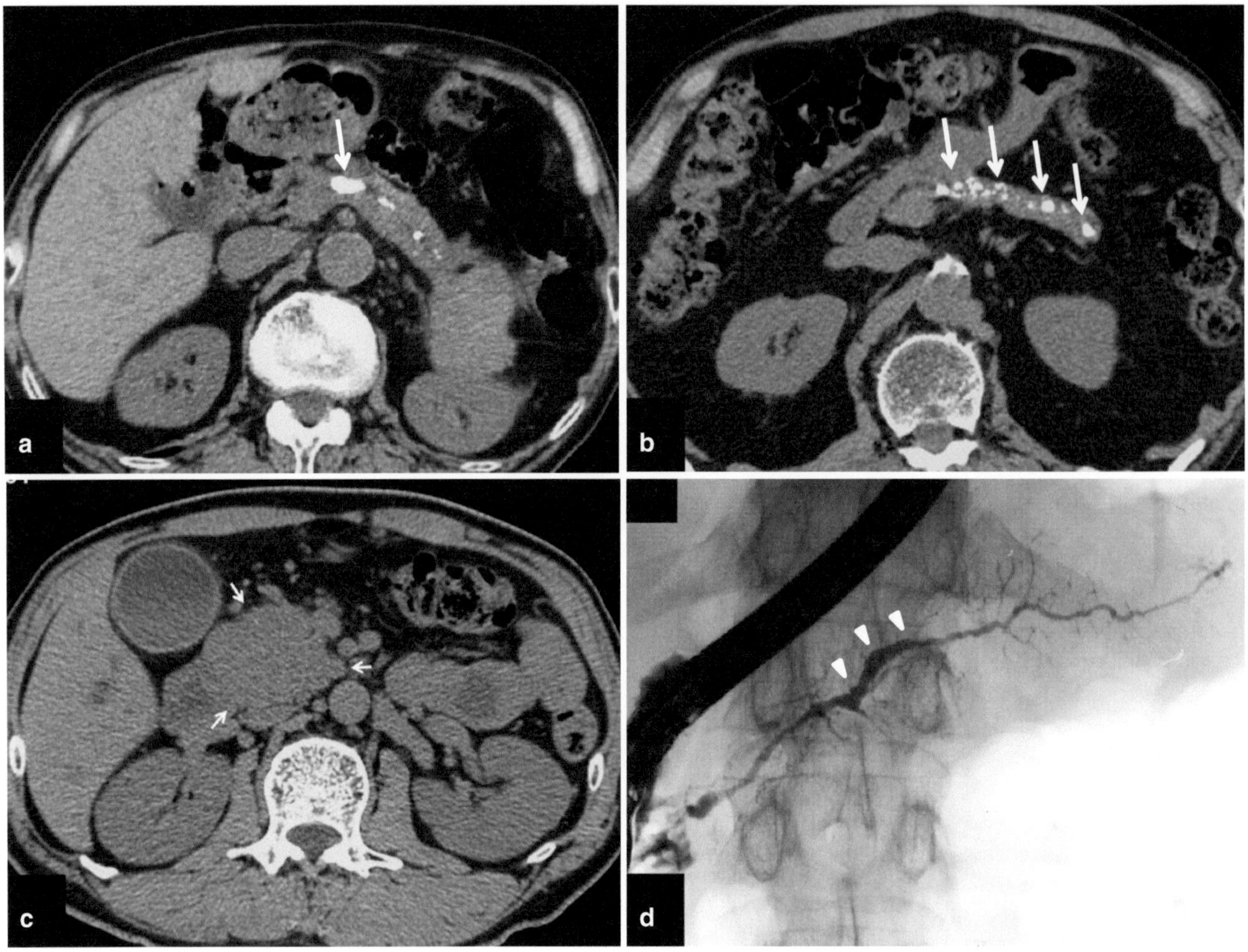

Fig. 25.2 CT of AIP showing definite imaging findings. (**a**) Stones in pancreatic ducts (*arrow*). (**b**) Multiple or numerous calcifications distributed throughout the pancreas (*arrows*). CT and ERCP findings of AIP showing independent risk factors for progression to confirmed chronic pancreatitis at diagnosis. (**c**) Pancreatic head swelling (*arrows*). (**d**) MPD non-narrowing in the pancreatic body (*arrowheads*) (From Ref. [23])

Period and Ratio of Progression to Chronic Pancreatitis

The median time from AIP diagnosis to chronic pancreatitis was 33 months (range, 16–124 months). Kaplan–Meier testing revealed that the progression rate to chronic pancreatitis was 10 % at 36 months, 20 % at 100 months, and 30 % at 124 months (Fig. 25.3a). Progression to chronic pancreatitis was not seen after 124 months, suggesting that disease development to the chronic stage occurs within 10 years of follow-up. Next, we performed stratification analysis for AIP progression to chronic pancreatitis using the two risk factors of pancreatic head swelling and MPD non-narrowing in the pancreatic body that were identified by multivariate analysis. Specifically, Kaplan–Meier testing was performed on three groups: the "zero risk factor" group (6 patients), the "one risk factor" group (45 patients), and the "two risk factor" group (21 patients). No AIP patients progressed to chronic pancreatitis in the "zero risk factor" group, whereas the "two risk factor" group showed a significantly higher progression rate compared with that of the "one risk factor" group ($P<0.001$, log-rank test) of 30 % at 3 years and 60 % at 10 years (Fig. 25.3b) [23]. Therefore, we infer that an effective regimen to prevent progression to chronic pancreatitis is necessary for patients with AIP who have two risk factors.

Mechanism of Autoimmune Pancreatitis Progressing to Chronic Pancreatitis

Based on our cumulative study results, we hypothesize a sequential progression mechanism of AIP to chronic pancreatitis. Namely, many cases of AIP show pancreatic head swelling during the acute stage, some of which induces long-standing narrowing of both the Wirsung and Santorini ducts in this region, which may cause pancreatic juice stasis in the

Table 25.4 Clinical features, laboratory tests, and pancreatic morphology at diagnosis

	Progression to CP ($n = 16$)	Nonprogression to CP ($n = 57$)	P value
Clinical features	Median (range)		
Observation period[a]	102 (37–165)	87 (36–230)	0.522
Age	66.5 (48–75)	65 (38–84)	0.989
Sex (M/F)	13/3	43/14	0.748
Alcohol (+/–)	6/10	29/28	0.405
PSL (+/–)	13/3	50/7	0.681
PSL maintenance therapy (+/–)	10/6	41/16	0.542
Relapse (+/–)	8/8	12/45	0.030*
Laboratory tests			
IgG	2140 (1166–3861)	2227 (892–7236)	0.509
IgG4	421 (146–1845)	663 (4–2970)	0.267
C3	100 (52–122)	98 (29–218)	0.551
C4	21.8 (12.4–37.7)	21.1 (1.1–47.3)	0.495
sIL2-R	726 (132–1845)	892 (257–4695)	0.053
CIC	5 (1.9–13.9)	5.7 (1.4–40)	0.219
Pancreatic morphology at diagnosis			
Pancreatic swelling (by CT)			
Head (+/–)	15/1	41/16	0.096
Body (+/–)	12/4	36/21	0.553
Tail (+/–)	10/6	37/20	1.000
Level 1/level 2[b]	8/8	30/27	1.000
Ductal narrowing in MPD (by ERP)			
Head (+/–)	13/3	44/13	1.000
Wirsung and Santorini (+/–)	11/5	34/23	0.573
Body (+/–)	3/13	37/20	0.001*
Tail (+/–)	12/4	42/15	1.000
Level 1/level 2[c]	6/10	17/40	0.558
Ductal dilatation in MPD (+/–)	9/7	7/50	0.001*

From Ref. [23]

CP chronic pancreatitis, *PSL* prednisolone, *sIL2-R* soluble interleukin 2 receptor, *CIC* circulating immune complex, *MPD* main pancreatic duct

*$P < 0.05$

[a]Period from AIP diagnosis to the most recent observation (months)

[b]Swelling was classified as level 1 (diffuse swelling) or level 2 (focal/segmental swelling) as defined by the International Consensus Diagnostic Criteria for Autoimmune Pancreatitis

[c]Pancreatic duct narrowing was classified as level 1 (long [segmental/diffuse] or multiple strictures) or level 2 (focal narrowing) as defined by the International Consensus Diagnostic Criteria for Autoimmune Pancreatitis

upstream pancreatic duct (Fig. 25.4a). These residual abnormalities may induce increased intrapancreatic duct pressure that is resistant to typical AIP-specific MPD narrowing in the pancreatic body, causing MPD non-narrowing in this region (Fig. 25.4b). These events in concert with relapse may finally result in severe calcification of the entire pancreas and pancreatic atrophy (Fig. 25.4c) [23].

Limitations and Future Perspectives

The limitations of our cumulative studies are as follows: Our earlier study designs included a limited number of patients and were mainly retrospective cohort designs; we applied Japanese diagnostic criteria for chronic pancreatitis with particular reference to imaging findings; and AIP patients were biased as type 1 defined by the International Consensus Diagnostic Criteria [24]. Because we primarily focused on imaging findings in our study, detailed analysis for exocrine or endocrine dysfunction and of pathological findings in advanced-stage AIP showing severe pancreatic calcification is needed for future study.

Conclusions

Over the last decade, it has been revealed that some patients with AIP could progress to pancreatic stone formation, pancreatic atrophy, and/or irregular dilatation of the MPD over a long-term course, which raised the question of whether AIP can progress to confirmed chronic pancreatitis or not. Our cumulative studies have clarified the following: (1) Pancreatic calcification in AIP is closely associated with disease recurrence; (2) the advanced stage

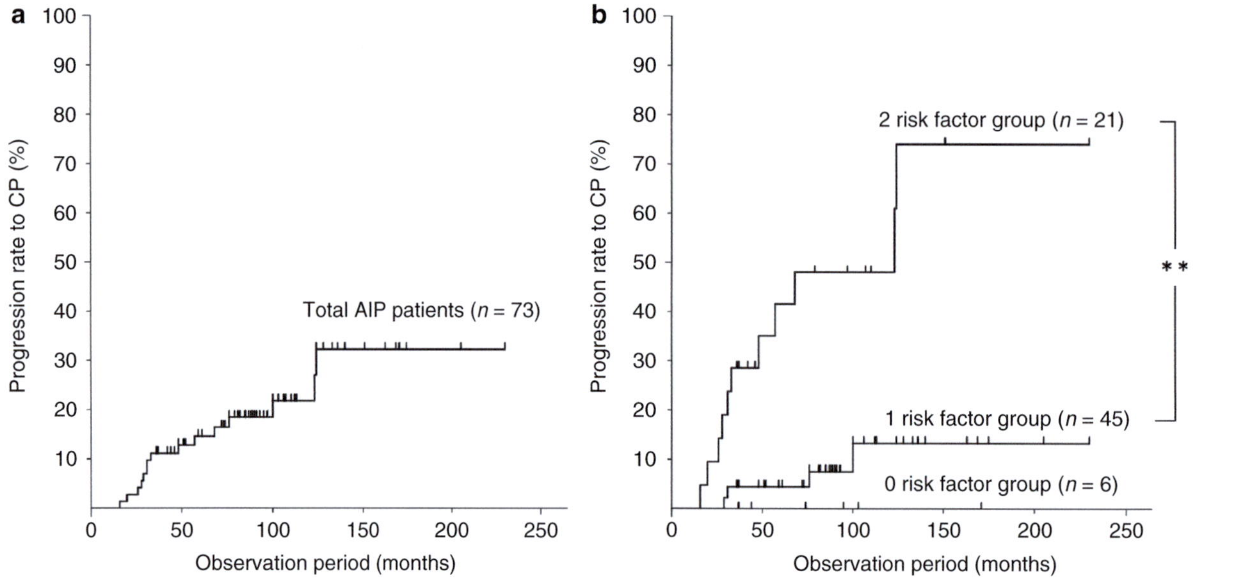

Fig. 25.3 (**a**) Kaplan–Meier analysis of the progression rate to confirmed chronic pancreatitis in 73 patients with AIP. (**b**) Kaplan–Meier analysis of the progression rate to confirmed chronic pancreatitis in AIP based on the risk factors of pancreatic head swelling and MPD non-narrowing in the pancreatic body. Comparison of the zero risk factor ($n=6$), 1 risk factor ($n=45$), and 2 risk factor ($n=21$) groups. $^{**}P<0.001$ (log-rank test) (From Ref. [23])

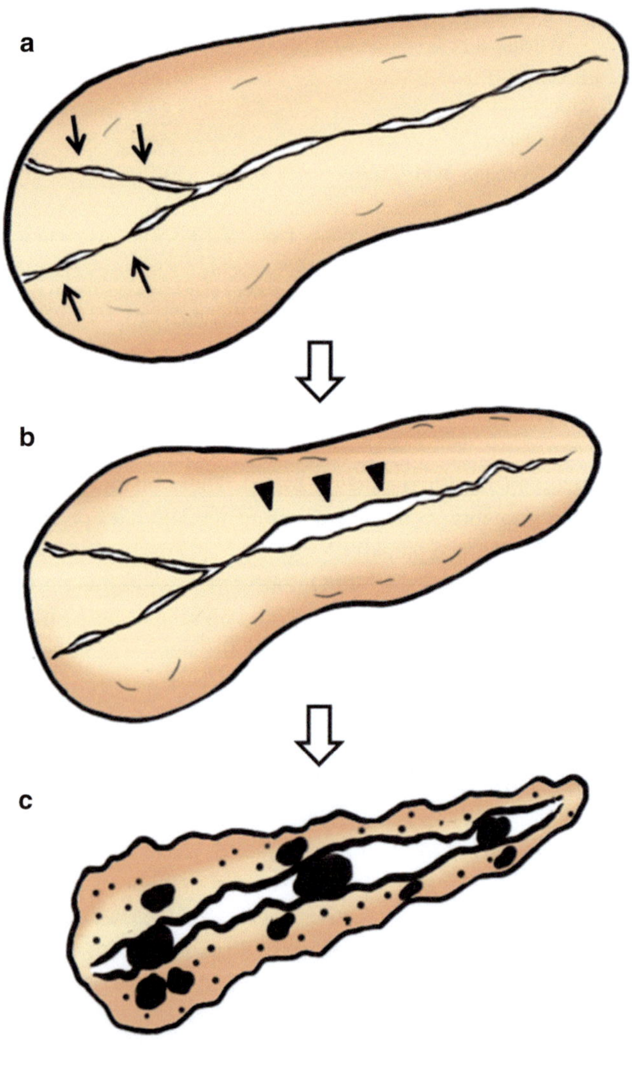

Fig. 25.4 Sequential progression mechanism of AIP to confirmed chronic pancreatitis. (**a**) Narrowing of both the Wirsung and Santorini ducts (*arrows*) by pancreatic head swelling causes pancreatic juice stasis in the upstream pancreatic duct. (**b**) Pancreatic juice stasis results in increased intrapancreatic duct pressure that is resistant to typical AIP-specific MPD narrowing in the pancreatic body region, leading to MPD non-narrowing in this region (*arrowheads*). (**c**) In concert with relapse, these events finally result in severe calcification (From Ref. [23])

of AIP formerly might have been included in other conditions of ordinary chronic pancreatitis; (3) approximately 40 % of patients with AIP progress to pancreatic stone formation over a long-term course, and their primary risk factor was narrowing of both the Wirsung and Santorini ducts; and (4) almost 20 % of AIP patients progress to confirmed chronic pancreatitis in terms of revised Japanese clinical diagnostic criteria, with independent risk factors of pancreatic head swelling and MPD non-narrowing in the pancreatic body. Finally, AIP can progress to severe pancreatic stone formation and confirmed chronic pancreatitis over a long-term course, which may be presumably caused by disease recurrence and pancreatic juice stasis. From these observations, we believe that it is necessary for patients with AIP to maintain a carefully devised follow-up regimen to prevent possible progression to chronic pancreatitis.

References

1. Kamisawa T, Shimosegawa T, Okazaki K, Nishino T, Watanabe H, Kanno A. Standard steroid treatment for autoimmune pancreatitis. Gut. 2009;58:1504–7.
2. Kamisawa T, Okazaki K, Kawa S, Shimosegawa T, Tanaka M. Japanese consensus guidelines for management of autoimmune pancreatitis: III. Treatment and prognosis of AIP. J Gastroenterol. 2010;45:471–7.
3. Hart PA, Kamisawa T, Brugge WR, Chung JB, Culver EL, Czako L, et al. Long-term outcomes of autoimmune pancreatitis: a multicentre, international analysis. Gut. 2013;62:1771–6.
4. Song MH, Kim MH, Lee SK, Seo DW, Lee SS, Han J, et al. Regression of pancreatic fibrosis after steroid therapy in patients with autoimmune chronic pancreatitis. Pancreas. 2005;30:83–6.
5. Ko SB, Mizuno N, Yatabe Y, Yoshikawa T, Ishiguro H, Yamamoto A. Corticosteroids correct aberrant CFTR localization in the duct and regenerate acinar cells in autoimmune pancreatitis. Gastroenterology. 2010;138:1988–96.
6. Takayama M, Hamano H, Ochi Y, Saegusa H, Komatsu K, Muraki T, et al. Recurrent attacks of autoimmune pancreatitis result in pancreatic stone formation. Am J Gastroenterol. 2004;99:932–7.
7. Kawa S, Hamano H, Ozaki Y, Ito T, Kodama R, Chou Y, et al. Long-term follow-up of autoimmune pancreatitis: characteristics of chronic disease and recurrence. Clin Gastroenterol Hepatol. 2009;7:S18–22.
8. Takuma K, Kamisawa T, Tabata T, Inaba Y, Egawa N, Igarashi Y. Short-term and long-term outcomes of autoimmune pancreatitis. Eur J Gastroenterol Hepatol. 2011;23:146–52.
9. Suzuki K, Itoh S, Nagasaka T, Ogawa H, Ota T, Naganawa S. CT findings in autoimmune pancreatitis: assessment using multiphase contrast-enhanced multisection CT. Clin Radiol. 2010;65:735–43.
10. Sah RP, Pannala R, Chari ST, Sugumar A, Clain JE, Levy MJ, et al. Prevalence, diagnosis, and profile of autoimmune pancreatitis presenting with features of acute or chronic pancreatitis. Clin Gastroenterol Hepatol. 2010;8:91–6.
11. Takada H, Nakazawa T, Ohara H, Ando T, Hayashi K, Naito I, et al. Role of osteopontin in calcification in autoimmune pancreatitis. Dig Dis Sci. 2009;54:793–801.
12. Nakazawa T, Ohara H, Sano H, Ando T, Imai H, Takada H, et al. Difficulty in diagnosing autoimmune pancreatitis by imaging findings. Gastrointest Endosc. 2007;65:99–108.
13. Nishino T, Toki F, Oyama H, Shimizu K, Shiratori K. Long-term outcome of autoimmune pancreatitis after oral prednisolone therapy. Intern Med. 2006;45:497–501.
14. Maire F, Le Baleur Y, Rebours V, Vullierme MP, Couvelard A, Voitot H, et al. Outcome of patients with type 1 or 2 autoimmune pancreatitis. Am J Gastroenterol. 2011;106:151–6.
15. Yoshida K, Toki F, Takeuchi T, Watanabe S, Shiratori K, Hayashi N. Chronic pancreatitis caused by an autoimmune abnormality. Proposal of the concept of autoimmune pancreatitis. Dig Dis Sci. 1995;40:1561–8.
16. Kawa S, Hamano H. Clinical features of autoimmune pancreatitis. J Gastroenterol. 2007;42 Suppl 18:9–14.
17. Muraki T, Hamano H, Ochi Y, Komatsu K, Komiyama Y, Arakura N, et al. Autoimmune pancreatitis and complement activation system. Pancreas. 2006;32:16–21.
18. Maruyama M, Arakura N, Ozaki Y, Watanabe T, Ito T, Yoneda S, et al. Risk factors for pancreatic stone formation in autoimmune pancreatitis over a long-term course. J Gastroenterol. 2012;47:553–60.
19. Hirano K, Tada M, Isayama H, Watanabe T, Saito T, Uchino R, et al. High alcohol consumption increases the risk of pancreatic stone formation and pancreatic atrophy in autoimmune pancreatitis. Pancreas. 2013;42(3):502–5.
20. Zhang X, Li W, Jiang L, Guo Y, Wang X. Clinical analysis of 36 cases of autoimmune pancreatitis in China. PLoS One. 2012;7:e44808.
21. Kawa S, Hamano H, Kiyosawa K. High serum IgG4 concentrations in patients with sclerosing pancreatitis. Reply. N Engl J Med. 2001;345:148.
22. Shimosegawa T, Kataoka K, Kamisawa T, Miyakawa H, Ohara H, Ito T, et al. The revised Japanese clinical diagnostic criteria for chronic pancreatitis. J Gastroenterol. 2010;45:584–91.
23. Maruyama M, Arakura N, Ozaki Y, Watanabe T, Ito T, Yoneda S, et al. Type 1 autoimmune pancreatitis can transform into chronic pancreatitis: a long-term follow-up study of 73 Japanese patients. Int J Rheumatol. 2013;2013:8.
24. Shimosegawa T, Chari ST, Frulloni L, Kamisawa T, Kawa S, Mino-Kenudson M, et al. International consensus diagnostic criteria for autoimmune pancreatitis: guidelines of the International Association of Pancreatology. Pancreas. 2011;40:352–8.

Occurrence of Malignant Neoplasms

26

Kyoko Shimizu

Introduction

The concept of autoimmune pancreatitis (AIP) was first proposed by Yoshida et al. in 1995 as a distinct type of chronic pancreatitis [1]. A clinicopathological profile associated with high serum IgG4 levels and an increased number of IgG4-positive plasma cells and presence of fibrosis in the pancreas and in other affected organs was identified as IgG4-related disease (IgG4-RD) [2–5]. The long-term prognosis of AIP remains unclear, but the diagnosis of various malignant neoplasms, including pancreatic cancer [6–15], colon cancer [16–18], gastric cancer [9, 16, 17], bile duct cancer [9, 17, 19], malignant lymphoma [20–30], and thyroid cancer [31], before the diagnosis of AIP, at the same time as the diagnosis of AIP was made, or several years later has been reported in several case studies and retrospective cohort studies. The process of chronic inflammation and fibrosis has generally been thought to increase the risk of cancer. Associations between chronic inflammation and malignancies have been recognized, for example, the association between the inflammation caused by chronic *Helicobacter pylori* infection and gastric carcinoma, between ulcerative colitis and adenocarcinoma of the colon, and between chronic hepatitis and hepatocellular carcinoma. The chronic inflammation in AIP was also originally thought to be a risk factor for pancreatic cancer [32–36], but the results of recent studies have suggested that AIP is a paraneoplastic syndrome [17].

K. Shimizu, MD, PhD
Department of Gastroenterology, Tokyo Women's Medical University, School of Medicine, Tokyo, Japan
e-mail: kyoko@ige.twmu.ac.jp

Incidence of Cancer in AIP

Four retrospective cohort studies have reported incidences of malignant neoplasms of 5.3–16.6 % in patients with IgG4-RD [9, 16–18]. The standardized incidence ratios (SIRs) for malignancies in IgG4-RD and in AIP have been reported to be 2.7 and 3.83, respectively [17, 18], meaning that the incidence of malignancies in both is higher than the incidence of malignancies in the general population. Interestingly, when the SIRs for malignancies were stratified according to the time after the diagnosis of AIP was made into the first year and subsequent years after the diagnosis of AIP, the SIRs were 6.1 (95 % confidence interval [CI] 2.3–9.9) and 1.5 (95 % CI 0.3–2.8), respectively [17]. The risk of malignancies in AIP patients at the time AIP was diagnosed relative to risk in age- and sex-matched control subjects who had a medical checkup that included a complete examination was 4.9 (95 % CI 1.7–14.9). The frequencies of extrapancreatic lesions of AIP were similar between AIP patients with and without cancer, but the incidence of retroperitoneal fibrosis was significantly higher in patients who had been simultaneously diagnosed with AIP and cancer than in AIP patients without cancer [17]. These results support the notion that AIP patients are at high risk of cancer, especially in the first year after the diagnosis of AIP.

Associations Between Malignant Neoplasms and AIP

Various types of malignant neoplasms have been found to be associated with AIP, and the most common cancer in AIP patients is gastric cancer (Table 26.1). The reason for the high incidence of gastric cancer in AIP patients is thought to

T. Kamisawa, J.B. Chung (eds.), *Autoimmune Pancreatitis*,
DOI 10.1007/978-3-642-55086-7_26, © Springer-Verlag Berlin Heidelberg 2015

be that the majority of AIP patients who were the subjects of the analyses in the studies shown in Table 26.1 have been Japanese and Korean, and the most common site of cancer in Japanese and Koreans is the stomach. In contrast, none of the patients in three retrospective cohort studies had pancreatic cancer [16–18]; however, five of the 1,064 AIP patients in one international study had pancreatic cancer [9]. If persistent inflammation in AIP is a risk factor for developing pancreatic cancer, then the AIP patients should have had a higher incidence of pancreatic cancer. The results of these studies seem to support the notion that the higher incidence of malignancy in AIP patients is not directly attributable to the underlying chronic inflammation in lymphoplasmacytic sclerosing pancreatitis (LPSP).

Several case reports [6, 7, 10–15] and two retrospective studies [8, 9] have documented synchronous and metachronous pancreatic cancer in AIP (Table 26.2). In six (40 %) of the 15 cases reported, the pancreatic cancer was detected within a year after the diagnosis of AIP, and histological examination of the cancers in all six cases revealed considerable IgG4-positive plasma cell infiltration around areas of invasive ductal adenocarcinoma but only a few IgG4-positive plasma cells in the noncancerous areas of the pancreas [11, 13, 15]. Pancreatic intraepithelial neoplasia (PanIN) lesions are common precursors of pancreatic cancer and are characterized by columnar to cuboidal cells with varying degrees of atypia [37–39]. KRAS mutations have been detected in more than 95 % of invasive pancreatic ductal adenocarcinomas (PDACs), and more than 90 % of PanIN lesions have been found to harbor a KRAS mutation, suggesting that KRAS activation is one of the earliest genetic events in PanIN [37, 40–43]. Kamisawa et al. [44] demonstrated KRAS mutations not only in the pancreas but also in the tissues of organs involved by IgG4-RD, including the major duodenal papilla, common bile duct, gallbladder epithelium, gastric mucosa, and colonic mucosa. A retrospective analysis of the surgically resected pancreata of AIP patients revealed PanIN lesions, including PanIN 2 and PanIN 3 lesions, in 82 % of AIP patients [8]. These findings support the notion that KRAS mutations and PanIN lesions are associated with the development of pancreatic cancer in AIP. In fact, it is questionable whether

Table 26.1 Incidence and SIR of malignancies in patients with AIP

	Nishino [16]	Hart [9]	Yamamoto [18]	Shiokawa [17]
Publication year	2006	2012	2012	2013
Number of pt. with AIP	12	1,064	106	108
Number of pt. with malignancy	2	57	11	15
Incidence of malignancies (%)	16.6	5.3	10.4	13.9
SIR			3.83	2.7
Types of malignant neoplasms				
Gastric	1	11		7
Lung		9	2	3
Prostate		7	1	2
Colorectal	1	5	2	2
Pancreatic		5		
Esophageal		4		
Cholangiocarcinoma		3		1
Leukemia		3		
Ovarian		2	1	
Renal		2	1	
Breast		1	1	
Lingual			1	
MALT			1	
NHL			1	2
Testicular		1		
Bladder		1		
Hepatocellular		1		
GIST		1		
Thyroid				1
Unknown primary		1		

pt patients, *SIR* standardized incidence ratio

persistent chronic inflammation due to LPSP induces cancer in AIP. While persistent subclinical inflammation without any signs of active AIP may have been present before the diagnosis of pancreatic cancer, many cases in which the diagnosis of pancreatic cancer was made at the same time as the diagnosis of AIP have been reported. Nevertheless, LPSP may not play a significant role in pancreatic carcinogenesis, and LPSP is more likely to be a paraneoplastic syndrome.

Several possible mechanisms to explain the association between AIP and malignant neoplasms have been suggested. The first possible mechanism that has been suggested is aging, because older age is a risk factor of cancer and AIP is found commonly among the elder population. The second possible mechanism is that widespread persistent IgG4-related fibroinflammation of the associated organs with abundant infiltration by T lymphocytes and Foxp3-positive cells may cause carcinogenesis in the various organs [11, 45, 46]. The third possible mechanism is that tumor cells may cause AIP by activating IgG4-related immune responses because tumor cells release various cytokines [47–50]. The fourth possible mechanism is that the dysregulation of B-lymphocytes associated with autoimmune disease may lead to abnormal B-lymphocyte proliferation and lymphoma [51]. Takahashi et al. [29] found that the SIR for malignant lymphoma in patients with IgG4-related disease was 16.0 (95 % CI: 3.3–45.5), suggesting that IgG4-RD is a risk factor for malignant lymphoma.

Although the mechanism underlying the development of malignant neoplasms in AIP patients has yet to be identified, it is important to examine AIP patients for malignant neoplasms when the diagnosis of AIP is made and during follow-up examinations.

In conclusion, all of the evidence that has accumulated thus far indicates that it is more likely that cancer induces the development of LPSP, that is, that LPSP develops as a paraneoplastic syndrome, than that LPSP induces cancer. Nevertheless, careful long-term follow-up of AIP patients is recommended because of their high incidence of malignant neoplasms.

Table 26.2 Reported cases of AIP with synchronous or metachronous onset of pancreatic cancer

Author	Publication year	Age	Sex	Synchronous/metachronous	Serum IgG4 (mg/dL)	Therapy for AIP
Kamisawa et al. [11]	2006	74	Female	Synchronous	433	(–)
Inoue et al. [10]	2006	62	Male	Synchronous	138	(–)
Ghazale [7]	2007	72	Male	5 years	NA	(–)
Fukui [6]	2007	80	Male	50 months	154	Steroid
Witkiewicz et al. [15]	2008	80	Male	Synchronous	NA	(–)
Motosugi et al. [13]	2009	59	Male	Synchronous	NA	(–)
Loos et al. [12]	2011	67	Female	18 months	NA	PPPD, steroid
Pezzilli et al. [14]	2011	70	Male	6 months	19	Azathioprine
Gupta et al. [8]	2013	73	Male	10 years	NA	PD
		69	Male	6 years	147	Steroid
Hart et al. [9]	2013	65–80	Male	4 cases: more than 3 years	NA	NA
				1 case: 9 months	NA	NA

NA not available, *PPPD* pylorus-preserving pancreatoduodenectomy, *PD* pancreatoduodenectomy

References

1. Yoshida K, Toki F, Takeuchi T, Watanabe S, Shiratori K, Hayashi N. Chronic pancreatitis caused by an autoimmune abnormality. Proposal of the concept of autoimmune pancreatitis. Dig Dis Sci. 1995;40:1561–8.
2. Deshpande V, Chicano S, Chiocca S, Finkelberg D, Selig MK, Mino-Kenudson M, Brugge WR, Colvin RB, Lauwers GY. Autoimmune pancreatitis: a systemic immune complex mediated disease. Am J Surg Pathol. 2006;30:1537–45.
3. Hamano H, Kawa S, Horiuchi A, Unno H, Furuya N, Akamatsu T, Fukushima M, Nikaido T, Nakayama K, Usuda N, Kiyosawa K. High serum IgG4 concentrations in patients with sclerosing pancreatitis. N Engl J Med. 2001;344:732–8.
4. Kamisawa T, Funata N, Hayashi Y, Eishi Y, Koike M, Tsuruta K, Okamoto A, Egawa N, Nakajima H. A new clinicopathological entity of IgG4-related autoimmune disease. J Gastroenterol. 2003;38:982–4.
5. Stone JH, Zen Y, Deshpande V. IgG4-related disease. N Engl J Med. 2012;366:539–51.
6. Fukui T, Mitsuyama T, Takaoka M, Uchida K, Matsushita M, Okazaki K. Pancreatic cancer associated with autoimmune pancreatitis in remission. Intern Med. 2008;47:151–5.
7. Ghazale A, Chari S. Is autoimmune pancreatitis a risk factor for pancreatic cancer? Pancreas. 2007;35:376.
8. Gupta R, Khosroshahi A, Shinagare S, Fernandez C, Ferrone C, Lauwers GY, Stone JH, Deshpande V. Does autoimmune pancreatitis increase the risk of pancreatic carcinoma?: a retrospective analysis of pancreatic resections. Pancreas. 2013;42:506–10.
9. Hart PA, Kamisawa T, Brugge WR, Chung JB, Culver EL, Czakó L, Frulloni L, Go VL, Gress TM, Kim MH, Kawa S, Lee KT, Lerch MM, Liao WC, Lör M, Okazaki K, Ryu JK, Schleinitz N, Shimizu K, Shimosegawa T, Soetikno R, Webster G, Yadav D, Zen Y, Chari ST. Long-term outcomes of autoimmune pancreatitis: a multicentre, international analysis. Gut. 2013;62:1771–6.
10. Inoue H, Miyatani H, Sawada Y, Yoshida Y. A case of pancreas cancer with autoimmune pancreatitis. Pancreas. 2006;33:208–9.
11. Kamisawa T, Chen PY, Tu Y, Nakajima H, Egawa N, Tsuruta K, Okamoto A, Hishima T. Pancreatic cancer with a high serum IgG4 concentration. World J Gastroenterol. 2006;12:6225–8.
12. Loos M, Esposito I, Hedderich DM, Ludwig L, Fingerle A, Friess H, Klöpel G, Bühler P. Autoimmune pancreatitis complicated by carcinoma of the pancreatobiliary system: a case report and review of the literature. Pancreas. 2011;40:151–4.
13. Motosugi U, Ichikawa T, Yamaguchi H, Nakazawa T, Katoh R, Itakura J, Fujii H, Sato T, Araki T, Shimizu M. Small invasive ductal adenocarcinoma of the pancreas associated with lymphoplasmacytic sclerosing pancreatitis. Pathol Int. 2009;59:744–7.
14. Pezzilli R, Vecchiarelli S, di Marco MC, Serra C, Santini D, Calculli L, Fabbri D, Rojas Mena B, Imbrogno A. Pancreatic ductal adenocarcinoma associated with autoimmune pancreatitis. Case Rep Gastroenterol. 2011;5:378–85.
15. Witkiewicz AK, Kennedy EP, Kennyon L, Yeo CJ, Hruban RH. Synchronous autoimmune pancreatitis and infiltrating pancreatic ductal adenocarcinoma: case report and review of the literature. Hum Pathol. 2008;39:1548–51.
16. Nishino T, Toki F, Oyama H, Shimizu K, Shiratori K. Long-term outcome of autoimmune pancreatitis after oral prednisolone therapy. Intern Med. 2006;45:497–501.
17. Shiokawa M, Kodama Y, Yoshimura K, Kawanami C, Mimura J, Yamashita Y, Asada M, Kikuyama M, Okabe Y, Inokuma T, Ohana M, Kokuryu H, Takeda K, Tsuji Y, Minami R, Sakuma Y, Kuriyama K, Ota Y, Tanabe W, Maruno T, Kurita A, Sawai Y, Uza N, Watanabe T, Haga H, Chiba T. Risk of cancer in patients with autoimmune pancreatitis. Am J Gastroenterol. 2013;108:610–7.
18. Yamamoto M, Takahashi H, Tabeya T, Suzuki C, Naishiro Y, Ishigami K, Yajima H, Shimizu Y, Obara M, Yamamoto H, Himi T, Imai K, Shinomura Y. Risk of malignancies in IgG4-related disease. Mod Rheumatol. 2012;22:414–8.
19. Oh HC, Kim JG, Kim JW, Lee KS, Kim MK, Chi KC, Kim YS, Kim KH. Early bile duct cancer in a background of sclerosing cholangitis and autoimmune pancreatitis. Intern Med. 2008;47:2025–8.
20. Cheuk W, Yuen HK, Chan AC, Shih LY, Kuo TT, Ma MW, Lo YF, Chan WK, Chan JK. Ocular adnexal lymphoma associated with IgG4+ chronic sclerosing dacryoadenitis: a previously undescribed complication of IgG4-related sclerosing disease. Am J Surg Pathol. 2008;32:1159–67.
21. Go H, Kim JE, Kim YA, Chung HK, Khwarg SI, Kim CW, Jeon YK. Ocular adnexal IgG4-related disease: comparative analysis with mucosa-associated lymphoid tissue lymphoma and other chronic inflammatory conditions. Histopathology. 2012;60:296–312.
22. Ishida M, Hodohara K, Yoshida K, Kagotani A, Iwai M, Yoshii M, Okuno H, Horinouchi A, Nakanishi R, Harada A, Yoshida T, Okabe H. Occurrence of anaplastic large cell lymphoma following IgG4-related autoimmune pancreatitis and cholecystitis and diffuse large B-cell lymphoma. Int J Clin Exp Pathol. 2013;6:2560–8.
23. Kanda G, Ryu T, Shirai T, Ijichi M, Hishima T, Kitamura S, Bandai Y. Peripheral T-cell lymphoma that developed during the follow-up of IgG4-related disease. Intern Med. 2011;50:155–60.
24. Kim T, Grobmyer SR, Dixon LR, Allan RW, Hochwald SN. Autoimmune pancreatitis and concurrent small lymphocytic lymphoma: not just a coincidence? J Gastrointest Surg. 2008;12:1566–70.
25. Kubota T, Moritani S, Yoshino T, Nagai H, Terasaki H. Ocular adnexal marginal zone B cell lymphoma infiltrated by IgG4-positive plasma cells. J Clin Pathol. 2010;63:1059–65.
26. Matsuo T, Ichimura K, Yoshino T. Local recurrence as immunoglobulin G4 (IgG4)-related disease 10 years after radiotherapy to ocular adnexal extranodal marginal zone B-cell lymphoma of mucosa-associated lymphoid tissue. J Clin Exp Hematop. 2011;51:125–33.
27. Mitsui T, Yokohama A, Koiso H, Ishizaki T, Uchiumi H, Saitoh T, Handa H, Hirato J, Karasawa M, Murakami H, Kojima M, Nojima Y, Tsukamoto N. Development of IgG4-related disease 10 years after chemotherapy for diffuse large B cell lymphoma and long-standing bronchial asthma. Int J Hematol. 2013;98:122–8.
28. Oshima Y, Usui R, Manabe S, Hasegawa N, Kakuta Y, Nitta K, Hatano M. IgG4-related tubulointerstitial nephritis and lymphadenopathy after therapy for malignant lymphoma. Intern Med. 2012;51:1221–6.
29. Takahashi N, Ghazale AH, Smyrk TC, Mandrekar JN, Chari ST. Possible association between IgG4-associated systemic disease with or without autoimmune pancreatitis and non-Hodgkin lymphoma. Pancreas. 2009;38:523–6.
30. Uehara T, Ikeda S, Hamano H, Kawa S, Moteki H, Matsuda K, Kaneko Y, Hara E. A case of Mikulicz's disease complicated by malignant lymphoma: a postmortem histopathological finding. Intern Med. 2012;51:419–23.
31. Ito M, Naruke Y, Mihara Y, So K, Miyashita T, Origuchi T, Nakashima M, Livolsi V. Thyroid papillary carcinoma with solid sclerosing change in IgG4-related sclerosing disease. Pathol Int. 2011;61:589–92.
32. Balkwill F, Mantovani A. Inflammation and cancer: back to Virchow? Lancet. 2001;357:539–45.
33. Bansal P, Sonnenberg A. Pancreatitis is a risk factor for pancreatic cancer. Gastroenterology. 1995;109:247–51.
34. Guerra C, Collado M, Navas C, Schuhmacher AJ, Hernández-Porras I, Cañamero M, Rodriguez-Justo M, Serrano M, Barbacid M. Pancreatitis-induced inflammation contributes to pancreatic cancer by inhibiting oncogene-induced senescence. Cancer Cell. 2011;19:728–39.

35. Lowenfels AB, Maisonneuve P, Cavallini G, Ammann RW, Lankisch PG, Andersen JR, Dimagno EP, Andrén-Sandberg A, Domellöf L. Pancreatitis and the risk of pancreatic cancer. International Pancreatitis Study Group. N Engl J Med. 1993;328:1433–7.
36. Yan L, Mcfaul C, Howes N, Leslie J, Lancaster G, Wong T, Threadgold J, Evans J, Gilmore I, Smart H, Lombard M, Neoptolemos J, Greenhalf W. Molecular analysis to detect pancreatic ductal adenocarcinoma in high-risk groups. Gastroenterology. 2005;128:2124–30.
37. Bardeesy N, Depinho RA. Pancreatic cancer biology and genetics. Nat Rev Cancer. 2002;2:897–909.
38. Hruban RH, Adsay NV, Albores-Saavedra J, Compton C, Garrett ES, Goodman SN, Kern SE, Klimstra DS, Klöpel G, Longnecker DS, Lütges J, Offerhaus GJ. Pancreatic intraepithelial neoplasia: a new nomenclature and classification system for pancreatic duct lesions. Am J Surg Pathol. 2001;25:579–86.
39. Takaori K, Hruban RH, Maitra A, Tanigawa N. Pancreatic intraepithelial neoplasia. Pancreas. 2004;28:257–62.
40. Collins MA, Bednar F, Zhang Y, Brisset JC, Galbá S, Galbá CJ, Rakshit S, Flannagan KS, Adsay NV, Pasca di magliano M. Oncogenic Kras is required for both the initiation and maintenance of pancreatic cancer in mice. J Clin Invest. 2012;122:639–53.
41. Hingorani SR, Petricoin EF, Maitra A, Rajapakse V, King C, Jacobetz MA, Ross S, Conrads TP, Veenstra TD, Hitt BA, Kawaguchi Y, Johann D, Liotta LA, Crawford HC, Putt ME, Jacks T, Wright CV, Hruban RH, Lowy AM, Tuveson DA. Preinvasive and invasive ductal pancreatic cancer and its early detection in the mouse. Cancer Cell. 2003;4:437–50.
42. Jones S, Zhang X, Parsons DW, Lin JC, Leary RJ, Angenendt P, Mankoo P, Carter H, Kamiyama H, Jimeno A, Hong SM, Fu B, Lin MT, Calhoun ES, Kamiyama M, Walter K, Nikolskaya T, Nikolsky Y, Hartigan J, Smith DR, Hidalgo M, Leach SD, Klein AP, Jaffee EM, Goggins M, Maitra A, Iacobuzio-Donahue C, Eshleman JR, Kern SE, Hruban RH, Karchin R, Papadopoulos N, Parmigiani G, Vogelstein B, Velculescu VE, Kinzler KW. Core signaling pathways in human pancreatic cancers revealed by global genomic analyses. Science. 2008;321:1801–6.
43. Kanda M, Matthaei H, Wu J, Hong SM, Yu J, Borges M, Hruban RH, Maitra A, Kinzler K, Vogelstein B, Goggins M. Presence of somatic mutations in most early-stage pancreatic intraepithelial neoplasia. Gastroenterology. 2012;142:730–3.
44. Kamisawa T, Horiguchi S, Hayashi Y, Yun X, Yamaguchi T, Tsuruta K, Sasaki T. K-ras mutation in the major duodenal papilla and gastric and colonic mucosa in patients with autoimmune pancreatitis. J Gastroenterol. 2010;45:771–8.
45. Okazaki K, Uchida K, Fukui T. Recent advances in autoimmune pancreatitis: concept, diagnosis, and pathogenesis. J Gastroenterol. 2008;43:409–18.
46. Zen Y, Fujii T, Harada K, Kawano M, Yamada K, Takahira M, Nakanuma Y. Th2 and regulatory immune reactions are increased in immunoglobin G4-related sclerosing pancreatitis and cholangitis. Hepatology. 2007;45:1538–46.
47. Apetoh L, Ghiringhelli F, Tesniere A, Obeid M, Ortiz C, Criollo A, Mignot G, Maiuri MC, Ullrich E, Saulnier P, Yang H, Amigorena S, Ryffel B, Barrat FJ, Saftig P, Levi F, Lidereau R, Nogues C, Mira JP, Chompret A, Joulin V, Clavel-Chapelon F, Bourhis J, André F, Delaloge S, Tursz T, Kroemer G, Zitvogel L. Toll-like receptor 4-dependent contribution of the immune system to anticancer chemotherapy and radiotherapy. Nat Med. 2007;13:1050–9.
48. Casares N, Pequignot MO, Tesniere A, Ghiringhelli F, Roux S, Chaput N, Schmitt E, Hamai A, Hervas-Stubbs S, Obeid M, Coutant F, Méivier D, Pichard E, Aucouturier P, Pierron G, Garrido C, Zitvogel L, Kroemer G. Caspase-dependent immunogenicity of doxorubicin-induced tumor cell death. J Exp Med. 2005;202:1691–701.
49. Granville CA, Memmott RM, Balogh A, Mariotti J, Kawabata S, Han W, Lopiccolo J, Foley J, Liewehr DJ, Steinberg SM, Fowler DH, Hollander MC, Dennis PA. A central role for Foxp3+ regulatory T cells in K-Ras-driven lung tumorigenesis. PLoS One. 2009;4:e5061.
50. Moo-Young TA, Larson JW, Belt BA, Tan MC, Hawkins WG, Eberlein TJ, Goedegebuure PS, Linehan DC. Tumor-derived TGF-beta mediates conversion of CD4+Foxp3+ regulatory T cells in a murine model of pancreas cancer. J Immunother. 2009;32:12–21.
51. Zintzaras E, Voulgarelis M, Moutsopoulos HM. The risk of lymphoma development in autoimmune diseases: a meta-analysis. Arch Intern Med. 2005;165:2337–44.

Part V

AIP in the World

International Survey of Autoimmune Pancreatitis

27

Terumi Kamisawa, Myung-Hwan Kim, and Jae Bock Chung

Introduction

Since the concept of autoimmune pancreatitis (AIP) was proposed by Yoshida et al. [1] in 1995, it has developed predominantly in Japan, with the diagnostic emphasis on the clinical phenotype. The characteristic histological finding of AIP is lymphoplasmacytic sclerosing pancreatitis (LPSP) [2]. From 2000, many AIP cases have been reported in Western countries and Korea, and AIP is now a distinct entity that is recognized worldwide [3, 4]. Another type of AIP, called idiopathic duct-centric pancreatitis (IDCP) [5] or AIP with granulocyte epithelial lesion (GEL) [6], was reported from Western countries in 2003 and 2004, respectively. Currently, AIP is classified into two subtypes: type 1 (LPSP) and type 2 (IDCP) [7].

In 2002, the "diagnostic criteria for autoimmune pancreatitis" [8] were established by the Japan Pancreas Society. These criteria were later revised in 2006 [9] and 2011 [10]. In 2006, diagnostic criteria for AIP were proposed from Korea [11] and the United States [12]. In 2008, Japanese and Korean pancreatologists developed the Asian diagnostic criteria for AIP [13]. In 2011, following several international consensus meetings, the international consensus diagnostic criteria (ICDC) were developed to incorporate the diagnostic strategies used in the different criteria, in consideration of the differences in clinical practice around the globe [14].

To clarify the global clinical and pathophysiological characteristics of AIP, international multicenter surveys of AIP have been performed three times.

T. Kamisawa, MD, PhD (✉)
Department of Internal Medicine,
Tokyo Metropolitan Komagome Hospital,
3-18-22 Honkomagome, Bunkyo-ku,
Tokyo 113-8677, Japan
e-mail: kamisawa@cick.jp

M.-H. Kim, MD, PhD
Department of Gastroenterology, Asan Medical Center,
University of Ulsan College of Medicine, Seoul, Korea

J.B. Chung, MD, PhD
Department of Internal Medicine, Yonsei University College of Medicine, Yonsei Institute of Gastroenterology,
Seoul, Republic of Korea

First International Survey of AIP

The first international survey of AIP was conducted in 10 centers of 5 Asian countries (Japan, Korea, Taiwan, China, and India) in 2009, with publication of the results in 2011 [15]. A total of 327 AIP cases (258 males, 69 females; average age 60.0 years) diagnosed by Asian diagnostic criteria [13] was enrolled.

The most frequent initial symptom was obstructive jaundice (46–74 %), followed by weight loss (4–51 %) and abdominal pain (19–44 %). Diffuse swelling of the pancreas was frequent in Japan (64 %) and Korea (81 %), but segmental swelling of the pancreas was more frequent in Taiwan (70 %) and China (72 %) ($p<0.01$). Increased serum IgG4 levels were seen in 58–100 % of cases in Japan, Korea, and Taiwan. Pathologically, almost all AIP cases in Asia were diagnosed as LPSP. The most frequent extrapancreatic lesion was sclerosing cholangitis (60–81 %). Steroid therapy was the major and effective therapeutic strategy in Japan, Korea, and Taiwan. However, the rate of resection or bypass operation was higher in Taiwan (40 %) and China (72 %) ($p<0.01$) (Table 27.1).

Japan, Korea, Taiwan, and China are geographically adjacent; their populations appear to share a common genetic background, and the features of AIP patients are fundamentally similar in these countries. Differences in the clinical and pathophysiological characteristics of AIP in these areas may be due to differences in the rates of recognition of this disease. Recognition of AIP should be more widespread in Asia to avoid unnecessary surgery.

T. Kamisawa, J.B. Chung (eds.), *Autoimmune Pancreatitis*,
DOI 10.1007/978-3-642-55086-7_27, © Springer-Verlag Berlin Heidelberg 2015

Table 27.1 Clinicopathological findings in the first international survey of AIP

	Japan	Korea	Taiwan	China
Number of patients	137	118	47	25
Average age (years)	62.2	57.2	64.9	54.0
Gender (% male)	109 (80 %)	85 (72 %)	42 (89 %)	22 (88 %)
Initial symptom				
Obstructive jaundice	62 (46 %)	64 (54 %)	35 (74 %)	18 (72 %)
Weight loss	5 (4 %)	41 (35 %)	24 (51 %)	10 (40 %)
Abdominal pain	26 (19 %)	34 (29 %)	8 (17 %)	11 (44 %)
Diffuse pancreatic swelling	87 (64 %)	96 (81 %)	14 (30 %)	7 (28 %)
Elevation of serum IgG4	95/111 (86 %)	50/86 (58 %)	28/28 (100 %)	0/0
Number of LPSP cases	21	30	23	10
Resected specimen	10	13	17	6
Biopsied specimen	11	17	6	4
Sclerosing cholangitis	82 (60 %)	95 (81 %)	35 (74 %)	18 (72 %)
Lower bile duct	78	84	35	18
Hilar bile duct	9	6	0	8
Intrahepatic bile duct	11	8	0	0
Sclerosing sialadenitis	30 (22 %)	8 (7 %)	0	1 (4 %)
Retroperitoneal fibrosis	9 (7 %)	15 (13 %)	0	1 (4 %)
Treatment				
Steroid	101 (74 %)	101 (86 %)	33 (70 %)	4 (16 %)
Resection	12 (9 %)	7 (6 %)	19 (40 %)	4 (16 %)
Bypass operation	5 (4 %)	6 (5 %)	0	14 (56 %)
Follow-up	22 (16 %)	4 (3 %)	0	3 (12 %)
Steroid responsiveness	101 (100 %)	101 (100 %)	23 (70 %)	4 (100 %)
Relapse after steroid	7/93 (8 %)	19/101 (19 %)	1/33 (3 %)	2/4 (50 %)

Redesigned from Ref. [15]

Second International Survey of AIP

The second international, multicenter survey of AIP was conducted in 15 institutes from eight countries (Japan, Korea, Taiwan, India, the United States, Germany, Italy, and the United Kingdom) in 2010 and was published in 2011 [16]. A total of 731 AIP cases was enrolled, with 204 cases confirmed histologically as LPSP and 64 cases confirmed as IDCP. The AIP cases were diagnosed according to Asian diagnostic criteria [13] in Japan, Korea, and Taiwan; according to the HISORt criteria [12] in the United States, the United Kingdom, and India; according to the Mannheim criteria [17] and Asian criteria [13] in Germany; and according to the Italian criteria [18] in Italy.

LPSP patients were approximately 16 years older than IDCP patients (average age of all patients in the cohorts, 61.6 years vs. 44.8 years, respectively). No sex difference was observed between the 2 groups. Obstructive jaundice was a more frequent presentation in LPSP than in IDCP (75 % vs. 47 %, $p<0.001$), whereas abdominal pain (41 % vs. 68 %, $p<0.001$) and acute pancreatitis (5 % vs. 34 %, $p<0.001$) were more frequent presentations in IDCP patients. Compared to IDCP patients, LPSP patients were more likely to have diffuse pancreatic swellings (40 % vs. 25 %, $p=0.037$), increased serum IgG4 levels (63 % vs. 23 %, $p<0.001$), retroperitoneal fibrosis (7 % vs. 0 %, $p=0.035$), salivary gland swelling (12 % vs. 0 %, $p=0.002$), and extensive lymphadenopathy (8 % vs. 0 %, $p=0.020$), but they were less likely to have ulcerative colitis (1 % vs. 16 %, $p<0.001$). IDCP patients more frequently underwent surgery (60 % vs. 78 %, $p=0.010$). Good therapeutic responses to steroid treatment were seen in both groups, but IDCP patients had a significantly lower relapse rate (36 % vs. 5 %, $p=0.007$). The clinical profiles of LPSP and IDCP patients were distinctly different. IDCP patients tended to have focal features, and they more frequently underwent surgical resection due to diagnostic difficulty (Table 27.2).

In non-histologically confirmed AIP patients, the average age at diagnosis ranged from 43.4 to 66.4 years, and the percentage of male patients ranged from 45 to 90 %. The most frequent initial symptom in six countries was obstructive jaundice, but it was less frequent in Italy (44 %) and Germany (13 %). Abdominal pain was the most frequent initial symptom in India (86 %) and Germany (63 %). Acute pancreatitis was seen frequently in Germany (66 %) and Italy (32 %). Diffuse pancreatic swelling was frequent in Korea (85 %), Japan (58 %), and the United States (57 %). However, segmental swelling of the pancreas was more frequent in the other five countries. Increased serum IgG4 levels were

Table 27.2 Comparison of clinical profiles of LPSP and IDCP patients in the second international survey

	LPSP	IDCP	*p* value
Number of cases	204	64	
Average age (years)	61.6	44.8	
Gender (% male)	151 (74 %)	47 (73 %)	
Initial symptom			
Jaundice	116/154 (75 %)	30 (47 %)	<.001
Abdominal pain	63/154 (41 %)	43 (68 %)	<.001
Acute pancreatitis	11/204 (5 %)	22 (34 %)	<.001
Diffuse pancreatic swelling	81 (40 %)	16 (25 %)	.037
Elevation of serum IgG4	100/160 (63 %)	11/47 (23 %)	<.001
Other organ involvement			
Total involved cases	85/190 (45 %)	24 (38 %)	
Proximal bile duct	45/153 (29 %)	15 (23 %)	
Renal lesions	13/153 (8 %)	2 (3 %)	
Retroperitoneal fibrosis	10/153 (7 %)	0	.035
Salivary (lacrimal) glands	18/153 (12 %)	0	.002
Extensive lymphadenopathy	12/153 (8 %)	0	.020
Ulcerative colitis	2/153 (1 %)	10 (16 %)	<.001
Histological examination			
Resection	123 (60 %)	50 (78 %)	.010
Biopsy	81 (40 %)	14 (22 %)	
Steroid therapy			
Steroid	90 (44 %)	21 (33 %)	
Response rate	100 %	100 %	
Relapse rate	32/90 (36 %)	1/21 (5 %)	.007

Redesigned from Ref. [16]

detected in 85–100 % of AIP patients in Japan, Taiwan, India, and the United States, but only in 50–61 % in other countries. Other organ involvement was present in 15–82 % of AIP patients. Other organ involvement was most frequently sclerosing cholangitis of the proximal bile duct in the United Kingdom (79 %), the United States (46 %), Germany (26 %), Taiwan (25 %), and India (19 %), salivary or lacrimal gland swelling in Japan (21 %), and retroperitoneal fibrosis in Korea (16 %). Italian AIP patients rarely showed other organ involvement, but they frequently had ulcerative colitis (30 %). Steroids were given in 69–100 % of AIP patients. The initial prednisolone dose was 1 mg/kg/day in three countries, 0.6 mg/kg/day in two countries, and 30–40 mg/day in the remaining three countries. This dose was tapered by 5 mg every 1–2 weeks. The time from initiation to cessation of steroid therapy ranged from 3 months to 2 years. All patients showed good responses to steroid treatment. The relapse rate in steroid-treated patients ranged from 15 to 64 % (Table 27.3).

Comparing the clinical profiles of non-histologically confirmed AIP patients among the eight countries, the profiles in the four Asian countries showed broad similarities. The United States and the United Kingdom showed similar profiles to those in Asia, except for a high rate of sclerosing cholangitis of the proximal bile duct in the United Kingdom. The clinical profiles seen in these six countries were similar to those of LPSP patients. However, Italian AIP patients had quite different clinical profiles, being younger with a relatively high proportion of women, a low prevalence of increased serum IgG4 levels, frequent associations with acute pancreatitis and ulcerative colitis, and rare involvement of other organs. German AIP patients were also younger with a high proportion of women and frequent association with abdominal pain and acute pancreatitis. The Italian and Mannheim criteria show a mixture of features of LPSP and IDCP, and they can diagnose both entities. The clinical profile of Italian AIP patients suggests that a fair proportion of Italian AIP patients have IDCP. German AIP patients also appear to include a mixture of LPSP and IDCP.

Due to the differences in the practice patterns with respect to the diagnostic tests used and their perceived accuracy for the diagnosis of AIP worldwide, the diagnostic approach to AIP shows significant heterogeneity.

Third International Survey of AIP

The third international, multicenter survey of AIP was conducted in 23 institutes from 10 countries (Japan, Korea, Taiwan, the United States, Germany, Italy, the United Kingdom, Hungary, Sweden, and France) in 2012, and its results were published in 2013 [19]. The patients who were

Table 27.3 Clinical, radiological, and serological features of non-histologically confirmed AIP patients in the second international survey

Country	Japan	Korea	Taiwan	India	The United States	Germany	Italy	The United Kingdom
Number of patients	127	86	33	36	28	38	87	28
Average age, years	64.7	59.0	66.4	NA	64.1	45.5	43.4	57.6
Gender (% male)	106 (83 %)	61 (71 %)	29 (90 %)	25 (69 %)	22 (79 %)	17 (45 %)	54 (62 %)	23 (82 %)
Initial symptom								
Jaundice	77 (61 %)	43 (50 %)	23 (70 %)	20 (56 %)	22 (79 %)	5 (13 %)	38 (44 %)	18 (64 %)
Abdominal pain	16 (13 %)	20 (23 %)	6 (18 %)	31 (86 %)	14 (50 %)	24 (63 %)	17 (20 %)	5 (18 %)
Acute pancreatitis	3 (2 %)	11 (13 %)	6 (18 %)	8 (22 %)	7 (25 %)	25 (66 %)	28 (32 %)	0
Diffuse pancreatic swelling	74 (58 %)	73 (85 %)	13 (39 %)	15 (41 %)	16 (57 %)	18 (47 %)	32 (37 %)	5 (18 %)
Elevation of serum IgG4	102/112 (91 %)	32/62 (52 %)	28/28 (100 %)	36/36 (100 %)	22/26 (85 %)	19/31 (61 %)	28/56 (50 %)	15/28 (54 %)
OOI								
Total involvement	80 (63 %)	35 (41 %)	(33 %)	11 (31 %)	21 (75 %)	17 (44 %)	13 (15 %)	23 (82 %)
Proximal bile duct	13 (10 %)	9 (10 %)	(25 %)	7 (19 %)	13 (46 %)	10 (26 %)	rare	22 (79 %)
Renal lesions	11 (9 %)	9 (10 %)	(4 %)	0	7 (25 %)	0	2 (2 %)	5 (18 %)
Retroperitoneal fibrosis	5 (4 %)	14 (16 %)	(4 %)	2 (6 %)	4 (14 %)	0	2 (2 %)	2 (7 %)
Salivary/lacrimal	27 (21 %)	7 (8 %)	(17 %)	1 (3 %)	2 (7 %)	1 (3 %)	4 (5 %)	3 (11 %)
Extensive LN	27 (21 %)	6 (7 %)	(17 %)	1 (3 %)	2 (7 %)	0	NA	5 (8 %)
Ulcerative colitis	4 (3 %)	3 (3 %)	0	2 (6 %)	3 (11 %)	0	26 (30 %)	4 (14 %)
Initial therapy								
Steroid	84 %	85 %	100 %	100 %	89 %	71 %	69 %	93 %
Response rate	100 %	100 %	100 %	100 %	100 %	100 %	100 %	100 %
Relapse rate	15 %	26 %	18 %	25 %	64 %	15 %	37 %	54 %

Redesigned from Ref. [16]
NA not available, *OOI* other organ involvement

diagnosed using the ICDC [14] were examined focusing on long-term outcomes, including organ involvement, treatments, relapse frequency, and long-term sequelae.

A total of 1,064 patients meeting the ICDC for type 1 ($n=978$) or type 2 ($n=86$) was included. The subjects' average ages at the time of diagnosis were 61.4 and 39.9 years for type 1 and type 2 subjects, respectively. The proportion of males was 77 % among type 1 subjects and 55 % among type 2 subjects ($p<0.001$). The proportion of patients diagnosed with type 2 AIP was lower in Asian countries (3.7 %) than in both European (12.9 %, $p<0.001$) and North American (13.7 %, $p<0.001$) countries.

The majority (74 %) of subjects with type 1 AIP were treated initially with steroids, rather than surgical or conservative treatments, while only 62 % of type 2 subjects were treated with steroids ($p=0.01$). Almost all subjects with types 1 and 2 AIP achieved remission. Prior to steroid treatment, biliary stenting was required for most subjects presenting with jaundice (type 1, 71 %; type 2, 77 %). In subjects with type 1 AIP, the most common indication was jaundice (63 %), followed by abdominal pain with or without biochemical pancreatitis. In subjects with type 2 AIP, the major indications were abdominal pain and inflammatory bowel disease (Table 27.4). In subjects with type 1 AIP and abnormal serum IgG4 levels ($n=446$) before steroid therapy, the serum IgG4 level decreased in 427 (95.7 %) and returned to being within normal limits in 204 (45.7 %).

Of the 978 subjects with type 1 disease, 302 (31 %) experienced at least one disease relapse, compared to 8 (9 %, $p<0.001$) with type 2 AIP. The vast majority of relapse episodes occurred in steroid-treated subjects after steroid discontinuation (67 %), rather than during the steroid taper (15 %) or during maintenance steroid therapy (18 %). Most relapses occurred in the biliary system or pancreas for type 1 AIP cases, while relapses in type 2 AIP cases were limited to the pancreas. Relapse occurred several times in type 1 AIP, but type 2 AIP relapsed only once (Table 27.5). Overall, 56.1 % (96/171) of subjects with IgG4-related SC had at least one relapse, while only 25.7 % (142/551) of subjects without IgG4-related SC relapsed. Steroid retreatment remained effective for inducing remission with or without alternative treatment, such as azathioprine.

Compared to subjects who never had a relapse, pancreatic duct stones were more likely in subjects with at least one relapse (14.4 % vs. 4.0 %, respectively). During follow-up, frequently occurring cancers included gastric ($n=11$), pulmonary ($n=9$), prostate ($n=7$), colonic ($n=5$), and pancreatic ($n=5$) cancers. Pancreatic cancer was diagnosed in five male patients at a median age of 77 years (range 65–80 years), and it occurred at a median of 5 years (range 0.7–7 years) from the time of AIP diagnosis.

Table 27.4 Initial treatment strategies and treatment details for those treated with steroids in the third international survey

	Type 1 AIP ($n=901$)		Type 2 AIP ($n=85$)		
	Successful remission, *n*	%	Successful remission, *n*	%	*p* value
Initial treatment:					
Steroids	681/684	99.6	48/52	92.3	NS
Surgical resection	125/127	98.4	17/25	68.0	NS
Palliative surgical bypass	22/23	95.7	1/2	50.0	NS
Conservative	37/67	55.2	4/6	66.7	NS

	Type 1 AIP ($n=724$)		Type 2 AIP ($n=53$)		
	n	%	*n*	%	*p* value
Indications for steroid treatment:					
Jaundice	458	63	13	25	<0.001
Pancreatitis/abdominal pain	198	27	34	64	<0.001
Inflammatory bowel disease	1	0.1	23	48	<0.001
Endoscopic management (for subjects with jaundice):					
Biliary stent placement	351/492	71	10/13	77	NS

Redesigned from Ref. [19]

Table 27.5 Relapse episodes, location and frequency in the third international survey

	Type 1 AIP		Type 2 AIP	
	Relapse, *n*	%	Relapse, *n*	%
Initial treatment				
Steroids	245/684	35.8	8/52	15.3
Surgical resection	35/116	30.2	0/25	0
Disease relapses following steroid treatment:				
Location of relapse:	*n=245 episodes*		*n=8 episodes*	
Biliary system	124	50.6	–	–
Pancreas	107	42.9	8	100
Salivary	18	7.3	–	–
Frequency per subject:				
1 relapse	189	77.1	8	100
2 relapses	39	15.9	–	–
3 relapses	13	5.3	–	–
≥4 relapses	4	1.6	–	–

Redesigned from Ref. [19]

Conclusion

International surveys of AIP showed the regional and ethnic differences in the pathological and clinical features of AIP and the quite different profiles of type 1 and type 2 AIP. To improve our understanding of this disease, further multinational collaborations are required.

References

1. Yoshida K, Toki F, Takeuchi T, Watanabe S, Shiratori K, Hayashi N. Chronic pancreatitis caused by an autoimmune abnormality. Proposal of the concept of autoimmune pancreatitis. Dig Dis Sci. 1995;40:1561–8.
2. Kawaguchi K, Koike M, Tsuruta K, Okamoto A, Tsuruta K, Fujita N. Lymphoplasmacytic sclerosing pancreatitis with cholangitis: a variant of primary sclerosing cholangitis extensively involving pancreas. Hum Pathol. 1991;22:387–95.
3. Kamisawa T, Takuma K, Egawa N, Tsuruta K, Sasaki T. Autoimmune pancreatitis and IgG4-related sclerosing disease. Nat Rev Gastroenterol Hepatol. 2010;7:401–9.
4. Kamisawa T, Chari ST, Lerch MM, Kim MH, Gress TM, Shimosegawa T. Recent advances in autoimmune pancreatitis: type 1 and type 2. Gut. 2013;62:1373–80.
5. Notohara K, Burgart LJ, Yadav D, Chari S, Smyrk TC. Idiopathic chronic pancreatitis with periductal lymphoplasmacytic infiltration. Clinicopathologic features of 35 cases. Am J Surg Pathol. 2003;27:1119–27.
6. Zamboni G, Luttges J, Capelli P, et al. Histopathological features of diagnostic and clinical relevance in autoimmune pancreatitis: a study on 53 resection specimens and 9 biopsy specimens. Virchows Arch. 2004;445:552–63.
7. Sah RP, Chari ST, Pannala R, et al. Differences in clinical profile and relapse rate of type 1 versus type 2 autoimmune pancreatitis. Gastroenterology. 2010;139:140–8.
8. Members of the Criteria Committee for Autoimmune Pancreatitis of the Japan Pancreas Society. Diagnostic criteria for autoimmune pancreatitis by the Japan Pancreas Society (in Japanese). Suizou. 2002;17:585–7.

9. Okazaki K, Kawa S, Kamisawa T, et al. Clinical diagnostic criteria of autoimmune pancreatitis: revised proposal. J Gastroenterol. 2006;41:626–31.
10. Shimosegawa T, Working Group Members of the Japan Pancreas Society; Research Committee for Intractable Pancreatic Disease by the Ministry of Labor. Health and welfare of Japan. Pancreas. 2012;41:1341–2.
11. Kim KP, Kim MH, Kim JC, et al. Diagnostic criteria for autoimmune chronic pancreatitis revised. World J Gastroenterol. 2006;12:2487–96.
12. Chari ST, Smyrk TC, Levy MJ, et al. Autoimmune pancreatitis: diagnosis using histology, imaging, serology, other organ involvement and response to steroids. Clin Gastroenterol Hepatol. 2006;4:1010–6.
13. Otsuki M, Chung JB, Okazaki K, et al. Asian diagnostic criteria for autoimmune pancreatitis: consensus of the Japan-Korea symposium on autoimmune pancreatitis. J Gastroenterol. 2008;43:403–8.
14. Shimosegawa T, Chari ST, Frulloni L, et al. International consensus diagnostic criteria for autoimmune pancreatitis: guidelines of the international association of pancreatology. Pancreas. 2011;40:352–8.
15. Kamisawa T, Kim MH, Liao WC, et al. Clinical characteristics of 327 Asian patients with autoimmune pancreatitis based on Asian diagnostic criteria. Pancreas. 2011;40:200–5.
16. Kamisawa T, Chari ST, Giday SA, et al. Clinical profile of autoimmune pancreatitis and its histological subtypes: an international multicenter survey. Pancreas. 2011;40:352–8.
17. Schneider A, Lohr JM, Singer MV. The M-ANNHEIM classification of chronic pancreatitis: introduction of a unifying classification system based on a review of previous classifications of the disease. J Gastroenterol. 2007;42:101–19.
18. Frulloni L, Scattolini C, Falconi M, et al. Autoimmune pancreatitis: differences between the focal and diffuse forms in 87 patients. Am J Gastroenterol. 2009;104:2288–94.
19. Hart PA, Kamisawa T, Brugge WR, et al. Long-term outcomes of autoimmune pancreatitis: a multicentre, international analysis. Gut. 2012;62:1771–6.

28 Autoimmune Pancreatitis in the USA

Raghuwansh P. Sah, Nazir Ahmed, Philip A. Hart, and Suresh T. Chari

Introduction

Autoimmune pancreatitis (AIP) is a fibroinflammatory disease of the pancreas which has been recognized and characterized predominantly in the last decade. Previous chapters in this book have introduced and extensively presented the features, associations, diagnosis, treatment, and prognosis of AIP. In this chapter, we aim to provide the readers with a historical account of recognition of AIP and developments regarding this disease in the USA. Further, we will summarize the profile of AIP patients in the USA and discuss clinical practice in the USA regarding their diagnosis and management highlighting the salient differences with respect to the Japanese and Korean practice guidelines.

Progress in AIP: A Historical Perspective

Earliest account of the fibrosclerosing disease of the pancreas with marked inflammatory infiltrate that retrospectively appears to be AIP can be traced back to 1960s by the French group of Sarles et al. [1, 2] which were grouped under chronic inflammatory pancreatitis in the 1988 Marseilles-Rome Pancreatitis Classification [3]. The term autoimmune pancreatitis was introduced in 1995 by Yoshida et al. based on autoimmune etiology-suggestive associations identified in their Japanese cohort [4]. In 1997, the term nonalcoholic duct destructive pancreatitis (NADDP) was used by Ectors et al. [5] in their European cohort. The Japanese formalized their experience with AIP with the development of JPS minimum diagnostic criteria by 2002 [6] after publication of several Japanese cohorts [7–11] including the recognition of serum immunoglobulin subtype 4 (IgG4) elevations [11].

In this section, we will continue the discussion on the historical developments in the USA. While we aim to highlight key contributions from the USA, this is by no means intended to undermine contributions from across the globe which have been extensively reviewed in the preceding chapters and the following chapter on AIP in Europe.

Early Reports of Multifocal Fibrosis from the USA

In 1963, Bartholomew et al. [12] described two cases from Mayo Clinic of sclerosing cholangitis with fibrosis affecting multiple organs. This report had first descriptions of steroid responsiveness and of the recognition that multiple affected organs were manifestations of a single systemic disease. Hache et al. [13] described a cohort of 20 patients from Mayo Clinic in 1962 with fibrosing mediastinitis noting lymphocytic and plasma cell infiltration in the fibrotic tissue. In 1965, another report of sclerosing cholangitis with involvement of other organs appeared which was novel in observing elevation of gamma globulin associated with this disease [14]. The term multifocal fibrosclerosis was introduced in 1967 by Comings et al. [15] emphasizing the association of sclerosing fibrotic disease of multiple organs. Reports of multifocal fibrosclerosis continued to appear in the subsequent years [16–18] including descriptions of pancreatitis in patients with Sjogren's syndrome (reports from the UK) [19, 20], pancreatic

R.P. Sah, MD • N. Ahmed, MD • P.A. Hart, MD
S.T. Chari, MD (✉)
Division of Gastroenterology and Hepatology, Mayo Clinic, Rochester, MN 55905, USA
e-mail: Chari.Suresh@mayo.edu

T. Kamisawa, J.B. Chung (eds.), *Autoimmune Pancreatitis*,
DOI 10.1007/978-3-642-55086-7_28, © Springer-Verlag Berlin Heidelberg 2015

pseudotumor [21], and pancreatic fibrosis in multifocal fibrosclerosis and of duct destructive pancreatitis [22]. Notably, these early reports from pre-AIP recognition era were keen on observing many of the key features of what is now recognized as IgG4-related disease (discussed below) including steroid responsiveness.

Surgical Resection of Pancreatic Mass Mimicking Pancreatic Cancer

Although the existence of AIP as a disease entity was not yet fully established among the US pancreatologists, the possibility of an autoimmune chronic pancreatitis was being increasingly appreciated by 2001. This is reflected in the inclusion of an autoimmune category in the TIGAR-O etiological classification of chronic pancreatitis proposed by Whitcomb et al. in 2001 [23]. It was in the year 2003 that the first sizeable cohorts of AIP were published in the USA from Mayo Clinic [24], Memorial Sloan Kettering Cancer Center [25], and Johns Hopkins Medical School [26].

It is now well recognized that the presentation of AIP mimics that of pancreatic cancer. Not surprisingly, most of the early work on AIP globally was based on retrospective analysis of pancreas resected for presumed pancreatic cancer which turned out noncancerous. The MSKCC cohort described 31 patients with LPSP identified from 1,287 pancreatic resections performed for presumed pancreatic cancer from 1985 to 2001 [25]. The Johns Hopkins cohort described 37 patients with LPSP identified from 1,648 pancreatic resections performed for presumed pancreatic cancer from 1992 to 2002 [26]. In the Mayo Clinic cohort, 35 patients with AIP were identified based on review of pancreatic resections between 1985 and 2002 [24].

Recognition of a New Disease

These first US cohorts of AIP published in 2003 [24–26] served to capture useful data on the clinical presentation, imaging features, histological features, and postsurgical prognosis. The relatively large cohort data [24–26] helped consolidate experiences of experts from multiple centers around the world regarding the existence of this new disease entity and its features. Although AIP was well accepted in Japan by 2003, the defining features of AIP were not fully established. With data from only small case series, there remained a significant risk of enthusiastic overdiagnosis including the dreaded mistake of misdiagnosing pancreatic cancer as AIP. This was well appreciated by the experts who debated the existence of this novel disease entity and its defining features at the American Pancreatic Association Meeting held in the same year (2003) [27]. A global consensus of recognition of AIP as a distinct disease entity emerged as a result [27]. Further, a preliminary set of the defining features of AIP was also agreed upon, with recognition of the need for caution in its diagnosis due to the dreaded consequences of misdiagnoses, and the need for further data [27].

Formulation of Criteria for Diagnosis

The minimum diagnostic criteria of Japanese Pancreatic Society (JPS) (2002) were based on parenchymal and ductal imaging and histology features [6]. Emerging data over the next few years showed multiple extrapancreatic organ involvement in AIP patients (termed other organ involvement), in association with elevated serum IgG4 levels and responsiveness to steroids [28]. Further, in the cohort of AIP defined by histological criteria at Mayo Clinic, wide spectrum of clinical and imaging features were seen which would otherwise not be captured by the minimum diagnostic criteria of JPS [28]. Based on this cohort of histologically confirmed cases at Mayo Clinic, the HISORt criteria were formulated in 2006 [28]. This included *H*istology, *I*maging (parenchymal), *S*erology (IgG4 elevation), *O*ther organ involvement and *R*esponse to *t*reatment with steroids. These criteria were validated in the Mayo Clinic cohort and demonstrated to identify the full spectrum of clinical presentation of AIP [28]. The HISORt criteria continue to form the backbone of AIP diagnosis in the USA which has also been utilized in multiple subsequent published AIP cohorts [29, 30].

Multiple other diagnostic criteria have subsequently emerged from Korea [31], Europe [32], revisions of JPS criteria [33], and combined Asian criteria [34]. These criteria reflect regional variations in practice patterns as well as possible differences in clinical profile and epidemiology. Existence of multiple diagnostic criteria increases the risk of misdiagnosis due to potential diagnostic loopholes as some criteria seem more relaxed and flexible [35]. Further, these criteria, including the HISORt criteria, were not aimed at differentiating the AIP subtypes which were subsequently recognized as described below. In 2009, the revised HISORt criteria were published to differentiate AIP from pancreatic cancer [36]. These criteria were validated in a cohort of AIP and pancreatic cancer patients.

With new developments in the field of AIP as described below which included consensus on the histological and clinical features of AIP subtypes (2009–2011) [37–39], a consensus on the diagnostic criteria for AIP was reached in 2011 [40]. The International Consensus Diagnostic Criteria (ICDC) [40] incorporates most of the features of the revised HISORt criteria [36] and combines the salient features of Asian/Japanese criteria [6, 34] that include ductal imaging (ERP/MRP) as well as ampullary biopsies with IgG4 staining. The ICDC provides a unified framework that allows for regional flexibility in establishing an institutional approach for diagnosing AIP based on available expertise and local practice pattern [40], as discussed in the clinical practice section.

Other Organ Involvement and Recognition of IgG4-Related Disease (IgG4-RD)

Multiple extrapancreatic organ involvement was consistently observed in AIP patients across all cohorts globally [41–45] including the first US cohorts of 2003 [24–26] and other studies published subsequently [28–30, 46–48]. While the syndrome of multifocal fibrosclerosis had been recognized as described earlier, the association between extrapancreatic organ involvement of AIP and multifocal fibrosclerosis was not clear.

The study of Notohara et al. in 2003 suggested that LPSP, but not ICDP (recognition of the two subtypes discussed below), was associated with multiple extrapancreatic manifestations which were likely related to the entity of multifocal fibrosclerosis recognized previously [24]. In the same year, Kamisawa et al. showed that the multiple extrapancreatic organs demonstrated infiltration with IgG4-positive plasma cells similar to that in the pancreas suggesting that AIP and multifocal fibrosclerosis were related [49, 50]. Subsequently, it became clear that distinct histological changes identical to LPSP are seen in the extrapancreatic organs affected in multifocal fibrosclerosis [51]. As the affected organs consistently demonstrate IgG4-rich lymphoplasmacytic infiltrate, the concept of IgG4-related systemic disease was proposed in 2004 by Kamisawa et al. [51, 52]. Multiple organ associations perhaps encompassing all major organs have now been reported with a variety of names [53]. A consensus on nomenclature and definitions has been reached in 2012 [54], which terms this newly characterized systemic disease as IgG4-related disease (IgG4-RD) of which type 1 AIP (histological counterpart, LPSP) is the pancreatic manifestation.

Differentiating AIP from Pancreatic Cancer

Unnecessary surgical treatment can be avoided with a correct and timely diagnosis of AIP. On the other hand, since pancreatic cancer is relatively more common, there is a risk of misdiagnosing pancreatic cancer as AIP which is of grave clinical consequence as discussed in the diagnostic criteria section. Recognition of serum IgG4 elevation in AIP led to this test being proposed for distinguishing AIP from pancreatic cancer [11]. The diagnostic utility of serum IgG4 levels in differentiating AIP from pancreatic cancer was examined by Ghazale et al. in the Mayo Clinic cohort in 2007 [55]. This study found that serum IgG4 elevations (>140 mg/dl) are seen in 70–80 % of AIP patients and also in 5 % of normal population and 10 % of pancreatic cancer making it an unsuitable single marker for diagnosis [55]. Meanwhile, a strategy of 2-week steroid trial was proposed by the Korean group to differentiate AIP from pancreatic cancer [56]. However, unrestricted use of steroid trial posed a serious risk of misdiagnosis [35].

The revised HISORt criteria were formed in 2009 [36], combining the diagnostic potential of serum IgG4 with other features of AIP, and incorporated strict criteria for diagnostic use of steroid trial. These criteria were validated in a cohort of AIP and pancreatic cancer patients with 100 % sensitivity and specificity for AIP [36]. Based on the criteria, a diagnostic strategy to differentiate AIP from pancreatic cancer was proposed in 2009 [36, 57]. As described earlier, the revised HISORt criteria were incorporated into ICDC and a revised diagnostic strategy based on ICDC for distinguishing AIP from pancreatic cancer has subsequently been published [58].

Recognition of AIP Subtypes

The cohort of Notohara et al. (2003) recognized two distinct histological patterns – 23 with LPSP and 13 with IDCP among the 35 patients [24]. Two histologically distinct groups based on presence of GELs (GEL-positive cases being identical to IDCP) were also reported in the European cohort of 53 patients published in the same year [43].

While multiple extrapancreatic manifestations had been recognized in AIP patients in Asian, European, and American cohorts, Notohara et al. noted that LPSP, but not IDCP, is associated with extrapancreatic organ involvement similar to multifocal fibrosis [24]. Further, IBD was noted to be associated with GEL-positive AIP (IDCP) in the European cohort [43].

As long-term follow-up data became available in the Mayo Clinic cohort published in 2010 [47], it was clear that LPSP but not IDCP is associated with frequent relapses. In addition, in this cohort, clinical features of these two subtypes were directly compared noting salient differences [47]. This study established that IgG4 elevations in the serum are seen in LPSP but not in IDCP, IgG4-related other organ involvement is seen in LPSP but not IDCP, and patients with IDCP are younger and are more likely to present with acute pancreatitis compared to LPSP and more likely to have focal findings on parenchymal imaging [47]. Thus, it was clear that distinct histological subtypes LPSP and IDCP had distinctive clinical correlates [47]. This was debated in the joint meeting of APA and JPS in 2009, leading to the consensus of recognizing two subtypes of AIP with the abovementioned clinical phenotypes termed type 1 and type 2 AIP, respectively [37].

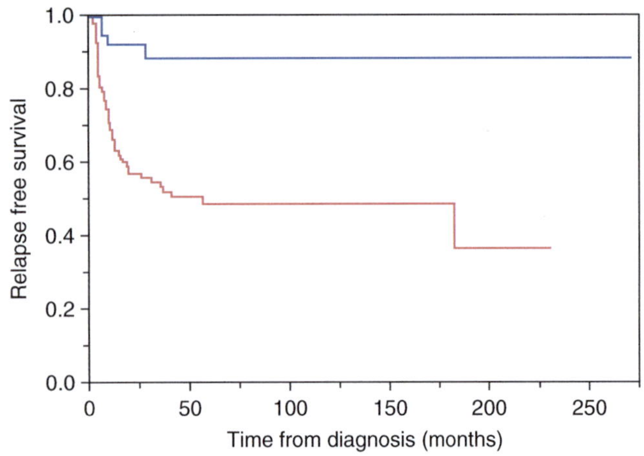

Fig. 28.1 Rates of relapse in type 1 and type 2 AIP. Kaplan-Meier survival curves for relapse-free survival following diagnosis for type 1 AIP (*red line*) compared to type 2 AIP (*blue line*) are shown. Relapse-free survival is significantly longer in those with type 2 AIP ($p<0.001$, using Wilcoxon test)

The histological diagnostic criteria for LPSP and IDCP were reviewed and consensus reached in 2010–2011 [37–39]. These paved way for the consensus diagnostic criteria of 2011 described previously [40].

Strategies for Treatment

The incidence of surgical resections has declined significantly after 2003 with increasing recognition of this disease [48]. However, strategies of steroid treatment have been highly variable across centers and regions. Our strategy of steroid treatment with short course followed by taper after disease remission (details discussed below) was optimized and validated in the Mayo Clinic cohort published in 2007 [59]. The use of immunomodulators for maintenance treatment for relapsing and use of rituximab for refractory disease or as steroid-sparing agent have been described in Hart et al. [60] recently and discussed elsewhere in this book.

Long-Term Follow-Up Results

Long-term follow-up data from the Mayo Clinic cohort were first published for the IgG4-associated cholangitis (IAC) cohort in 2008 [46] and for AIP cohort in 2010 [47] and 2012 [48]. These studies showed that relapses are common in type 1 AIP but not in type 2 AIP, and patients with IAC (or proximal bile duct involvement) have a much higher risk of relapse. An updated data on relapse rates in AIP in our cohort is shown in Fig. 28.1. Importantly, when long-term survival of AIP patients was compared to matched general population, no differences were found which for the first time showed the benign long-term prognosis of both subtypes of AIP [47]. Cumulative incidence of malignancies was observed in the recent international multicenter cohort of AIP [48] but no matched controls were available to compare the cumulative risk of cancer. Another recent study from the Mayo Clinic cohort showed no increase in immediate pre- or post-diagnosis risk of cancers compared to matched controls [61].

Profile of AIP in the USA

The profile of AIP patients in the Mayo Clinic cohort is presented in Table 28.1. A comparison to the profile of AIP cohorts from across the world, performed in an international survey [62], is presented in detail in the previous chapter.

Clinical Practices Regarding AIP in the USA

In this section, we summarize the salient differences in clinical practices regarding diagnosis and management of AIP in the USA as compared to Asian/Japanese strategy described in separate chapters in this book.

Diagnosis of AIP

One important difference in the diagnosis strategy lies in the utility of pancreatic core biopsies. EUS-guided pancreatic core biopsies are routinely performed at our center [63] and have also been routinely done at many other centers in the USA [64]. These are included in the HISORt criteria [28, 36]. In contrary, core biopsies are not performed frequently in Japan and thereby not required in the Asian and Japanese criteria [6, 34].

Another major contention is in the use of ductal imaging (ERP/MRP). The HISORt criteria [28, 36] does not require for ERP/MRP, while the Asian and Japanese criteria require pancreatic duct imaging by ERP/MRP [6, 34]. In the USA, routine ERP/MRP is not performed of obstructive jaundice. The diagnostic utility of ERP from the diagnosis of AIP and differentiating it from pancreatic cancer in the USA was not satisfactory in contrary to that observed in the Japanese centers [65].

The ICDC [40] includes ERP as an additional option which could supplement evidence in favor of AIP to qualify patients for a steroid trial who would otherwise need to be subjected to core biopsy. This is applicable to patients who do not have highly supportive parenchymal imaging and have some collateral evidence (other organ involvement or serum IgG4 elevations) but not sufficient for meeting criteria [40]. In our experience, only 10 % of patients would fall in this category who could be subjected to ductal imaging or

Table 28.1 Clinical profile of type 1 and type 2 AIP

Variable	Type 1 AIP (n=116)	Type 2 AIP (n=44)	p value
Age at diagnosis, mean (SD)	63.4 (13.3)	37.0 (19.2)	<0.01[a]
Male gender, n (%)	93 (80.2)	26 (59.1)	<0.01
Presenting symptoms:			
Jaundice	75 (64.7)	18 (40.9)	<0.01
Pancreatic mass	48 (41.4)	14 (31.8)	0.27
Pancreatitis	13 (11.2)	24 (54.5)	<0.01
Others	8 (6.9)	2 (4.5)	0.72[b]
Serum IgG4 status:			
>ULN, n (%)	71/99 (71.7)	2/33 (6.1)	<0.01
>2xULN, n (%)	41/99 (41.4)	0/33	<0.01
Parenchymal imaging at presentation:			
Diffuse enlargement	49 (30.6)	11 (25.0)	0.04
Focal enlargement	20 (17.2)	6 (13.6)	0.64[b]
Indeterminate (includes atypical)	27 (23.3)	23 (52.3)	<0.01
N/A	20 (17.2)	4 (9.1)	
Biliary involvement at presentation:			
Distal only	54 (46.7)	20 (45.4)	0.90
Proximal ± distal	30 (25.9)	–	<0.01[b]
None	32	24	<0.01
Other organ involvement (excluding IBD)	58 (50.4)	0	<0.01
# of relapses per patient:			–
0	63	40	
1	35	4	
≥2	18	0	
Duration of initial prednisone course, median (IQR)	2.8, 2.3–4.6	2.8, 2.1–3.1	0.94
Duration of f/u, months (SD)	57.3 (48.8)	75.9 (11.3)	0.13
Duration of f/u, years (SD)	4.8 (4.1)	6.3 (6.2)	0.13

Data of patients in the Mayo Clinic Rochester cohort of AIP patients (1986–2013) are presented here. All data are displayed as n (%), unless otherwise indicated. Comparisons are performed using chi-squared test, unless otherwise indicated

[a]Comparison using the paired t-test

[b]Comparisons using Fisher's exact t-test

core biopsy for diagnosis by ICDC thereby allowing for regional flexibility. About 20 % of patients do not have any collateral evidence and histological diagnosis is mandated in these patients regardless of parenchymal or ductal imaging.

Treatment and Follow-Up of AIP

Our protocol for initial steroid treatment is as follows: prednisone 40 mg/day for 4 weeks and tapering off by 5 mg/week to complete a course of 11 weeks. Treatment response is objectively monitored by clinical follow-up, follow-up imaging, and biochemical tests (LFT). Steroid taper is started once response to treatment is confirmed objectively [59, 60].

In our experience, about half of type 1 AIP patients do not relapse after short course of steroid treatment [60]. No maintenance therapy is necessary in these patients [60]. The major difference from Asian strategy is the need for maintenance steroid therapy [66]. Centers in Japan routinely use a prolonged maintenance therapy for up to 3 years with the logic that most patients relapse within 3 years [66]. In a multicenter study from Japan, it was shown that maintenance therapy reduced the relapse rate to 23 % from 34 % in those who weaned off steroids [66]. In our experience, the risks of universal use of maintenance steroid therapy outweigh the benefits in AIP.

Our strategy for follow-up for relapses involves close monitoring of symptoms with radiological and biochemical confirmation of relapse if symptomatic [60]. Early detection of relapses and prompt institution of treatment are recommended. Steroid retreatment with or without immunomodulators, rituximab treatment, and maintenance therapy with these agents may be necessary in 30–40 % of AIP patients with frequent relapses or refractory disease or steroid intolerance [60]. Details of treatment of relapses and maintenance therapy options are discussed extensively in an earlier chapter.

Conclusion

AIP is a fibroinflammatory disease affecting the pancreas which has recently been characterized. We have described the historical aspects, clinical profile, and practice patterns regarding AIP in the USA.

References

1. Sarles H, Sarles JC, Muratore R, et al. Chronic inflammatory sclerosis of the pancreas – an autonomous pancreatic disease? Am J Dig Dis. 1961;6:688–98.
2. Sarles H, Sarles JC, Camatte R, et al. Observations on 205 confirmed cases of acute pancreatitis, recurring pancreatitis, and chronic pancreatitis. Gut. 1965;6(6):545–59.
3. Sarles H, Adler G, Dani R, et al. The pancreatitis classification of Marseilles-Rome 1988. Scand J Gastroenterol. 1989;24(6):641–2.
4. Yoshida K, Toki F, Takeuchi T, et al. Chronic pancreatitis caused by an autoimmune abnormality. Proposal of the concept of autoimmune pancreatitis. Dig Dis Sci. 1995;40(7):1561–8.
5. Ectors N, Maillet B, Aerts R, et al. Non-alcoholic duct destructive chronic pancreatitis. Gut. 1997;41(2):263–8.
6. Society MotCCfAPotJP. Diagnostic criteria for autoimmune pancreatitis by the Japan Pancreas Society. J Jpn Pancreas Soc. 2002;17:585–7.
7. Uchida K, Okazaki K, Konishi Y, et al. Clinical analysis of autoimmune-related pancreatitis. Am J Gastroenterol. 2000;95(10):2788–94.
8. Okazaki K, Uchida K, Ohana M, et al. Autoimmune-related pancreatitis is associated with autoantibodies and a Th1/Th2-type cellular immune response. Gastroenterology. 2000;118(3):573–81.
9. Tanaka S, Kobayashi T, Nakanishi K, et al. Corticosteroid-responsive diabetes mellitus associated with autoimmune pancreatitis. Lancet. 2000;356(9233):910–1.
10. Ito T, Nakano I, Koyanagi S, et al. Autoimmune pancreatitis as a new clinical entity. Three cases of autoimmune pancreatitis with effective steroid therapy. Dig Dis Sci. 1997;42(7):1458–68.
11. Hamano H, Kawa S, Horiuchi A, et al. High serum IgG4 concentrations in patients with sclerosing pancreatitis. N Engl J Med. 2001;344(10):732–8.
12. Bartholomew LG, Cain JC, Woolner LB, et al. Sclerosing cholangitis: its possible association with Riedel's struma and fibrous retroperitonitis. Report of two cases. N Engl J Med. 1963;269:8–12.
13. Hache L, Woolner LB, Bernatz PE. Idiopathic fibrous mediastinitis. Dis Chest. 1962;41:9–25.
14. Wenger J, Gingrich GW, Mendeloff J. Sclerosing cholangitis – a manifestation of systemic disease. Increased serum gammaglobulin, follicular lymph node hyperplasia, and orbital pseudotumor. Arch Intern Med. 1965;116(4):509–14.
15. Comings DE, Skubi KB, Van Eyes J, et al. Familial multifocal fibrosclerosis. Findings suggesting that retroperitoneal fibrosis, mediastinal fibrosis, sclerosing cholangitis, Riedel's thyroiditis, and pseudotumor of the orbit may be different manifestations of a single disease. Ann Intern Med. 1967;66(5):884–92.
16. Case records of the Massachusetts General Hospital. Weekly clinicopathological exercises. Case 6-1982. A 55-year-old man with eight months of obstructive jaundice. N Engl J Med. 1982;306(6):349–58.
17. Meijer S, Hoitsma HF, Scholtmeijer R. Idiopathic retroperitoneal fibrosis in multifocal fibrosclerosis. Eur Urol. 1976;2(5):258–60.
18. Meyer S, Hausman R. Occlusive phlebitis in multifocal fibrosclerosis. Am J Clin Pathol. 1976;65(3):274–83.
19. Waldram R, Kopelman H, Tsantoulas D, et al. Chronic pancreatitis, sclerosing cholangitis, and sicca complex in two siblings. Lancet. 1975;1(7906):550–2.
20. Sood S, Fossard DP, Shorrock K. Chronic sclerosing pancreatitis in Sjogren's syndrome: a case report. Pancreas. 1995;10(4):419–21.
21. Clark A, Zeman RK, Choyke PL, et al. Pancreatic pseudotumors associated with multifocal idiopathic fibrosclerosis. Gastrointest Radiol. 1988;13(1):30–2.
22. Scully KA, Li SC, Hebert JC, et al. The characteristic appearance of non-alcoholic duct destructive chronic pancreatitis: a report of 2 cases. Arch Pathol Lab Med. 2000;124(10):1535–8.
23. Etemad B, Whitcomb DC. Chronic pancreatitis: diagnosis, classification, and new genetic developments. Gastroenterology. 2001;120(3):682–707.
24. Notohara K, Burgart LJ, Yadav D, et al. Idiopathic chronic pancreatitis with periductal lymphoplasmacytic infiltration: clinicopathologic features of 35 cases. Am J Surg Pathol. 2003;27(8):1119–27.
25. Weber SM, Cubukcu-Dimopulo O, Palesty JA, et al. Lymphoplasmacytic sclerosing pancreatitis: inflammatory mimic of pancreatic carcinoma. J Gastrointest Surg. 2003;7(1):129–37; discussion 37–9.
26. Hardacre JM, Iacobuzio-Donahue CA, Sohn TA, et al. Results of pancreaticoduodenectomy for lymphoplasmacytic sclerosing pancreatitis. Ann Surg. 2003;237(6):853–8; discussion 8–9.
27. Pearson RK, Longnecker DS, Chari ST, et al. Controversies in clinical pancreatology: autoimmune pancreatitis: does it exist? Pancreas. 2003;27(1):1–13.
28. Chari ST, Smyrk TC, Levy MJ, et al. Diagnosis of autoimmune pancreatitis: the Mayo Clinic experience. Clin Gastroenterol Hepatol. 2006;4(8):1010–6; quiz 934.
29. Raina A, Yadav D, Krasinskas AM, et al. Evaluation and management of autoimmune pancreatitis: experience at a large US center. Am J Gastroenterol. 2009;104(9):2295–306.
30. Clark CJ, Morales-Oyarvide V, Zaydfudim V, et al. Short-term and long-term outcomes for patients with autoimmune pancreatitis after pancreatectomy: a multi-institutional study. J Gastrointest Surg. 2013;17(5):899–906.
31. Kim MH, Kwon S. Diagnostic criteria for autoimmune chronic pancreatitis. J Gastroenterol. 2007;42 Suppl 18:42–9.
32. Schneider A, Lohr JM, Singer MV. The M-ANNHEIM classification of chronic pancreatitis: introduction of a unifying classification system based on a review of previous classifications of the disease. J Gastroenterol. 2007;42(2):101–19.
33. Okazaki K, Kawa S, Kamisawa T, et al. Japanese consensus guidelines for management of autoimmune pancreatitis: I. Concept and diagnosis of autoimmune pancreatitis. J Gastroenterol. 2010;45(3):249–65.
34. Otsuki M, Chung JB, Okazaki K, et al. Asian diagnostic criteria for autoimmune pancreatitis: consensus of the Japan-Korea Symposium on Autoimmune Pancreatitis. J Gastroenterol. 2008;43(6):403–8.
35. Gardner TB, Levy MJ, Takahashi N, et al. Misdiagnosis of autoimmune pancreatitis: a caution to clinicians. Am J Gastroenterol. 2009;104(7):1620–3.
36. Chari ST, Takahashi N, Levy MJ, et al. A diagnostic strategy to distinguish autoimmune pancreatitis from pancreatic cancer. Clin Gastroenterol Hepatol. 2009;7(10):1097–103.
37. Chari ST, Kloeppel G, Zhang L, et al. Histopathologic and clinical subtypes of autoimmune pancreatitis: the Honolulu consensus document. Pancreas. 2010;39(5):549–54.
38. Kloppel G, Detlefsen S, Chari ST, et al. Autoimmune pancreatitis: the clinicopathological characteristics of the subtype with granulocytic epithelial lesions. J Gastroenterol. 2010;45(8):787–93.
39. Levy MJ, Smyrk TC, Takahashi N, et al. Idiopathic duct-centric pancreatitis: disease description and endoscopic ultrasonography-guided trucut biopsy diagnosis. Pancreatology. 2011;11(1):76–80.
40. Shimosegawa T, Chari ST, Frulloni L, et al. International consensus diagnostic criteria for autoimmune pancreatitis: guidelines of the International Association of Pancreatology. Pancreas. 2011;40(3):352–8.
41. Frulloni L, Scattolini C, Falconi M, et al. Autoimmune pancreatitis: differences between the focal and diffuse forms in 87 patients. Am J Gastroenterol. 2009;104(9):2288–94.
42. Church NI, Pereira SP, Deheragoda MG, et al. Autoimmune pancreatitis: clinical and radiological features and objective response to steroid therapy in a UK series. Am J Gastroenterol. 2007;102(11):2417–25.
43. Zamboni G, Luttges J, Capelli P, et al. Histopathological features of diagnostic and clinical relevance in autoimmune pancreatitis: a

study on 53 resection specimens and 9 biopsy specimens. Virchows Arch. 2004;445(6):552–63.

44. Ryu JK, Chung JB, Park SW, et al. Review of 67 patients with autoimmune pancreatitis in Korea: a multicenter nationwide study. Pancreas. 2008;37(4):377–85.
45. Maire F, Le Baleur Y, Rebours V, et al. Outcome of patients with type 1 or 2 autoimmune pancreatitis. Am J Gastroenterol. 2011;106(1):151–6.
46. Ghazale A, Chari ST, Zhang L, et al. Immunoglobulin G4-associated cholangitis: clinical profile and response to therapy. Gastroenterology. 2008;134(3):706–15.
47. Sah RP, Chari ST, Pannala R, et al. Differences in clinical profile and relapse rate of type 1 versus type 2 autoimmune pancreatitis. Gastroenterology. 2010;139(1):140–8; quiz e12–3.
48. Hart PA, Kamisawa T, Brugge WR, et al. Long-term outcomes of autoimmune pancreatitis: a multicentre, international analysis. Gut. 2013;62(12):1771–6.
49. Kamisawa T, Funata N, Hayashi Y, et al. Close relationship between autoimmune pancreatitis and multifocal fibrosclerosis. Gut. 2003;52(5):683–7.
50. Kamisawa T. IgG4-positive plasma cells specifically infiltrate various organs in autoimmune pancreatitis. Pancreas. 2004;29(2):167–8.
51. Kamisawa T, Funata N, Hayashi Y. Lymphoplasmacytic sclerosing pancreatitis is a pancreatic lesion of IgG4-related systemic disease. Am J Surg Pathol. 2004;28(8):1114.
52. Kamisawa T, Nakajima H, Egawa N, et al. IgG4-related sclerosing disease incorporating sclerosing pancreatitis, cholangitis, sialadenitis and retroperitoneal fibrosis with lymphadenopathy. Pancreatology. 2006;6(1–2):132–7.
53. Stone JH, Zen Y, Deshpande V. IgG4-related disease. N Engl J Med. 2012;366(6):539–51.
54. Stone JH, Khosroshahi V, Deshpande V. IgG4-related disease: recommendations for the nomenclature of this condition and its individual organ system manifestations. Arthritis Rheum. 2012;64(10):3061–7.
55. Ghazale A, Chari ST, Smyrk TC, et al. Value of serum IgG4 in the diagnosis of autoimmune pancreatitis and in distinguishing it from pancreatic cancer. Am J Gastroenterol. 2007;102(8):1646–53.
56. Moon SH, Kim MH, Park DH, et al. Is a 2-week steroid trial after initial negative investigation for malignancy useful in differentiating autoimmune pancreatitis from pancreatic cancer? A prospective outcome study. Gut. 2008;57(12):1704–12.
57. Sugumar A, Chari ST. Distinguishing pancreatic cancer from autoimmune pancreatitis: a comparison of two strategies. Clin Gastroenterol Hepatol. 2009;7(11 Suppl):S59–62.
58. Sah RP, Chari ST. Autoimmune pancreatitis: an update on classification, diagnosis, natural history and management. Curr Gastroenterol Rep. 2012;14(2):95–105.
59. Ghazale A, Chari ST. Optimising corticosteroid treatment for autoimmune pancreatitis. Gut. 2007;56(12):1650–2.
60. Hart PA, Topazian MD, Witzig TE, et al. Treatment of relapsing autoimmune pancreatitis with immunomodulators and rituximab: the Mayo Clinic experience. Gut. 2013;62(11):1607–15.
61. Hart PA, Law RJ, Dierkhising RA, et al. Risk of cancer in autoimmune pancreatitis: a case-control study and review of the literature. Pancreas. 2014;43(3):417–21.
62. Kamisawa T, Chari ST, Giday SA, et al. Clinical profile of autoimmune pancreatitis and its histological subtypes: an international multicenter survey. Pancreas. 2011;40(6):809–14.
63. Levy MJ, Reddy RP, Wiersema MJ, et al. EUS-guided trucut biopsy in establishing autoimmune pancreatitis as the cause of obstructive jaundice. Gastrointest Endosc. 2005;61(3):467–72.
64. Levy MJ. Endoscopic ultrasound-guided trucut biopsy of the pancreas: prospects and problems. Pancreatology. 2007;7(2–3):163–6.
65. Sugumar A, Levy MJ, Kamisawa T, et al. Endoscopic retrograde pancreatography criteria to diagnose autoimmune pancreatitis: an international multicentre study. Gut. 2011;60(5):666–70.
66. Kamisawa T, Shimosegawa T, Okazaki K, et al. Standard steroid treatment for autoimmune pancreatitis. Gut. 2009;58(11):1504–7.

Autoimmune Pancreatitis in Europe

29

Georg Beyer, Julia Mayerle, and Markus M. Lerch

Autoimmune Pancreatitis in Europe: the Beginning

Although the first description of chronic sclerosing pancreatitis with increased serum immunoglobulin came from the group of Henri Sarles in Marseilles [1, 2], the concept of autoimmune pancreatitis as a distinct disease entity [3] as well as the early case series originated from Japan, and it took almost half a century until AIP was established as a separate variety of chronic pancreatitis in Europe.

Reports of European patients with nonalcoholic pancreatitis and pancreatitis in the context of extrapancreatic autoimmune disease from the late 1990s describe histological features which, in retrospect, are known to be characteristic for AIP [4, 5], and it became obvious that AIP could also be found among Western patients [6–9].

A large study by Klöppel et al. that included 54 specimens from pancreatic resections collected from Germany, Belgium, and Italy highlighted macroscopic and microscopic features which later found their way into various diagnostic guidelines [10], namely, narrowing of the pancreatic duct and common bile duct without upstream dilatation, lack of calcifications or pseudocysts, and the dense lymphoplasmacytic infiltrate and periductal fibrosis that can involve the exocrine tissue. It is noteworthy that in a number of these cases, "granulocytic-epithelial" lesions (GELs) were described, which were later defined as a hallmark of idiopathic duct-centric chronic pancreatitis (IDCP), the histological subtype of type 2 AIP [11].

In another series involving 53 resection specimens and nine biopsy specimens from Germany, the United States, and Italy, two subtypes could be distinguished by the presence or absence of GELs [12]. When these histological findings were correlated to the clinical characteristics, it turned out that patients with GEL-positive AIP were younger, more likely to be female and often had associated IBD. This already suggested not only a histologically but clinically distinct subtype of AIP. Curiously, these findings seemed to be unique to Western patients as GEL-positive AIP could only rarely be detected in Asian cohorts.

An additional review of the combined series, now including 88 resection specimens in 2010, concluded that AIP with GELs resembles IDCP, whereas the absence of GELs is typically found in patients with lymphoplasmacytic sclerosing pancreatitis (LPSP) which also has prominent IgG4-positive plasma cells [13]. The prevalence of AIP with GELs/IDCP was 38 % in this series of European patients. It is, however, important to realize that this number is likely to be an overestimation due to a selection bias, because the prevalence of a focal mass is higher among patients with AIP type 2, and thus this group is more likely to undergo surgery for presumed malignancy [14].

The European AIP Cohort

Over the course of the last decade, several series of AIP cases from all over Europe have been reported, giving valuable insight into the affected population (Table 29.1). Variations in study design, inclusion criteria, diagnostic criteria, and reported characteristics unfortunately limit the comparability between cohorts and with studies from other parts of the world.

In most series, the diagnosis was based on the Mayo Clinic's HISORt criteria [15, 16] or histological features of resection specimens. The overall gender distribution shows a male predominance of 65 % (50–100 %), and the median age was 51 years, thus lying within the margins of large international multicenter studies [14, 17]. The average age and percentage of male patients with proven LPSP/AIP type 1, however, were higher in these international cohorts (61 years; 74–77 % male), suggesting that the reported European cases

G. Beyer, MD • J. Mayerle, MD • M.M. Lerch, MD, FRCP (✉)
Department of Medicine A, University Medicine, Ernst-Moritz-Arndt-University Greifswald, Ferdinand-Sauerbruchstraße, Greifswald 17475, Germany
e-mail: lerch@uni-greifswald.de

T. Kamisawa, J.B. Chung (eds.), *Autoimmune Pancreatitis*,
DOI 10.1007/978-3-642-55086-7_29, © Springer-Verlag Berlin Heidelberg 2015

Table 29.1 European case series of autoimmune pancreatitis

Author name	Year	*N*	Country	Diagnostic criteria	Male	%	Age	Age (range)	AIP Type 1	%	AIP Type 2	%	OOI	%	IBD	%
Zamboni et al. [12]	2004	53	Italy	Resection specimens	35	66.04	56	56 (14–77)	–		–		10	18.9	6	11.3
van Buuren et al. [41]	2006	10	The Netherlands	Histology	10	100	55	55 (19–80)	–		–		10	100	0	0
Kleeff et al. [42]	2006	17	Germany	Resection specimens	15	88.24	42	42 (16–78)	–		–		–		–	
Church et al. [35]	2007	11	The United Kingdom	–	11	100	53	53 (28–78)	–		–		10	90.9	2	18.2
Detlefsen et al. [20]	2009	26	Germany/Denmark	HISORt	16	61.54	51	51 (10–79)	–		–		8	30.8	1	3.85
de Castro et al. [22]	2010	24	The Netherlands	Resection specimens	18	75	57	57	–		–		–		–	
Frulloni et al. [28]	2009	87	Italy	Verona	54	62.07	43	43	–		–		46	52.9	26	29.9
Maire et al. [19]	2011	44	France	HISORt	22	50	38	38 (19–73)	28	63.6	16	36.4	7	15.9	6	13.6
Czakó et al. [18]	2011	17	Hungary	HISORt/GEL	9	52.94	43	43 (16–74)	11	64.7	6	35.3	8	47.1	5	29.4
Detlefsen [37]	2012	114	Germany, Italy, Belgium, Denmark, Austria, Switzerland, Croatia	HISORt	70	61.4	–	(11–81)	63	55.3	51	44.7	39	34.2	16	14
Total		403			260	64.52	51		102		73		138	50.7	62	22.8

include a significant proportion of patients with AIP type 2 that were not identified as belonging to that subtype. Two more recent reports from France and Hungary consistently report a proportion of AIP type 2 of greater than 33 % among their study population [18, 19], and the percentage of GEL-positive AIP was reported to be as high as 38.5 % in another study using core biopsy specimens [20]. Taken together, these data suggest that the prevalence of AIP type 2 in Europe is higher than the international average, and the published international surveys underestimate the importance of AIP type 2. Although the quality of the summarized European studies is variable and none of them uses the International Consensus Diagnostic Criteria introduced by the IAP in 2011 [21], the results warrant caution when dealing with suspected cases of AIP in clinical practice as patients from Europe could be younger and the female proportion higher than previously assumed.

Other features of AIP among European cohorts seem to be in keeping with what is published in international surveys. The radiological appearance varies widely with the presence of a pancreatic mass in 27–96 % and diffuses swelling in 23–72 % of the cases. Obstructive jaundice is a common clinical feature that has been reported in 56 % of cases, and an association with inflammatory bowel disease was noted in 25 % of the patients in the studies that recorded this characteristic organ involvement.

The overall prevalence and incidence of AIP in Europe remains elusive. In two single-center retrospective analyses from the Netherlands, a total of 913 patients underwent a pancreaticoduodenectomy for presumed malignancy, of which 30 (3.3 %) turned out to have AIP [22, 23]. On one hand, this indicates that AIP remains a rare diagnosis despite the increasing attention among various clinical specialties but also suggests a rather high prevalence among certain subgroups of patients. In another single center's experience from Italy, about 5 % of all chronic pancreatitis patients had AIP [24].

Diagnostic Approaches

The correct diagnosis of AIP remains a clinical challenge. Especially the high prevalence of type 2 AIP in Europe and North America, with its lack of elevated serum IgG4 concentrations, a broader age spectrum, and a higher proportion of mass-forming lesions that mimic malignant disease, prevented a European adoption of the early diagnostic guidelines, which were based on the experience in Japan [25].

To our knowledge, the only set of diagnostic criteria for AIP from Europe was proposed by the group from Verona. In contrast to the Japanese and Asian consensus criteria (imaging of pancreatic parenchyma and duct appearance, elevated serum IgG4/autoantibodies, LPSP with IgG4-positive plasma cells) [26, 27] or the American HISORt criteria (histology showing LPSP/IDCP, suggestive imaging, elevated serum IgG4, other organ involvement, response to steroids) [15], the Italian criteria do not consider serological changes as diagnostic, reflecting the high prevalence of IgG4-negative AIP type 2 among their study cohort. They emphasize the importance of a steroid response as proof of diagnosis, when clinically justified and also suggested that of the following four criteria, three had to be fulfilled to allow the diagnosis of AIP [28]:

- Suggestive radiological features on CT or MRI (no ERCP required)
- Association with autoimmune disease
- Consistent histology (lymphoplasmacytic infiltration and GELs)
- Response to steroid therapy (clinically and on imaging)

The diagnostic work-up that used these Italian criteria initially distinguished between diffuse "sausage-shaped" swelling of the pancreas and a focal, hypodense mass that mimics malignancy [29]. In cases of diffuse swelling, acute pancreatitis was considered the principal differential diagnosis, which can be easily ruled out by the absence of elevated serum pancreatic enzyme activity, absence of pancreatic necrosis, and only mild abdominal symptoms. In combination with associated autoimmune disease and a response to steroids, the diagnosis can be made without the need of pancreatic biopsies according to the authors' experience. In the case of a focal mass, the histological exclusion of malignancy by EUS-guided biopsy would be the first step. If the sample is suggestive for AIP, a steroid trail can complete the diagnosis.

The International Consensus Diagnostic Criteria, which were introduced in 2011, combine the different approaches and allow to establish the diagnosis of AIP in accordance to regional needs and preferences [21]. For example, ductal imaging is no longer required to make the definitive diagnosis for AIP type 1 as diagnostic ERP is not commonly used in Western countries. In equivocal cases, it remains, however, permitted.

But even with these diagnostic criteria and proposed diagnostic work-up in place, the definitive diagnosis of AIP type 2 remains challenging. The group from the Mayo Clinic has emphasized the importance of histological evidence and championed the use of pancreatic true-cut biopsies [30]. Unfortunately, this method is still not everywhere available, and the more commonly used EUS-guided FNA has limitations due to the sampling technique [31]. It therefore remains common practice in Europe to refer patients with suspected AIP to specialized centers.

The authors of this chapter have previously stressed that the role of ductal imaging for the diagnosis of AIP in Western patients might be underestimated [32], especially for patients with IgG4-negative AIP type 2. In a 2-phase interventional study, Sugumar et al. have demonstrated that the analysis of pancreatograms by trained physicians can lead to a sensitivity of 71 % and specificity of 83 % (higher when selected criteria are combined) for the diagnosis of AIP including AIP type 2 [33]. Thus, ERCP can be helpful in establishing the diagnosis of AIP in IgG4-negative patients and in distinguishing it from pancreatic cancer when diagnostic tissue material is hard to obtain or nondiagnostic. The German S3-guideline for management of chronic pancreatitis therefore explicitly allows for the use of diagnostic ERCP in cases of suspected AIP [34] when other imaging modalities are non-conclusive. Alternatively, MRCP can be used to assess the configuration of the pancreatic duct, although a formal evaluation of the "Sugumar criteria" for the use by MRCP has still to be conducted.

Treatment Strategies

The first-line therapy for both types of AIP is corticosteroids, and virtually, all cases show a satisfactory initial response. However, treatment regimens differ greatly between countries. Whereas studies from the United Kingdom and France report fixed prednisolone doses of 30–40 mg over a period of 4 weeks [19, 35], 1 mg/kg prednisolone for 2–3 weeks was given in an Italian study [36] and is commonly used in Germany [31]. In all of these trials, steroids were tapered off over a period of 2–3 months and eventually discontinued (Table 29.2). These approaches are similar to what has been reported from the European centers participating in the largest international follow-up study [17]. Also the relapse rate after a steroid taper or discontinuation was similar to the international average (33 % vs. 34 %). A study that enrolled 102 patients from several European centers that underwent surgical treatment found an overall relapse rate of 26 % [37] which is, again, comparable to the international average, which was reported to be 30 %.

In the case of relapsing disease, most authors used a repeat course of steroids with or without steroid-sparing drugs. The most commonly used immunomodulator was Azathioprine [17, 19, 35].

The studies by Maire et al. and Detlefsen et al. also compared the outcome between the different subtypes of AIP. While no difference was seen in the smaller French cohort, the relapse rate after surgery was less than half in patients with AIP type 2 (15.4 %) when compared to AIP type 1 (41.2 %) [19, 37]. This difference in the probability of recurrence between the clinical subtypes appears to be universal, as it is found in non-European cohorts as well [17, 38].

In summary, in European centers, steroids are widely used as first-line treatment for AIP of both types, although the doses administered and length of treatment differ between regions. The relapse rate does not differ from other parts of the world, and recurrence must be expected in roughly 30 % of cases. Retreatment with steroids and immunomodulators is used in recurrent disease. From Asian studies, we know that long-term treatment with low-dose steroids can reduce the relapse rate [26]. Therefore, some European experts suggest the use of steroid maintenance therapy and or immunomodulators in patients at high risk for relapse [39, 40].

Table 29.2 Treatment regimens and outcome of AIP in Europe

Author name	Year	*N*	Country	Diagnostic criteria	Steroids	Surgery	untreated	Steroid dose	Steroid taper	Maintanenance	Relapse	%	Management of relapse
Church et al. [35]	2007	11	The United Kingdom	–	11	–	–	30 mg	2–3 months	yes (in 9 cases)	6	55	Steroids and Azathioprine
Frulloni et al. [36]	2010	21	Italy	Verona	21	–	–	1 mg/kg	2–3 months	no	–		–
Maire et al. [19]	2010	44	France	HISORt	26	12	6	40 mg	2 months	no	12	27	Steriods and Azathioprine
Detlefsen [37]	2012	102	Germany, Italy, Belgium, Denmark, Austria, Switzerland, Croatia	HISORt	–	102	–	–	–	–	27	26	Steroids and Azathioprine

References

1. Sarles H, Sarles JC, Camatte R, et al. Observations on 205 confirmed cases of acute pancreatitis, recurring pancreatitis, and chronic pancreatitis. Gut. 1965;6:545–59.
2. Sarles H, Sarles JC, Muratore R, Guien C. Chronic inflammatory sclerosis of the pancreas–an autonomous pancreatic disease? Am J Dig Dis. 1961;6:688–98.
3. Yoshida K, Toki F, Takeuchi T, et al. Chronic pancreatitis caused by an autoimmune abnormality. Proposal of the concept of autoimmune pancreatitis. Dig Dis Sci. 1995;40:1561–8.
4. Ectors N, Maillet B, Aerts R, et al. Non-alcoholic duct destructive chronic pancreatitis. Gut. 1997;41:263–8.
5. Sood S, Fossard DP, Shorrock K. Chronic sclerosing pancreatitis in Sjögren's syndrome: a case report. Pancreas. 1995;10:419–21.
6. Abisi S, Morris-Stiff G, Hill SM, et al. Autoimmune pancreatitis: an underdiagnosed condition in Caucasians. J Hepatobiliary Pancreat Surg. 2005;12:332–5.
7. Kim K-P, Kim M-H, Lee SS, et al. Autoimmune pancreatitis: it may be a worldwide entity. Gastroenterology. 2004;126:1214.
8. Sutton R. Autoimmune pancreatitis–also a Western disease. Gut. 2005;54:581–3.
9. Varadarajulu S, Cotton PB. Autoimmune pancreatitis: is it relevant in the west? Gastroenterology. 2003;125:1557.
10. Klöppel G, Lüttges J, Löhr M, et al. Autoimmune pancreatitis: pathological, clinical, and immunological features. Pancreas. 2003;27:14–9.
11. Chari ST, Kloeppel G, Zhang L, et al. Histopathologic and clinical subtypes of autoimmune pancreatitis: the honolulu consensus document. Pancreatology. 2010;10:664–72.
12. Zamboni G, Lüttges J, Capelli P, et al. Histopathological features of diagnostic and clinical relevance in autoimmune pancreatitis: a study on 53 resection specimens and 9 biopsy specimens. Virchows Arch. 2004;445:552–63.
13. Klöppel G, Detlefsen S, Chari ST, et al. Autoimmune pancreatitis: the clinicopathological characteristics of the subtype with granulocytic epithelial lesions. J Gastroenterol. 2010;45:787–93.
14. Kamisawa T, Chari ST, Giday SA, et al. Clinical profile of autoimmune pancreatitis and its histological subtypes: an international multicenter survey. Pancreas. 2011;40:809–14.
15. Chari ST. Diagnosis of autoimmune pancreatitis using its five cardinal features: introducing the Mayo Clinic's HISORt criteria. J Gastroenterol. 2007;42 Suppl 18:39–41.
16. Chari ST, Smyrk TC, Levy MJ, et al. Diagnosis of autoimmune pancreatitis: the Mayo Clinic experience. Clin Gastroenterol Hepatol. 2006;4:1010–6; quiz 934.
17. Hart PA, Kamisawa T, Brugge WR, et al. Long-term outcomes of autoimmune pancreatitis: a multicentre, international analysis. Gut. 2013;62:1771–6.
18. Czakó L, Gyökeres T, Topa L, et al. Autoimmune pancreatitis in Hungary: a multicenter nationwide study. Pancreatology. 2011;11:261–7.
19. Maire F, Le Baleur Y, Rebours V, et al. Outcome of patients with type 1 or 2 autoimmune pancreatitis. Am J Gastroenterol. 2011;106:151–6.
20. Detlefsen S, Mohr Drewes A, Vyberg M, Klöppel G. Diagnosis of autoimmune pancreatitis by core needle biopsy: application of six microscopic criteria. Virchows Arch. 2009;454:531–9.
21. Shimosegawa T, Chari ST, Frulloni L, et al. International consensus diagnostic criteria for autoimmune pancreatitis: guidelines of the International Association of Pancreatology. Pancreas. 2011;40:352–8.
22. De Castro SMM, de Nes LCF, Nio CY, et al. Incidence and characteristics of chronic and lymphoplasmacytic sclerosing pancreatitis in patients scheduled to undergo a pancreatoduodenectomy. HPB (Oxford). 2010;12:15–21.
23. Van Heerde MJ, Biermann K, Zondervan PE, et al. Prevalence of autoimmune pancreatitis and other benign disorders in pancreatoduodenectomy for presumed malignancy of the pancreatic head. Dig Dis Sci. 2012;57:2458–65.
24. Andren-Sandberg A, Hardt PD. Giessen international workshop on interactions of exocrine and endocrine pancreatic diseases. Castle of Rauischholzhausen of the Justus-Liebig-University, Giessen, Germany. J Pancreas. 2005;6:382–405.
25. Chari ST, Longnecker DS, Klöppel G. The diagnosis of autoimmune pancreatitis: a Western perspective. Pancreas. 2009;38:846–8.
26. Okazaki K, Kawa S, Kamisawa T, et al. Japanese clinical guidelines for autoimmune pancreatitis. Pancreas. 2009;38:849–66.
27. Otsuki M, Chung JB, Okazaki K, et al. Asian diagnostic criteria for autoimmune pancreatitis: consensus of the Japan-Korea Symposium on Autoimmune Pancreatitis. J Gastroenterol. 2008;43:403–8.
28. Frulloni L, Scattolini C, Falconi M, et al. Autoimmune pancreatitis: differences between the focal and diffuse forms in 87 patients. Am J Gastroenterol. 2009;104:2288–94.
29. Frulloni L, Amodio A, Katsotourchi AM, Vantini I. A practical approach to the diagnosis of autoimmune pancreatitis. World J Gastroenterol. 2011;17:2076–9.
30. Levy MJ, Smyrk TC, Takahashi N, et al. Idiopathic duct-centric pancreatitis: disease description and endoscopic ultrasonography-guided trucut biopsy diagnosis. Pancreatology. 2011;11:76–80.
31. Pickartz T, Mayerle J, Lerch MM. Autoimmune pancreatitis. Nat Clin Pract Gastroenterol Hepatol. 2007;3:314–23.
32. Lerch MM, Mayerle J. The benefits of diagnostic ERCP in autoimmune pancreatitis. Gut. 2011;60:565–6.
33. Sugumar A, Levy MJ, Kamisawa T, et al. Endoscopic retrograde pancreatography criteria to diagnose autoimmune pancreatitis: an international multicentre study. Gut. 2011;60:666–70.
34. Hoffmeister A, Mayerle J, Beglinger C, et al. S3-Consensus guidelines on definition, etiology, diagnosis and medical, endoscopic and surgical management of chronic pancreatitis German Society of Digestive and Metabolic Diseases (DGVS). Z Gastroenterol. 2012;50:1176–224.
35. Church NI, Pereira SP, Deheragoda MG, et al. Autoimmune pancreatitis: clinical and radiological features and objective response to steroid therapy in a UK series. Am J Gastroenterol. 2007;102:2417–25.
36. Frulloni L, Scattolini C, Katsotourchi AM, et al. Exocrine and endocrine pancreatic function in 21 patients suffering from autoimmune pancreatitis before and after steroid treatment. Pancreatology. 2010;10:129–33.
37. Detlefsen S, Zamboni G, Frulloni L, et al. Clinical features and relapse rates after surgery in type 1 autoimmune pancreatitis differ from type 2: a study of 114 surgically treated European patients. Pancreatology. 2012;12:276–83.

38. Sah RP, Chari ST, Pannala R, et al. Differences in clinical profile and relapse rate of type 1 versus type 2 autoimmune pancreatitis. Gastroenterology. 2010;139:140–8; quiz e12–13.
39. Frulloni L, Lunardi C. Serum IgG4 in autoimmune pancreatitis: a marker of disease severity and recurrence? Dig Liver Dis. 2011;43:674–5.
40. Beyer G, Menzel J, Krüger P-C, et al. Autoimmune pancreatitis. Dtsch Med Wochenschr. 2013;138:2359–74.
41. Van Buuren HR, Vleggaar FP, Willemien Erkelens G, et al (2006) Autoimmune pancreatocholangitis: a series of ten patients. Scand J Gastroenterol Suppl. 70–78.
42. Kleeff J, Welsch T, Esposito I, et al (2006) Autoimmune pancreatitis–a surgical disease?. Chirurg. 77:154–165.

Part VI

Future Perspective

Future Perspective

30

Tsutomu Chiba, Masahiro Shiokawa, and Yuzo Kodama

The concept of autoimmune pancreatitis (AIP) was first reported in 1995 by Yoshida K et al. [1]. Even before this report, cases of AIP or chronic pancreatitis with other organ involvement such as the lacrimal glands, retroperitoneum, and biliary ducts had begun to accumulate in the literature [2–5]. Then in 2001, Hamano et al. [6] reported high serum IgG4 levels in patients with AIP, which is now a hallmark of type 1 AIP/IgG4-related disease (RD). In 2002, Yamamoto Y et al. [7] reported that patients with so-called Mikulicz's disease, the disease ignored for nearly 50 years [8], also had high serum IgG4 levels. Then, through extensive discussion and communications among experts from different clinical fields, finally, a new concept of IgG4-RD was established by combining AIP, Mikulicz's disease, and other diseases [9–12]. Since the concept of AIP was introduced in 1995 [1], cases of AIP have been identified not only in Japan but also in other countries, and interesting differences have been observed between AIP cases from Asia and Western countries [13–15]. In brief, AIP in Western countries occurs equally between males and females in a relatively young population and is frequently associated with inflammatory bowel disease. Importantly, no such cases had elevated serum IgG4 levels. These features are quite distinct from AIP with high serum IgG4 levels seen in Japan. After extensive discussion, a consensus statement on Asian diagnostic criteria for AIP [16] and international consensus diagnostic criteria (ICDC) for AIP [17] were created, and now, these two types of AIP are referred to as type 1 and type 2 AIP. Diagnosis of type 1 AIP is well established, whereas that of type 2 AIP mainly depends on histological findings, and none of specific serum markers have been identified. Fortunately, both types of AIP generally respond well to corticosteroid treatment. A consensus for treatment of AIP, however, has not yet been established. More importantly, the pathophysiology of AIP is largely unknown.

Although the pathogenesis of AIP remains a mystery, establishing both an accurate diagnosis and appropriate and effective treatments is currently the most important goal. Great progress has been made in diagnostic imaging such as computed tomography, endoscopic ultrasonography, and endoscopic retrograde pancreatography, but high serum IgG4 levels and dense infiltration of IgG4-positive plasma cells in the affected tissues are the core comprehensive diagnostic criteria for type 1 AIP/IgG4-RD [11, 17]. But, obtaining tissue samples is difficult in some patients with AIP; thus, diagnosis of type 1 AIP often depends on high serum IgG4 levels together with typical images and clinical manifestations. While a high serum IgG4 level is a very sensitive and specific marker for type 1 AIP, type 1 AIP patients with normal IgG4 and IgG levels are occasionally encountered. Thus, more universal serum markers for diagnosing type 1 AIP are needed, such as the specific autoantibodies for other autoimmune diseases. Although the histopathologic and clinical features are quite distinct for type 2 AIP [13–15], which is more prevalent in Western countries than in Asian countries, no characteristic immunologic changes have been detected in the serum or the tissues to date.

As for treatment, both types of AIP are very sensitive to corticosteroid administration, and indeed, many patients have been successfully treated with corticosteroids. There is currently no consensus, however, regarding the treatment regimen for induction or maintenance or therapeutic end points. Now, clinical trials are in progress in patients with IgG4-RD/type 1 AIP to establish a consensus for corticosteroid treatment regarding the initial dose, duration of treatment, and therapeutic end point. Importantly, it has been increasingly recognized that a considerable number of patients relapse after a decrease or cessation of corticosteroid administration [18, 19]. Therefore, at first, a treatment method for maintaining long-term remission must be established. Indeed, relapse may be prevented altogether by careful and long-term use of low-dose corticosteroids.

T. Chiba, MD, PhD (✉) • M. Shiokawa, MD, PhD
Y. Kodama, MD, PhD
Department of Gastroenterology and Hepatology, Graduate School of Medicine, Kyoto University, Shogoin, Kawahara-cho 54, Sakyo, Kyoto 606-8507, Japan
e-mail: chiba@kuhp.kyoto-u.ac.jp

T. Kamisawa, J.B. Chung (eds.), *Autoimmune Pancreatitis*,
DOI 10.1007/978-3-642-55086-7_30, © Springer-Verlag Berlin Heidelberg 2015

Immunomodulators such as azathioprine and 6-mercaptopurine may have a role in maintaining remission in relapsing type 1 AIP. Recent reports also demonstrated a very potent therapeutic effect of anti-CD20 antibody, rituximab, on refractory IgG4-RD, including type 1 AIP [18–20]. Interestingly, the effect of anti-CD20 antibody appears to persist over time. This is a bit surprising but very interesting findings. Although the precise mechanism underlying the effect of CD20 antibody on pathophysiology of AIP is not clear, it may be noted that in addition to the decrease of B cells and IgG4 plasma cells [20], this antibody appears to induce significant reduction of T-cell infiltration in the affected tissues, suggesting a B-cell-T-cell interaction in the pathophysiology of type I AIP/IgG4-RD [21].

To develop more precise diagnostic methods and treatment options, elucidation of the pathophysiology of the disease is essential. Infection, allergic reaction, and autoimmune mechanisms are proposed to be involved in the pathophysiology of AIP. Despite intensive research, however, the pathogenesis and pathophysiology of both types 1 and 2 AIP remain unknown in most part. But, there are several clues in considering its pathophysiology particularly for type 1 AIP/IgG4-RD. A hallmark of type 1 AIP/IgG4-RD is a very high serum IgG4 concentration with dense IgG4-positive plasma cell infiltration in the affected tissues. In contrast to the generalized hypergammaglobulinemia associated with many other inflammatory or autoimmune diseases, type 1 AIP/IgG4-RD is characterized by high IgG1 and high IgE levels with normal or even low serum IgM and IgA levels in the serum [22]. Also, although IgG4 is known to have a critical role in the pathophysiology of some diseases, even in such diseases, the total IgG4 levels are not high [23, 24]. Therefore, distinct mechanisms for an IgG4 class switch must be involved in this disease. Early studies demonstrated an increase in Th2 cytokines such as interleukin (IL) 4 and transforming growth factor β in type 1 AIP/IgG4-RD [25], but recent reports demonstrated increase in several other cytokines as well, including IL10, a proliferation-inducing ligand (APRIL), and B-cell activating factor (BAFF), which might contribute to the increase in IgG4 plasma cells and high serum IgG4 levels [26, 27]. The data may also suggest the involvement of regulatory T cells and innate immune cells [25]. Nevertheless, it is unknown why these cytokines in particular are increased in this disease.

Whether the high IgG4 has a pathogenic role is an interesting question. In this regard, IgG4 autoantibodies have a critical pathogenic role in primary membranous glomerulonephropathy [23] and pemphigus vulgaris [24]. In contrast, because IgG4 is incapable of inducing complement activation [28], it is generally believed that IgG4 does not have a pathogenic role. However, the fact that IgG4 is deposited together with IgG1 and C3 and occasionally with C1q and C4 in the tubular basal membrane in IgG4-related nephropathy [29, 30] suggests a pathogenic role of IgG4 in this disease. Curiously, many patients with type 1 AIP/IgG4-RD have low C3 and C4 levels [30], suggesting complement activation. Alternatively, because IgG4 binds other immunoglobulins through their Fc regions [31], IgG4 deposition in the affected tissues might merely reflect its binding to other IgG subclasses such as IgG1 within the tissue.

Careful observation of patients with type 1 AIP/IgG4-RD reveals several interesting characteristic features as well. First, similar to Behcet's disease or sarcoidosis, this disease rarely overlaps with other inflammatory or autoimmune diseases. For example, different from type 2 AIP, type 1 AIP is rarely associated with ulcerative colitis (UC) or primary sclerosing cholangitis (PSC). Although colitis is reported to be associated with type 1 AIP/IgG4-RD [32], this appears to be a manifestation of the disease itself rather than an overlap with other diseases [33]. Another point is that few familial cases have been reported [34]. This fact might contradict the idea of the involvement of genetic or environmental factors in the development of the disease, but the association of some genetic factors including MHC class II gene with type 1 AIP/IgG4-RD has been reported [35]. As recently reported, B-cell depletion by rituximab, a CD20 antibody, has a potent therapeutic effect on refractory type 1 AIP/IgG4-RD [19, 21], and this effect is associated with a reduction of not only serum IgG4 and infiltrating IgG4 plasma cells in the affected tissues but also T cells infiltrated in the tissues. These results might suggest not only an important regulatory function of B cells on T cells but also critical roles of T cells in the pathophysiology of type 1 AIP/IgG4-RD. In relation to this, whether or not tissues infiltrated with lymphocytes may serve as an effector site or an induction site requires clarification.

Another interesting issue is the relationship between type 1 AIP/IgG4-RD and cancer. Yamamoto et al. [36] and Shiokawa et al. [37] reported a high risk of cancer in patients with Mikulicz's disease and AIP, respectively. Indeed, Shiokawa et al. found that among 108 AIP patients, 15 patients (13.9 %) had cancer during a median follow-up of 3.3 years, with a relative risk of cancer of 4.9 at the time of AIP diagnosis. It is well established that inflammation promotes cancer development, such as gastric cancer and liver cancer [38]. On the other hand, several cancers are known to induce paraneoplastic syndrome, such as dermatomyositis and pemphigus vulgaris. Notably, however, Shiokawa et al. found no pancreatic cancer in their patients. Moreover, the risk of cancer was highest within the first year after AIP diagnosis, and only few cases of AIP recurred after successful treatment of coexisting cancers, while relapse often occurred in patients without cancer cure. These data may favor the notion that some cases with AIP develop as a paraneoplastic syndrome, but further investigation is clearly required to obtain a final conclusion. Interestingly, previous studies suggested important roles of IgG4 autoantibodies in the pathophysiology of some paraneoplastic syndromes [23, 24].

In conclusion, type 1 AIP/IgG4-RD is a new disease entity characterized by numerous infiltrating IgG4 plasma cells in affected tissues and high serum IgG4 levels. As described, the pathophysiology of type 1 AIP/IgG4-RD is mainly unknown, and very few studies of the pathogenesis of type 2 AIP are reported. Although corticosteroid treatment is very effective for both types 1 and 2 AIP, there is currently no consensus for the treatment of AIP, including maintenance and relapse therapies. Further studies are required to elucidate the precise pathophysiology of AIP and to establish more appropriate treatment strategies.

References

1. Yoshida K, Toki F, Takeuchi T, et al. Chronic pancreatitis caused by an autoimmune abnormality. Proposal of the concept of autoimmune pancreatitis. Dig Dis Sci. 1995;40:1561–8.
2. Nakano S, Takeda I, Kitamura K, et al. Chronic pancreatitis complicated with Sjogren's syndrome. Vanishing tumor of the abdomen in a patient with Sjogren's syndrome. Dig Dis. 1978;23(Suppl):75–9.
3. Nishimori I, Okazaki K, Yamamoto Y, et al. Specific cellular immune responses to pancreatic antigen in chronic pancreatitis and Sjogren's syndrome. J Clin Immunol. 1993;13:265–71.
4. Nakazawa T, Ohara H, Yamada T, et al. Atypical primary sclerosing cholangitis cases associated with unusual pancreatitis. Hepatogastroenterology. 2001;48:625–30.
5. Hamano H, Kawa S, Ochi Y, et al. Hydronephrosis associated with retroperitoneal fibrosis and sclerosing pancreatitis. Lancet. 2002;359:1403–4.
6. Hamano H, Kawa S, Horiuchi A, et al. High serum IgG4 concentrations in patients with sclerosing pancreatitis. N Engl J Med. 2001;344:732–8.
7. Yamamoto M, Takahashi H, Sugai S, et al. Clinical and pathological characteristics of Mikulicz's disease (IgG4-related plasmacytic exocrinopathy). Autoimmun Rev. 2005;4:195–200.
8. Morgan WS, Castleman B. A clinicopathologic study of "Mikulicz's disease". Am J Pathol. 1953;29:471–503.
9. Kamisawa T, Okamoto A. Autoimmune pancreatitis: proposal of IgG4-related sclerosing disease. J Gastroenterol. 2006;41:613–25.
10. Umehara H, Okazaki K, Masaki Y, et al. A novel clinical entity, IgG4-related disease (IgG4RD): general concept and details. Mod Rheumatol. 2012;22:1–14.
11. Umehara H, Okazaki K, Masaki Y, et al. Comprehensive diagnostic criteria for Ig4-related disease (IgG4-RD), 2011. Mod Rheumatol. 2012;22:21–30.
12. Stone H, Khosroshahi A, Deshpande V, et al. Recommendations for the nomenclature of IgG4-related disease and its individual organ system manifestations. Arthritis Rheum. 2012;64:3061–7.
13. Pearson RK, Longnecker DS, Chari ST, et al. Controversies in clinical pancreatology: autoimmune pancreatitis. Does it exist? Pancreas. 2003;27:1–13.
14. Notohara K, Burgart LJ, Yadav D, et al. Idiopathic chronic pancreatitis with periductal lymphoplasmacytic infiltration: clinicopathologic features of 35 cases. Am J Surg Pathol. 2003;27:1119–27.
15. Zamboni G, Luttges J, Capelli P, et al. Histopathological features of diagnostic and clinical relevance in autoimmune pancreatitis: a study on 53 resection specimens and 9 biopsy specimens. Virchows Arch. 2004;445:552–63.
16. Otsuki M, Chung JB, Okazaki K, et al. Asian diagnostic criteria for autoimmune pancreatitis: consensus of the Japan-Korea symposium on autoimmune pancreatitis. J Gastroenterol. 2008;43:403–8.
17. Shimosegawa T, Chari ST, Frulloni L, et al. International consensus diagnostic criteria for autoimmune pancreatitis: guidelines of the international association of pancreatology. Pancreas. 2011;40:352–8.
18. Kosroshahi A, Bloch DB, Deshpande V, et al. Rituximab leads to rapid decline of serum IgG4-related systemic disease. Arthritis Rheum. 2010;62:1755–62.
19. Hart PA, Topazian MD, Witzig TE, et al. Treatment of relapsing autoimmune pancreatitis with immunomodulators and rituximab: the Mayo Clinic experience. Gut. 2013;62:1607–15.
20. Khosroshahi A, Carruthers MN, Deshpande V, et al. Rituximab for the treatment of IgG4-related disease. Medicine. 2012;91:57–66.
21. Stone JH. B cell depletion in IgG4-related disease. In: Umehara H, Okazaki K, Stone JH, Kawa S, Kawano M, editors. IgG4-related disease. Tokyo: Springer; 2012. p. 51–7.
22. Taguchi M, Kihara Y, Nagashio Y, et al. Decreased production of immunoglobulin M and A in autoimmune pancreatitis. J Gastroenterol. 2009;44:1133–9.
23. Beck LH, Bonegio RGB, Lambeau G, et al. M-type phospholipase A2 receptor as target antigen in idiopathic membranous nephropathy. N Engl J Med. 2009;361:11–21.
24. Bhol K, Natarajan K, Nagarwalla N, et al. Correlation of peptide specificity and IgG subclass with pathogenic and nonpathogenic autoantibodies in pemphigus vulgaris: A model for autoimmunity. Proc Natl Acad Sci U S A. 1995;92:5239–43.
25. Zen Y, Fujii T, Harada K, et al. Th2 and regulatory immune reactions are increased in immunoglobulin G4-related sclerosing pancreatitis and cholangitis. Hepatology. 2007;45:1538–46.
26. Watanabe T, Yamashita K, Fujikawa S, et al. Involvement of activation of toll-like receptors and nucleotide-binding oligomerization domain-like receptors in enhanced IgG4 responses in autoimmune pancreatitis. Arthritis Rheum. 2012;64:914–24.
27. Kiyama K, Kawabata D, Hosono Y, et al. Serum BAFF and APRIL levels in patients with IgG4-related disease and their clinical significance. Arthritis Res Ther. 2012;14:R86.
28. Aalberse RC, Schuurman J. IgG4 breaking the rules. Immunology. 2002;105:9–19.
29. Yamaguchi Y, Kanetsuna Y, Honda K, et al. Characteristic tubulointerstitial nephritis in IgG4-related disease. Hum Pathol. 2012;43:536–49.
30. Kawano M, Mizushima I, Yamaguchi Y, et al. Immunohistochemical characteristics of IgG4-related tubulointerstitial nephritis: detailed analysis of 20 Japanese cases. Int J Rheumatol. 2012;609795.
31. Zack DJM, Stempniak M, Wong AL. Localization of an Fc-binding reactivity to the constant region of human IgG4: implications for the pathogenesis of rheumatoid arthritis. J Immunol. 1995;155:5057–63.
32. Ueno K, Watanabe T, Kawata Y, et al. IgG4-related autoimmune pancreatitis involving the colonic mucosa. Eur J Gastroenterol Hepatol. 2008;20:1181–21.
33. Koizumi S, Kamisawa T, Kuruma S, et al. Immunoglobulin G4-related gastrointestinal diseases, are they immunoglobulin G4-related disease? World J Gastroenterol. 2013;19:5769–74.
34. Watanabe T, Maruyama M, Ito T. Two siblings with type 1 autoimmune pancreatitis. Intern Med. 2013;52:895–9.
35. Kawa S, Ota M, Yoshizawa K, et al. HLA DRB10405-DQB10401 haplotype is associated with autoimmune pancreatitis in the Japanese population. Gastroenterology. 2002;122:1264–9.
36. Yamamoto M, Takahashi H, Tabeya T, et al. Risk of malignancies in IgG4-related disease. Mod Rheumatol. 2012;22:414–8.
37. Shiokawa M, Kodama Y, Yoshimura K, et al. Risk of cancer in patients with autoimmune pancreatitis. Am J Gastroenterol. 2013;108:610–7.
38. Chiba T, Marusawa H, Ushijima T. Inflammation-associated cancer development in digestive organs: mechanisms and roles for genetic and epigenetic modulation. Gastroenterology. 2012;143:550–63.

MIX
Papier aus verantwortungsvollen Quellen
Paper from responsible sources
FSC® C105338

If you have any concerns about our products, you can contact us on
ProductSafety@springernature.com

In case Publisher is established outside the EU, the EU authorized representative is:
Springer Nature Customer Service Center GmbH
Europaplatz 3, 69115 Heidelberg, Germany

Printed by Libri Plureos GmbH
in Hamburg, Germany